Case Studies
in Pediatric
Infectious Diseases

Case Studies in Pediatric Infectious Diseases

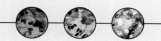

Frank E. Berkowitz, BSc MBBCh, FCP(Paed)(SA), MPH

Professor of Pediatrics
Department of Pediatrics
Emory University School of Medicine
Atlanta, Georgia, USA

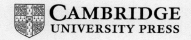

CAMBRIDGE UNIVERSITY PRESS

Cambridge, New York, Melbourne, Madrid, Cape Town, São Paulo, Delhi

Cambridge University Press
32 Avenue of the Americas, New York, NY 10013–2473, USA

www.cambridge.org
Information on this title: www.cambridge.org/9780521697613

First published 2007

Printed in the United States of America

A catalog record for this book is available from the British Library

Library of Congress Cataloging in Publication Data

Berkowitz, Frank E. (Frank Ellis), 1948-
Case studies in pediatric infectious diseases / Frank E. Berkowitz.
p. ; cm.
Includes bibliographical references.
ISBN-13: 978-0-521-69761-3 (pbk.)
ISBN-10: 0-521-69761-1 (pbk.)
1. Communicable diseases in children – Case studies.   I. Title.
[DNLM: 1. Infection – Case Reports.   2. Bacterial Infections – Case Reports.
3. Child.   4. Infant.   5. Mycoses – Case Reports.   6. Parasitic Diseases – Case Reports.
7. Virus Diseases – Case Reports. WC 195 B513c 2007] I. Title.
RJ401.B47 2007
618.92′9–dc22   2007009668

ISBN 978-0-521-69761-3

*This book is dedicated
to the memory of my father,*

Abraham Philip Berkowitz,

*who first introduced me to the concept
of infectious diseases.*

Contents

Preface

THE PURPOSE of this book is to provide the pediatric practitioner with an approach to the diagnosis and management of patients suspected of suffering from an infection through the use of teaching case exercises.

These cases have been designed as teaching exercises in clinical infectious diseases. Their sources are as follows:

(i)   The majority are derived from my own clinical experience. Because this experience covers a period of 30 years, many of these are reconstructed from memory, and therefore some of the details, especially the child's age and sex, may not be accurate.

(ii)   Three cases are based on reports in the Morbidity and Mortality Weekly Reviews (MMWR).

(iii) Several cases are composites of different cases from my experience.

(iv) The remainder of the cases are hypothetical, based on current knowledge of the clinical manifestations of a particular illness. These include cases in which I have constructed a clinical scenario to match a photograph.

Where names of the cases have been used, they are not the patients' real names, but they contain clinically important information.

Although these cases cover a wide range of infections, they do not necessarily include cases of commonly encountered infections. They do, however, include cases of uncommon infections. I make no apology for this because the goal of the exercises is to encourage thought about diagnostic possibilities, both within and outside the range of the usual clinical encounters in the United States.

The first chapter addresses general principles in the diagnosis and management of patients suspected of suffering from an infectious disease.

In the second chapter the cases are presented and discussed. The emphasis of the discussions is on clinical evaluation based on history, particularly on risk factors, and on physical examination. This evaluation consists mainly of considerations of diagnostic possibilities and of physiologic disturbances. There is little mention of broad-spectrum laboratory testing such as blood counts because it is my view that these seldom help in differentiating between the different diagnostic possibilities. The discussions often include noninfectious diseases, because patients do not present waving a flag that they have an infectious disease.

Management is discussed mainly as it relates to principles. Details of management are not discussed for the following reasons: (i) optimal antimicrobial therapy changes over time and is influenced by susceptibility patterns of organisms in a particular location; (ii) one should consult a handbook for the dosages of drugs that one does not prescribe frequently.

Most cases have reading or references applicable to that case. These are mostly recent review articles. A list of books that should be consulted as reference sources is given in Chapter 3.

ACKNOWLEDGMENTS

I wish to acknowledge the following individuals who, over many years, have stimulated my interest in and taught me microbiology and infectious diseases: Hendrik J. Koornhof, Benny Miller, James H.S. Gear, Barry Schoub, Walter O. Prozesky, Myron Levin, Mimi Glode, James Todd, and Brian Lauer.

I also wish to thank Dr. Carlos Abramowsky and Dr. Robert Jerris for providing me with some of the pictures, and the librarians of the Grady Memorial Hospital branch of the Emory University School of Medicine library for their help in obtaining literature. Finally, I wish to thank W. Dean Wilcox for all his encouragement.

Part One

INTRODUCTION

THE NATURE OF THE PRACTICE OF INFECTIOUS DISEASES

The practice of infectious diseases depends on the application of information, knowledge, skills, and judgment related to three areas, namely epidemiology, clinical medicine, and clinical microbiology. This book is intended to provide insights into infectious diseases in children, emphasizing the importance of these considerations.

The goal of clinical practice is to cure patients or, at least, to ameliorate their condition. The ultimate goal lies in a good or beneficial outcome, not only for the individual patient but also for the public. The outcome depends to a large extent on some kind of action being taken. For the individual this is usually therapeutic. For the public the action might entail tracing of exposed contacts, quarantining of exposed individuals, and providing vaccination or chemoprophylaxis. The action to be taken often, but not always, depends on an accurate diagnosis being made. It is important to remember that the ultimate goal does not lie in making an accurate diagnosis, nor in taking some action, but in obtaining a favorable outcome. There are circumstances in which the accurate diagnosis in an individual patient is not as important to that patient, for whom there may be no available therapy, as to the community.

COMPONENTS OF A DIAGNOSIS

Giving appropriate therapy often depends on making an accurate diagnosis. The diagnosis, like ancient Gaul, is divided into three parts (omnis diagnosis in tres partes divisa est):

1. Anatomic diagnosis, for example, the lung, the middle ear, the urinary tract.

2. Physiologic diagnosis. This describes functional disturbances, for example, respiratory failure, shock.

The physiologic diagnosis is important for determining what supportive care the patient requires. In patients with severe illness providing appropriate supportive care is more urgent than is providing antimicrobial therapy. For example, in a patient with septic shock, the most urgent matter is to restore adequate perfusion; in a patient with respiratory failure complicating pneumonia, the most urgent matter is to ensure adequate ventilation and oxygenation.

Making an anatomical and physiological diagnosis depends on the history, physical examination, and sometimes on laboratory and imaging tests.

3. Pathologic and/or etiologic diagnosis, for example, inflammation caused by *Streptococcus pneumoniae* or purpura fulminans caused by *Neisseria meningitidis*.

In the case of infectious diseases, the etiological diagnosis is represented by the microbiological diagnosis.

MICROBIOLOGICAL DIAGNOSIS

In infectious diseases making an etiologic or microbiological diagnosis is very important because specific therapy, where available, entails use of an antimicrobial agent.

The microbiological diagnosis can often be made based on the anatomic diagnosis. For example, if the diagnosis is otitis media, we can assume, based on previous studies of middle ear fluid of children with otitis media, that the likely causative organism is one of the following: *Streptococcus pneumoniae*, *Haemophilus influenzae*, or *Moraxella catarrhalis*. This principle can be applied to an infection at any anatomic site. An etiological diagnosis is usually difficult to make in the absence of an anatomic diagnosis.

RISK FACTORS FOR INFECTION

The microbiological diagnosis also depends on the **risk factors** that the patient has for acquiring a particular infection. Such risk factors can be considered in terms of (a) genetic factors, for example, sickle cell disease, and (b) environmental factors or the epidemiological circumstances in which the patient's infection was acquired. This constitutes the patient's **exposures**.

A list of possible exposures that should be inquired about is shown in Table 1. When obtaining a history about exposures, I have found it useful to explain to patients (or their parents) the purpose of the apparently bizarre questions that I intend to ask.

■TAB. 1: Types of exposures to infectious agents.

Sick human beings	family, friends, day care, shelter for the homeless, immigrants, visitors from abroad, prison, military
Maternal infections	intrauterine (transplacental), intrapartum, postnatal
Animals	vertebrates – fish, amphibians, reptiles, birds, mammals arthropods – ticks, mosquitoes, fleas, lice, flies, mites
Travel	foreign or domestic; foreign-sounding names or accents should prompt enquiry about foreign travel
Occupation of patient or parents Recreational activities	sports, hobbies, sexual activity, drug abuse
Hospitalizations and visits to health care facilities	
Injections Surgery, foreign body insertions Immunizations Antimicrobial therapy Food and water sources	legal and illicit, blood transfusions, vascular catheters

There is an aphorism used in clinical medicine in the United States regarding the likelihood of a particular disease among a differential diagnosis: "when you hear hoofbeats, think of horses, not zebras." One of the messages of this book is:

"Think about zebras as well as horses, because whether horses or zebras are more likely depends on where you come from!" (Figure 1).

Furthermore, zebras are found in groups. Therefore, when individuals are exposed to exotic diseases, they may be exposed to more than one disease at the same time.

Patients with defects in their host defenses (genetic or acquired) are at risk for infections caused by certain microorganisms that are unlikely to infect normal hosts. Different host defense defects predispose to different kinds of infections. Table 2 lists some host defense defects and infections to which they predispose.

METHODS FOR MAKING A MICROBIOLOGICAL DIAGNOSIS

There are several different methods for confirming a microbiological diagnosis, which are summarized in Table 3. They can be divided into (a) direct methods, in which the organism is visualized, cultured, or a component of

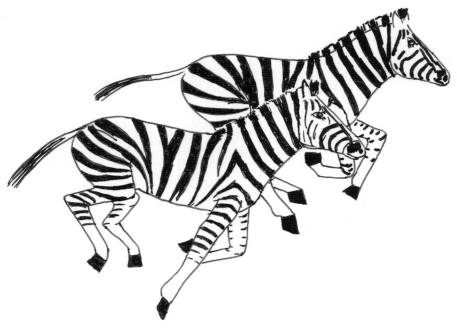

FIG. 1 Zebras.

the organism is detected, for example, antigen, DNA; and (b) indirect methods, which depend on the host's response to the infection (i.e. serological methods). The direct methods are undergoing significant changes due to the rapid advances being made in our ability to detect microbial nucleic acid.

In making a microbiological diagnosis, the optimal site for obtaining material for diagnosis is from the site of infection, when possible. Although this may seem intuitive, it is remarkable how frequently this principle is not followed. This principle is frequently referred to as "Sutton's Law," named for the bank robber, Willie Sutton, who, when asked why he robbed banks, replied, "Because that's where the money is."

In the diagnosis of infections, in general, the sicker the patient is, the less room there is for making an error in diagnosis, and consequently the more important it is to make a microbiological diagnosis. This may necessitate invasive procedures. For example a normal child with otitis media does not require a myringotomy to obtain middle ear fluid for culture. Most children with this condition recover with or without antimicrobial therapy. On the other hand, a child who has recently undergone bone marrow transplantation and has a rapidly progressive pneumonia might need to undergo an invasive procedure such as a bronchoalveolar lavage or a lung biopsy in order to determine the causative organism, considering the wide variety of possible pathogens and the toxicity of some of the therapeutic agents that might be indicated.

■**TAB. 2: Host defense defects and infections to which they predispose.**

Defect	Infection/Organism
Skin	
Atopic dermatitis	*Staphylococcus aureus*, *Streptococcus pyogenes*
Burn	*Staph. aureus*, *Strep. pyogenes*, *Pseudomonas aeruginosa*
Varicella	*Strep. pyogenes*, *Staph. aureus*
Vascular catheter	staphylococci, *Candida* sp., enterococci, enteric bacilli
Endotracheal intubation	pharyngeal flora, Gram-negative bacilli
Urinary catheter	Gram-negative bacilli, enterococci, *Candida* spp.
Blood diseases	
Sickle cell disease	*Streptococcus pneumoniae* sepsis, salmonella osteomyelitis
Iron overload	enteric rod sepsis, especially *Yersinia enterocolitica*
Cancer chemotherapy with neutropenia	staphylococci, streptococci, Gram-negative rods, fungi
Transplant	herpes group viruses, adenovirus, many different bacteria, including mycobacteria and *Nocardia* spp., *Listeria monocytogenes*, fungi, *Pneumocystis jiroveci*, and *Toxoplasma gondii*
Congenital Immunodeficiencies	
Immunoglobulin deficiencies	pyogenic bacterial infections, pneumonia, sinusitis
Combined immunodeficiencies	bacterial infections, severe viral infections, *Pneumocystis jiroveci*
Chronic granulomatous disease	infections with staphylococci, Gram-negative bacilli, mycobacteria, fungi
HIV infection	*Pneumocystis jireveci*, mycobacteria, *Candida* spp., Cytomegalovirus, bacteremia

PRINCIPLES OF MANAGEMENT OF PATIENTS WITH INFECTIOUS DISEASES

The following five main principles should be considered in the management of patients with infections, not all of them necessarily applying to all cases:

Supportive care. This is the most important aspect to consider, and, in patients with life-threatening infections, it is the aspect that must be addressed immediately. For example, in a patient with shock due to severe bacterial infection, the most important first step in management is to ensure adequate tissue perfusion with intravenous fluid. In a patient with respiratory failure due to pneumonia, the most important first step in management is to ensure adequate oxygenation and ventilation.

■**TAB. 3: Methods for making a microbiological diagnosis.**

A. Direct visualization of the organism

Electron microscopy for viruses	seldom performed
Gram stain for bacteria	very useful; rapid, cheap, semi-quantitative
Wet preparations	bacteruria, *Trichomonas vaginalis*
unstained, mixed with saline	*Entamoeba histolytica*, ova, fungi
dark field	spirochetes
cleared with 10%KOH	fungi
Acid-Fast stain	Mycobacteria

Cytology	
Papanicolaou stain	viral inclusions, viral cytopathic effects
Silver stain	*Pneumocystis jiroveci*, fungi
Gram stain	bacteria
Immunostaining	viruses, bacteria, fungi, parasites
Blood smears (stained with a	*Plasmodium* spp., *Trypanosoma* spp., *Babesia* spp.,
Romanowsky stain – Wright's, Leishman's,	relapsing fever *Borrelia* spp., morula of *Ehrlichia* spp.,
Giemsa)	*Bartonella bacilliformis*, microfilaria

Histology – sections stained with hematoxylin
and eosin and the above-mentioned stains

B. Culture of the organism – this is the "gold" standard for detection of many organisms,
especially bacteria and viruses

Tissue culture	viruses, *Chlamydia* spp., *Rickettsia* spp.
Nutrient-containing agar and broths	bacteria, fungi
Living tissue e.g. eggs	viruses, *Rickettsia* spp.
Animal inoculation	this is very seldom performed

C. Detection of microbial antigens in body fluids and tissues

D. Detection of nucleic acid in body fluids and tissues, by signal amplification, nucleic acid
amplification (e.g. polymerase chain reaction), and several other methods

E. Serology – this detects the host's response to the infection, that is the presence of antibodies. Although
not the optimal way in which to diagnose an infection, in some infections it is the only way. There are
many different methods for detecting antibody responses to infection. These include the following:
Neutralization
Complement fixation
ELISA
Immunofluorescence
Hemagglutination

READING: Winn WC Jr, Allen SD, Janda WM, Koneman EW, Procop GW, Schreckenberger PC, Woods GL: Molecular Microbiology. Chapter 4 in Koneman's Color Atlas and Textbook of Diagnostic Microbiology. 6th edition. Lippincott William and Wilkins, Philadelphia, 2006, pp. 132–165.

Antimicrobial therapy. This is specifically intended to kill or inhibit the growth of invading microorganisms. For many patients with infections, especially viral infections, there is currently no available antimicrobial therapy. The principles for choosing antimicrobial agents are discussed below.

Surgery. This may be necessary for therapy or for diagnostic purposes. It includes aspirating or biopsying infected lesions to obtain material for staining, culture, or histology, and draining of abscesses.

Addressing the interests of the community. The community may be the family, friends, school attendees, other patients in a hospital or clinic, or members of the broader community of the city, country, or world. For example, when a case of tuberculosis is diagnosed, the local health department should be informed so that contact tracing can be instituted. When a child with a contagious illness is admitted to hospital, specific isolation precautions should be instituted.

Prevention. For the most part this entails immunization. Although this will have failed if a patient is diagnosed with a preventable disease, making such a diagnosis should lead to an examination of the possible reasons why this failure occurred and how the problem can be rectified to prevent other patients acquiring the same illness.

The Gram Stain

Remember, Oh! The Gram stain test.
It's quick, it's cheap, it is the best!

Whenever you have secretions,
Exudates or draining lesions.
If its closed, suck some juice,
Then a diagnosis you'll deduce.

Make a smear (not too high),
On a slide, and let it dry.
After each step you must rinse,
Purple, brown – it's a cinch.
Clear (few secs), then safranin.
Wash and dry: now examine.
Optimize the light. For vision
Use the oil immersion.

Cells are red, and germs – all kind
Purple (pos), Pink (neg) – you will find.

Remember, Oh! To hold in awe
The verity of Sutton's Law,
Which from a robber may sound funny
In diagnostics:
GO FOR THE MONEY!

Don't throw pus, sputum, or pee down the drain
Until you have first done –
A GRAM STAIN
With some purple, then brown; then red after alcohol
You can Gram stain anything, ANYTHING,
ANYTHING AT ALL.

PRINCIPLES OF CHOOSING ANTIMICROBIAL THERAPY

Antimicrobial therapy is different from other forms of medical therapy in that its goal is to affect a biological process in an invading microorganism, thus inhibiting its growth or resulting in its death. The goals of other forms of medical therapy are directed at influencing a physiologic process in the patient. The use of antimicrobial agents can result in microorganisms developing resistance to such agents. Microorganisms in an individual patient can spread from that individual to colonize or infect another individual. Any antimicrobial resistance that has developed among microorganisms within this host will thus be carried to the new host. Thus antimicrobial resistance can be spread to other members of the community and, in fact, to other generations of hosts. Therefore prescribing antimicrobial agents carries with it an awesome responsibility and should be carried out judiciously.

Once it has been determined that the patient has or probably has an infection, AND that antimicrobial therapy is indicated, the main questions to be answered are

1. What is (are) the most likely causative organism(s)?
2. What are their most likely antimicrobial susceptibilities?

These are the most important questions to ask, and the most challenging to answer, particularly in situations in which a specific diagnosis has not been made (a frequent situation in pediatrics). The answer to question 1 lies in the diagnosis, discussed above. The answer to the question regarding antimicrobial susceptibilities is determined by local epidemiology and the patient's history of prior exposure to antimicrobial agents. The antimicrobial susceptibilities may vary from country-to-country, community-to-community, hospital-to-hospital, and ward-to-ward. For example ampicillin might be indicated for empiric treatment of a patient with an *E. coli* infection acquired in a community where the resistance rate of *E. coli* to ampicillin is 5%, whereas it would not be indicated for someone with the same infection acquired in a hospital ward where the resistant rate is 70%. Once a causative organism has been isolated and its antimicrobial susceptibilities are known, antimicrobial therapy usually becomes fairly simple.

The next question to be asked is:

3. What is the most appropriate agent to use?

In actually choosing a specific antimicrobial agent, several factors must be considered. The overriding principle in choosing therapy, however, is the following: USE AS NARROW A SPECTRUM AGENT AS POSSIBLE.

The other factors that should be taken into account are as follows:

1. *Spectrum of antimicrobial activity.* The drug must have the necessary spectrum as determined by questions 1 and 2 above.

2. *Severity of infection.* This determines the balance of risks between treatment and no treatment or between treatment with one drug and another, which is, in turn, determined by the adverse effect profile of the drugs. The severity of the infection also determines the speed with which an effect is necessary and, therefore, also influences the route of drug administration. For example, it would not be appropriate to use chloramphenicol, which has the rare side effect of causing aplastic anemia, to treat a patient with simple otitis media, but it might be appropriate to use it for treating a patient with a brain abscess. Similarly it would not be appropriate to use intravenous cefotaxime for treating a child with simple otitis media thought to be caused by *Streptococcus pneumoniae*, but it would be appropriate to use such therapy in a toxic-appearing patient with lobar pneumonia suspected to be caused by the same organism.

3. *The pharmacokinetics of the drug.*

    (a) *The distribution of the drug.* The drug must attain an adequate concentration at the site of infection to eliminate the infection. Because different drugs penetrate different tissues to different degrees, infections caused by the same organism but at different sites might necessitate the use of different drugs. For example, clindamycin would be suitable for treating a patient with a lung abscess but not for a patient with meningitis caused by the same organism because it does not enter the cerebrospinal fluid in a significant concentration.

    (b) *The elimination of the drug by metabolism or excretion.* Dysfunction of the liver or kidney might interfere with the elimination of certain drugs. In such cases the drug might accumulate to toxic concentrations. This might prevent the drug from being used safely.

4. *The route of administration.* This is usually determined by the severity of infection (see 2 above) and the possible routes for administration of the specific drug. Several drugs, especially those used for treating patients

with severe illness, can be given only intravenously, for example, vancomycin. This places a constraint on the use of this drug.

1. *Drug–drug interactions.* Many patients, especially those with underlying illnesses, receive multiple drugs. Several drugs, including "over-the-counter" preparations, interfere with the pharmacokinetics of other drugs, resulting in their blood levels being inadequate or excessive. The general mechanisms by which these interactions occur are as follows:

   (a) Interference with oral absorption, for example, antacids, such as aluminum hydroxide, interfere with the absorption of fluoroquinolones.
   (b) Interference with hepatic metabolism. This applies particularly to drugs that are metabolized by the cytochrome P450 enzyme systems. Drugs that induce hepatic enzymes, for example, rifamycins and anticonvulsants, speed up the metabolism of some other drugs, for example, corticosteroids and warfarin, resulting in reduced effects. Some drugs, for example, erythromycin, inhibit the metabolism of other drugs, for example, theophylline, resulting in them reaching toxic levels in the blood.

   Antimicrobial agents that are frequently associated with drug–drug interactions include the rifamycins, imidazole antifungal agents, macrolides, and antiretroviral protease inhibitors.
   (c) Additive injury to the kidney, resulting in decreased excretion of the drug, for example, a combination of an aminoglycoside and vancomycin.

2. *Cost.* When multiple drugs are equivalent in the above characteristics, the cheapest option should be used.

PRINCIPLES OF ADDRESSING PUBLIC HEALTH INTERESTS

Members of a community often have an interest in the diagnosis of an infection in an individual because they may be at risk for acquiring the same infection. There are several situations in which this may occur, but essentially there are two main reasons for community interest:

(a) the patient may be the index case of a broader outbreak or represent a sentinel case, indicating the local presence of the disease. For example, a child is generally the victim of tuberculosis spread from an adult. Therefore the diagnosis of tuberculosis in a child indicates the presence of an adult source who must be sought, so that he or she can be treated, so that spread to additional individuals is interrupted, and so that other individuals already infected can be identified and treated. The diagnosis of certain infections in an individual indicates that several individuals might harbor the causative agent and spread it without being ill or prior to becoming ill. When the agent causes serious disease, prevention of disease is highly desirable, for example, in the cases of *Neisseria meningitidis*, *Haemophilus influenzae* type b, and *Bordetella pertussis*. In such situations antimicrobial prophylaxis should be provided to high-risk contacts such as members of the household.

(b) the patient is the potential source of spread of the infection to others, such as in the case of a sexually transmitted disease, or measles.

Children admitted to hospital with a wide variety of infections should be isolated or nursed with precautions designed to prevent the spread of infection to other individuals.

There are four main types of isolation precautions, which should be used on the **presumption** of the relevant diagnosis.

1. Standard (universal) precautions, which should be used in dealing with all patients, entail washing hands after all patient contacts and wearing gloves when there is a risk of having contact with body fluids. Hands should be washed even if gloves have been worn.

2. Droplet precautions, which entails wearing a mask when within 3 feet of the patient and are indicated for all viral respiratory tract infections (except respiratory syncytial virus and parainfluenza virus infections (see below)), *Streptococcus pyogenes*, *Neisseria meningitidis*, *Bordetella pertussis*, and invasive *Haemophilus influenzae* infections.

3. Contact precautions, which entails wearing gloves and a gown and are indicated when one comes into contact with patients who have infected skin lesions or wound infections, who have diarrhea or other enteric-transmitted infections, such as enteroviral meningitis, or who have respiratory syncytial virus or parainfluenza virus infection.

4. Airborne precautions, which entails nursing the patient in a room with negative air pressure and the door closed (except when people are entering and leaving). It is used for patients with tuberculosis (in which case an appropriate mask should be worn by those entering the room), and for measles and varicella (in which case nonimmune individuals should not enter the room).

Individual clinicians can seldom perform the contact tracing and management necessary for addressing community interests. Therefore cases of specific infections must be reported to the local health department, whether city, county, or state. The urgency with which this should be done depends on the nature of the infection.

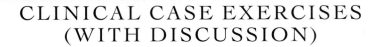

Part Two

CLINICAL CASE EXERCISES
(WITH DISCUSSION)

The sources of these cases are as follows:

(i)   The majority are derived from my own clinical experience. Because this experience covers a period of 30 years, many of these are reconstructed from memory, and therefore some of the details, especially the child's age and sex, may not be accurate.

(ii) Three cases are based on reports in the Morbidity and Mortality Weekly Reviews (MMWR). This is indicated by "(MMWR)" with the number of the case and in the reference.

(iii) Several cases are composites of different cases from my experience. These are indicated by ("COMP").

(iv) The remainder of the cases are hypothetical, based on current knowledge of the clinical manifestations of a particular illness. These include cases in which I have constructed a clinical scenario to match a photograph. These are indicated by ("HYP").

Where names of the cases have been used, they are not the patients' real names, but they contain clinically important information.

CASE 1. A previously well 13-year-old girl presents with a history of nausea, anorexia, abdominal pain , and dark urine for 3 days. On examination she has mild right upper quadrant discomfort. Jaundice cannot be detected. The rest of the examination is normal.

- *What is your differential diagnosis?*
- *What quick (2-minute) test can you do to help you?*
- *What further studies might you do?*

The differential diagnosis in this patient includes the following:

1. acute hepatitis
2. cholecystitis, cholangitis, cholelithiasis
3. gastritis and peptic ulcer disease
4. pancreatitis
5. pyelonephritis
6. hepatic sludging/sequestration if she has sickle cell disease
7. liver abscess

The clinical features of nausea, anorexia, and right upper quadrant tenderness suggest disease of the liver or gallbladder, and the dark urine suggests the possibility of bilirubinuria, which results from conjugated hyperbilirubinemia. The most likely cause of acute liver disease in a previously normal teenager is acute hepatitis. Although cholecystitis is the most common disease of the gallbladder in a teenager, it is rare in the absence of an underlying hemolytic disorder such as sickle cell disease.

The tests that can help to localize the site of disease are (a) the urinalysis, which can be performed very quickly and can demonstrate evidence of urinary tract infection (leukocyturia, hematuria, bacteruria) and evidence of conjugated hyperbilirubinemia (bilirubinuria); conjugated hyperbilirubinemia occurs in hepatitis as a result of the swollen hepatocytes compressing the bile cannaliculi; and (b) the serum bilirubin (direct and indirect) and the hepatic transaminases levels. These are elevated in hepatitis. They may also be elevated in cholelithiasis, but generally the transaminases are not elevated to levels greater than 1000 IU/ml in this condition, whereas they may reach levels of several thousand in hepatitis. The other main causes of markedly elevated transaminase levels are hepatic ischemia and drug/toxin-induced hepatic injury.

An abdominal ultrasound can be helpful in diagnosing disease of the gallbladder and of the biliary tract.

This patient had bilirubinuria and a mildly elevated conjugated serum bilirubin, and her transaminases (alanine aminotransferase (ALT) and aspartate aminotransferase (AST)) were elevated to approximately 1500 IU/dl. Acute hepatitis was diagnosed.

Hepatitis implies inflammation of the liver. Although it may occur as part of many systemic viral infections, it is usually caused by one of several specific viral infections that primarily affect the liver. In the initial stages these may not be clinically distinguishable, but they differ epidemiologically, and their outcomes may be very different. They are compared in Table 1.1.

Hepatitis A is the most likely cause of acute hepatitis in this patient. Hepatitis B and hepatitis C would be considerations if she were sexually

■TAB. 1.1: Comparison of viral hepatitides.

Virus		Transmission route	Incubation period	Potential for chronicity
Hepatitis A	RNA	fecal–oral	15–50 days	–
Hepatitis B	DNA	parenteral	28–160 days	+
Hepatitis C	RNA	parenteral	14–160 days	+
Hepatitis D	DNA	parenteral coinfection with hepatitis B	variable	+
Hepatitis E	RNA	fecal–oral	15–45	–

active, engaged in intravenous drug abuse, or had received a blood transfusion. Hepatitis E is very uncommon in the United States, but is particularly prevalent in Asia.

Patients with viral hepatitis may be asymptomatic or they may present with fever, anorexia, right upper quadrant discomfort or pain, and dark urine. On examination they have jaundice and tender hepatomegaly. Hepatitis B may be associated with a prodromal illness characterized by arthralgias and a rash. The clinical illness of hepatitis may take one of several courses: (a) mild-to-moderate illness with recovery over several weeks; (b) severe illness associated with hepatic failure (fulminant hepatitis). This may be associated with death, unless liver transplantation can be performed. Patients with hepatitis B or C may develop chronic infection that may lead to cirrhosis and hepatocellular carcinoma.

The diagnosis of hepatitis should be considered in terms of (a) Is there hepatitis? (b) What is the cause of the hepatitis, the answer to which has important public health implications?, and (c) Is there evidence of liver decompensation?

The differential diagnosis of the causes of acute hepatitis and the tests used to diagnose or differentiate between them are shown in Table 1.2.

Management of acute viral hepatitis

This consists essentially of supportive care, directed at ensuring adequate hydration, blood glucose concentration, and overall nutrition, and of monitoring the patient for the development of liver failure. Tests of liver

■TAB. 1.2: Differential diagnosis of the causes of acute hepatitis, and the tests used to diagnose them.

Etiology	Diagnostic test
Viral hepatitis	
A	anti-HAV IgM
B	anti-HBV core IgM, HBV surface antigen
C	HCV RNA
D	anti-HDV; genome detection
E	anti-HEV IgM
EBV	anti-EBV early antigen, anti-EBV VCA IgM
CMV	anti-CMV IgM, urine culture for CMV, serum CMV PCR or antigen
Bacterial hepatitis	
Q fever (*Coxiella burnetii*)	serology
Leptospirosis (*Leptospira interrogans*)	serology
Drugs and Toxins	exposure history
Isoniazid	exposure history
Acetaminophen	exposure history, serum level may or may not be helpful
Mushrooms	exposure history
Metabolic disease	
Wilson's disease	serum ceruloplasmin concentration, liver copper content

synthetic function, in particular the prothrombin time, are important in this regard. The management of liver failure and of chronic liver disease is beyond the scope of this discussion.

Antiviral therapy is not generally used in cases of acute hepatitis, but there is some evidence of the benefit of a combination of ribavirin and interferon in cases of acute hepatitis C.

The decisions about management of chronic hepatitis B with nucleotide analogues such as lamivudine, together with interferon, and of chronic hepatitis C with ribavirin and interferon should be made in consultation with a hepatologist.

Public health issues

Hepatitis A: Since the spread is fecal–oral, often from a child who is asymptomatic, once this diagnosis is made the local public health department should be notified. Therefore it is important to confirm a diagnosis of hepatitis A rapidly, by demonstration of antihepatitis A IgM in the blood. Immune globulin should be offered to family contacts and may be indicated for day-care contacts. Hepatitis A vaccine should be used routinely in high prevalence areas and before travel to countries where the risk is high.

The epidemiology and clinical features of hepatitis A are summarized in the following song:

When your stomach's feeling funny
And right up you want to throw
But your bu-bu is not runny
And your liver starts to grow

Chorus:

Hepatitis gives your skin a yellow sheen
Your stool the color cream
Your liver turning green
If your food or water are not clean
Or you have poor hygiene

In most cases it is mild
And especially in a child
But it may be fulminant
So it's something to prevent

Chorus

Hepatitis B: Hepatitis B vaccine should be given routinely to all children. Unimmunized sexual contacts of acute cases should be given hepatitis B immune globulin (HBIG) and active immunization should be initiated. Infants born to women infected with hepatitis B virus have an extremely high risk of developing chronic liver disease. Therefore such infants should receive HBIG and hepatitis B vaccine at birth. This vaccine has resulted in a marked reduction in the incidence of hepatitis B and hepatocellular carcinoma in areas where it has been widely used. It is the first vaccine to reduce the incidence of a cancer in human beings.

Readings:

Beckingham RSD: Acute hepatitis. Br Med J 2001; 322: 151–153.

Aggarwal R, Krawczynski K: Hepatitis E: an overview and recent advances in clinical and laboratory research. J Gasteroenterol Hepatol 2000; 15: 9–20.

Hochman JA, Balistreri WF: Chronic viral hepatitis: always be current! Pediatr Rev. 2003; 24: 399–410.

Lauer GM, Walker BD: Hepatitis C virus infection. N Engl J Med 2001; 345: 41–52.

Ganem D, Prince AM: Hepatitis B virus infection – natural history and clinical consequences. N Engl J Med 2004; 350: 1118–1129.

CASE 2. An 18-month-old child presents with a history of fever, cough, and red eyes for 4 days.

He is shown in the picture (Figure 2.1).

- *What is your differential diagnosis?*
- *What would you do?*

The main differential diagnosis is:

Measles
Adenovirus infection
Kawasaki disease

The constellation of symptoms and signs in this child are highly suggestive of measles. Questions about prior immunization against the infection and possible risk factors, such as foreign travel, can help to make the diagnosis. Adenoviral infections can cause conjunctivitis and respiratory tract infection and rarely a rash. Kawasaki disease is generally not associated with significant respiratory symptoms, which are very prominent in measles. In Kawasaki disease the rash occurs earlier in the febrile illness than it does in measles, and the conjunctival inflammation is primarily bulbal with perilimbic sparing and is not associated with discharge. In measles the conjunctival inflammation is tarsal as well as bulbal, and there is a conjunctival discharge. Drug eruption is not associated with a cough, and in Stevens–Johnson syndrome the mucosal disease is associated with pseudomembrane formation, which

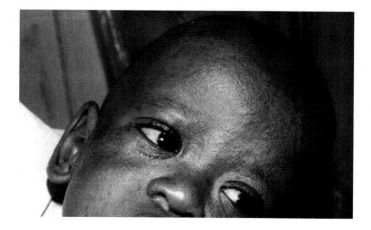

FIG. 2.1.   Child with fever, cough, and rash.

does not occur in measles. Characteristic of measles, early in the infection (1–2 days) is the presence of Koplik spots on the buccal mucosa (see below), and late in the infection (4–7 days) is the development of the rash that is almost confluent and that becomes darker with time.

This child had measles.

Measles is one of the most contagious and terrible diseases of humankind. It has an attack rate of almost 100%, and in some areas of the world, it is associated with a case fatality rate of up to 20%. Fortunately it has been eliminated from many parts of the world and has the potential to be totally eradicated. It is spread by the airborne route and has an incubation period of about 10 days.

The virus is spread systemically but also throughout the respiratory tract, where it can wreak havoc. It can also cause profound immunosuppression, which can last for several weeks. Most of the complications (discussed below) affect the respiratory tract.

Clinical manifestations: there is a prodromal illness (10th day from infection) of fever, cough, coryza, and conjunctival inflammation. About 2 days later (12th day) Koplik spots appear. These are tiny white raised spots on the very red background of the buccal mucosa including the gingival sulcus. They have the appearance of salt sprinkled on red velvet.

The whole buccal mucosa is fiery red. The whole face is running. A vague papular rash might be present at this time. (This is not the main measles rash.) The patient looks very miserable. (The origin of the name "measles" is from the Latin "misellus," which means miserable.) The measles rash appears 2 days later (14th day). This is a maculopapular rash, beginning behind the ears and descending to cover the whole body, including the palms and soles (Figure 2.2).

The spots are not very discreet, and become slightly confluent. In the early stages this rash can be difficult to see on a dark skin. However, after a few days, it becomes darker and more readily visible (Figure 2.3).

Of particular importance among the clinical manifestations is the prominence of cough.

Over the ensuing few days the rash becomes darker and desquamates. The acute illness lasts about 7 days. However, the resulting debilitation, resulting from the severe catabolic nature of the infection and its complications, may last much longer.

Organs affected/complications:

1. The whole respiratory tract can be affected, resulting in

    (a) otitis media

    (b) laryngotracheobronchitis (croup) – although initially caused by the virus, this may be complicated by bacterial superinfection

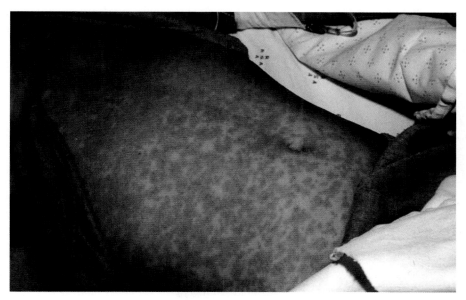

FIG. 2.2.   The rash of measles infection.

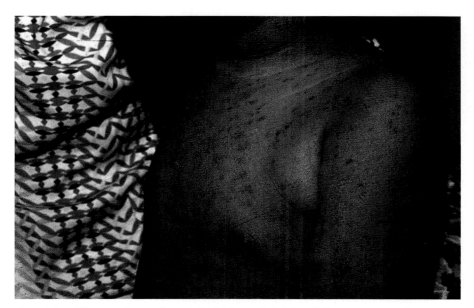

FIG. 2.3.   The measles rash in a dark-skinned child with late stage measles.

(c) bronchitis – this may lead to bronchiectasis

(d) pneumonia – this is the main cause of death from measles. It can result in chronic lung disease from obliterative bronchiolitis and bronchiectasis. Measles virus itself causes pneumonia (Figure 2.4).

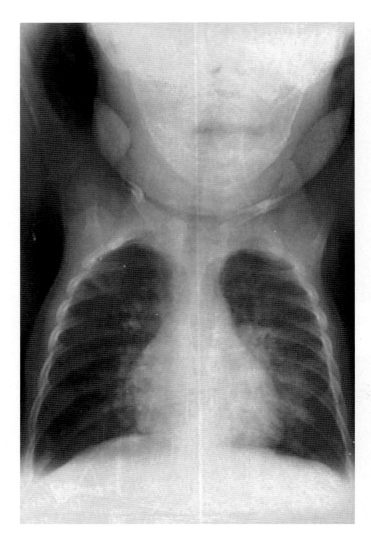

FIG. 2.4.   Chest X ray showing perihilar infiltrates due to measles pneumonia.

Because histologically this demonstrates syncytial cells (see below), it is called measles "giant cell" pneumonia.

The patient with measles is susceptible to secondary infection of the lung due to the denuded respiratory epithelium and immunosuppression. Hospitalization further exposes the patient to a variety of pathogens that might be highly antibiotic resistant. The secondary pneumonia is caused by other viruses, in particular adenovirus and herpes simplex virus, and bacteria, including *Staphylococcus aureus*, *Streptococcus pneumoniae*, *Haemophilus influenzae*, and enteric rods, in particular *Klebsiella pneumoniae* (Figure 2.5). Tuberculosis can also be reactivated during measles.

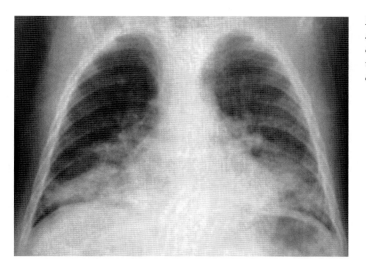

FIG. 2.5.   Chest X ray showing bronchopneumonia complicating measles. This was ultimately fatal in this child.

■TAB. 2.1:   Causes of altered mental status in individuals with measles.

Metabolic
    Hypoxia due to a respiratory complication
    Hypoglycemia due to starvation or due to kwashiorkor
    Hyponatremia due to malnutrition or diarrhea
    Reye's syndrome
Encephalitis
Meningitis complicating bacterial pneumonia

2. *Brain*:   Measles is associated with several different types of encephalitis.

  (a) *Acute encephalitis*: This occurs during or within a few weeks of the infection. In most cases it probably represents parainfectious encephalitis, or what is now called acute disseminated encephalomyelitis (ADEM). When nonselected children with measles have had electroencephalograms performed or cerebrospinal fluid (CSF) examined, these have frequently been found to be abnormal. Whether this represents mild encephalitis is unclear. Not all patients with altered mental status associated with measles have encephalitis. Other causes of altered mental status are shown in Table 2.1.

  (b) *Progressive encephalitis in immunocompromised individuals (e.g. those receiving cancer chemotherapy)*: This has its onset about 6 months after the infection. It is relentless and ultimately fatal.

  (c) *Subacute sclerosing panencephalitis (SSPE) (also called Dawson's encephalitis)*: This is a very rare complication that begins to manifest more than 1 year after the infection. It is characterized by personality changes and gradual intellectual deterioration and is ultimately fatal.

3. *Malnutrition*: Being a severely catabolic event, measles results in malnutrition. It can also be associated with diarrhea. In individuals with a borderline nutritional status, measles can precipitate overt malnutrition such as kwashiorkor. One of the nutrients whose blood concentrations decreases during measles is vitamin A. Therapy with this vitamin can reduce the fatality rate very significantly (see below).

4. *Eye*: Measles causes a punctate keratitis. In the face of vitamin A deficiency, keratitis can progress to keratomalacia and corneal perforation (Figure 2.6).

5. *Heart*: Myocarditis.

Diagnosis of measles: This should be suspected clinically in an individual with fever, cough, conjunctivitis, and a rash, especially if he or she has been in an area or in contact with someone from an area in which the disease is prevalent. In the United States, presently all cases of measles are imported. The main differential diagnosis is adenovirus infection. Kawasaki disease shares several features with measles (fever, conjunctivitis, and rash), but it is not associated with respiratory tract symptoms (see above). In the United States, it is useful to consult older practitioners who are likely to have experience in managing patients with measles. For public health reasons it is important to confirm the diagnosis of measles. This is done by demonstrating the presence of measles IgM in the blood. Other tests that might be helpful if the results can be obtained sooner than those of the IgM include the following: cytopathology of a buccal scraping, which may show multinucleate giant cells (Figure 2.7), and immunofluorescent staining for the virus of a buccal scraping or of urinary sediment.

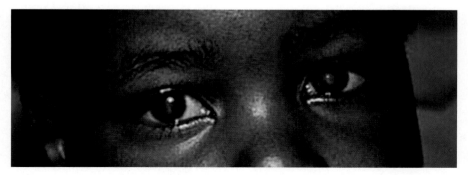

FIG. 2.6.   *A child with bilateral corneal perforations caused by measles keratitis.*

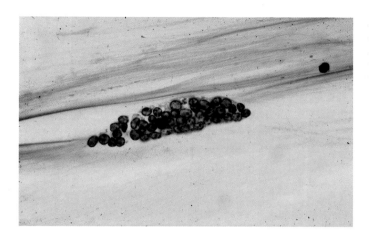

FIG. 2.7.   A Papanicolaou stained smear of a buccal scraping from a child with measles showing a multinucleate giant cell.

Management: The diagnosis of measles represents a public health emergency, because this is a highly contagious disease with a significant morbidity and mortality rate. Therefore the local health department must be contacted immediately so that contacts can be traced and managed (see below).

The management of the patient is supportive. In most patients this should be done in the home. This should entail ensuring adequate hydration and observing for complications. There is no currently available antiviral therapy for measles. In individuals with malnutrition or borderline nutritional status, or in those living in communities in which malnutrition is prevalent, vitamin A should be administered, in the dosage of 100,000–200,000 units orally. If significant complications develop for which hospitalization is necessary, the patient should be nursed with airborne isolation, and nonimmune individuals should not enter the room.

Patients who develop complications should be treated as necessary for those complications. This often entails antibiotics for presumed bacterial superinfections.

Prevention: Measles can readily be prevented by active immunization. The vaccine, which is a live, attenuated vaccine, is highly effective. Low concentrations of immune globulin that infants have acquired transplacentally from their mothers (or that children could have received from infusions of blood products) can inactivate the vaccine. In the United States, the vaccine is given routinely twice, at 12 months and at 4 years of age. In countries where the risk of measles is higher, it is given earlier. If American children are visiting such countries, they should be given the vaccine earlier (as early as 6 months of age). Although this will not be considered as the first dose for official purposes, it may be protective.

Postexposure prophylaxis for a susceptible individual: if the exposure is less than 72 hours earlier, then vaccine should be given; if more than 72 hours earlier then immune globulin should be given (0.25 ml/kg intramuscularly for normal hosts, 0.5 ml for immunocompromised hosts); HIV-infected and HIV-exposed individuals of unknown infection status should receive immune globulin irrespective of their immunization status.

Reading:

Duke T, Mgone CS: Measles: not just another viral exanthema. Lancet 2003; 361: 763–773.

Mulholland EK: Measles in the United States, N Engl J Med. 2006; 355: 440–442.

CASE 3. A 4-month-old infant presents with a runny nose, cough, and rapid breathing 5 days after receiving his 4-month immunizations. On examination he has a temperature of 38.6°C, a respiratory rate of 60/minute, and he has a diffuse expiratory wheeze.

- *What is your diagnosis?*
- *How did he get this illness?*
- *How would you treat him?*

The likely diagnosis is bronchiolitis.

This is a common pediatric condition in which there is inflammation of the small airways. The pathogenesis involves a combination of respiratory viral infection and the host's immune response to the infection. The physiological effect is narrowing of the bronchioles, resulting in air-trapping. The most common viral cause is respiratory syncytial virus (RSV), but other viral pathogens, including parainfluenza virus, may cause this disease. This disease affects primarily children younger than 1 year, although RSV infection occurs in older individuals. Affected children present with fever and cough (often following a short illness with rhinorrhea) and pulmonary findings of varying degrees of severity: tachypnea, intercostal and subcostal retractions, expiratory wheeze, and crackles. The lower edge of the liver may be displaced inferiorly (the vertical span of the liver is normal), and normal cardiac dullness to percussion may be absent, both these findings indicating hyperinflation. The clinical course of the illness lasts 1–2 weeks. Children with bronchiolitis may have concurrent pneumonia. There is a wide range of severity of disease. Most infants do not require hospitalization, a few require hospitalization, and very few develop respiratory failure.

Diagnosis: Most infants with bronchiolitis can be diagnosed clinically. Chest radiography is seldom helpful or necessary. If performed, it may show hyperinflation (Figure 3.1).

The only value of knowing whether RSV is the cause of the illness is for infection control precautions for hospitalized infants (contact isolation for those with RSV and parainfluenza infections, and droplet isolation for those with all other respiratory viral infections).

Differential diagnosis: In an infant with fever and tachypnea, the other main cause of illness is pneumonia. This may be present concurrently in children with bronchiolitis. (RSV is also the commonest cause of pneumonia in infants). In children with wheezing, asthma is a consideration. It may be difficult to differentiate bronchiolitis from asthma for the following reasons: (a) the clinical findings of tachypnea, wheezing, and hyperinflation occur in both conditions; (b) acute exacerbations of asthma are often precipitated by viral respiratory infections that cause fever and rhinorrhea. The diagnosis of

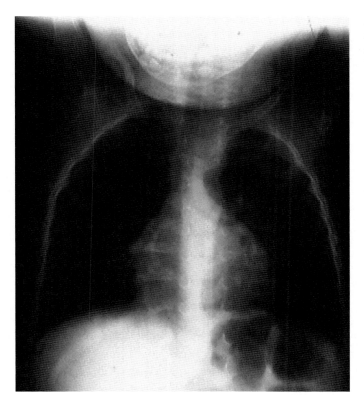

FIG. 3.1.   A chest X ray of a child with bronchiolitis, showing hyperinflation of the lungs.

bronchiolitis is more likely in patients younger than 1 year and in whom this is the first episode of wheezing.

Management is primarily supportive: it consists of ensuring adequate oxygenation and hydration (but not excessive hydration). Bronchodilator therapy with a β-agonist may be of value in some patients but has not been shown to result in improved pulmonary function in large studies. Corticosteroids are not of value, and antiviral therapy with inhaled ribavirin is of doubtful value. Two groups of children are at high risk for severe morbidity or mortality from infections with RSV, namely those with chronic lung disease resulting from prematurity (formerly called bronchopulmonary dysplasia) and those with cyanotic congenital heart disease. These children should receive anti-RSV prophylaxis with specific immune globulin (palivizumab), which is given intramuscularly once per month during the RSV season (October through March in the United States).

Reading:

Smyth RL, Openshaw PJM: Bronchiolitis. Lancet 2006; 368: 312–322.

Wohl ME, Chernick V: Treatment of acute bronchiolitis. N Engl J Med: 2003; 349: 82–83.

Breese Hall C: Respiratory syncytial virus and parainfluenza virus. N Engl J Med 2001; 344: 1917–1928.

CASE 4. A 3-week-old infant is admitted to hospital in May 1998 because of fever. On examination she has a temperature of 38°C, a red right conjunctiva, and no other abnormalities. Cerebrospinal fluid reveals 50 leukocytes per microliter, of which the majority are lymphocytes, with protein and glucose concentrations of 120 and 60 mg/dl, respectively.

- *What is your differential diagnosis?*
- *What else would you like to know?*
- *What would you do?*

This infant has meningitis or meningoencephalitis. Although bacterial meningitis is possible, it is unlikely given the predominance of lymphocytes and the normal glucose concentration in the cerebrospinal fluid. It is very likely that the infant has a viral meningitis or meningoencephalitis. The most important viruses to consider are herpes simplex virus (HSV), which can cause very severe brain damage and against which treatment is available, and enteroviruses, which usually cause benign disease and against which treatment is currently not available.

Examination of the eye might give useful information. If there is a corneal ulcer, it would strongly suggest HSV infection. HSV infection in the neonate is usually acquired from the mother during the birth process. A maternal history of genital sores at the time of delivery would raise the likelihood of HSV infection significantly, but lack of this history would not exclude this possibility. The risk of HSV infection in a baby born vaginally to a mother with a primary genital HSV infection at the time of delivery is about 60%, while the risk if the mother has a recurrence of this infection is only about 2%.

Although rare, neonatal HSV infection is a very severe disease because it can result in death or very severe brain damage. There are three main forms of the infection.

(a) *Skin, eye, and mouth disease*: The skin lesions are vesicles with a red base, which progress to pustules, often in clusters. They can occur anywhere but are most frequent at the presenting site or where a break in the skin might have occurred. Therefore the scalp, including the site of a scalp fetal monitor probe, is often affected. When typical skin or mucosal lesions are present, the diagnosis can be readily made clinically. Such lesions should nevertheless be cultured. However, these lesions are present in only about one-third of cases of neonatal HSV infection. Therefore the possibility of HSV infection should be entertained in any newborn with fever or evidence of serious disease for which there is no other obvious explanation.

Other cutaneous lesions that can resemble HSV vesicles are (i) varicella – this is a generalized rash; (ii) bullous impetigo due to *Staphylococcus aureus*. These are larger than herpetic vesicles, are often in different parts of the body, and a Gram stain of a smear of the lesion fluid shows numerous polymorphonuclear leukocytes and Gram-positive cocci in clusters. (iii) Candida infection – these are usually confined to the diaper area and inner thighs, and a Gram stain of fluid from the lesions shows yeasts. (iv) Other bullous diseases of childhood, such as epidermolysis bullosa. These lesions are much larger than those of HSV infection. (v) Aplasia cutis: HSV infection acquired in utero can cause loss of skin that gives the appearance of aplasia cutis.

The mouth lesions are similar to those on the skin.

The ocular disease usually manifests as conjunctivitis or keratitis. The typical herpetic corneal lesion is a dendritic ulcer, which has a serpiginous border. (The name for herpes is derived from the Greek word for "creeping thing").

(b) *Brain disease (encephalitis):* This often manifests with seizures and a change in level of consciousness. However, early on in the herpetic infection there may not be any specific neurological manifestation. Most infants with perinatally acquired HSV encephalitis present between 15 and 19 days of age. The differential diagnosis includes several metabolic diseases, such as hypoglycemia, hyponatremia, hypocalcemia, hypomagnesemia, pyridoxine deficiency, inborn errors of metabolism, hypoxic injury, hemorrhage, and other infections, including bacterial meningitis and enteroviral meningoencephalitis. Differentiating HSV from enterovirus infection in infants with CSF pleocytosis is a major challenge. The differences are shown in Table 4.1. The main differences are that the cell count tends to be much higher and the protein concentration much lower in enteroviral meningitis. Despite these differences, I treat all neonates with CSF pleocytosis and with a negative Gram stain for bacteria, for the possibility of HSV encephalitis, pending the results of further studies (see below). HSV encephalitis, even in infants who have been appropriately treated, is associated with a very low probability for normal neurological outcome.

(c) *Disseminated disease:* This manifests with features of the sepsis syndrome, with fever, and progressive evidence of multiorgan dysfunction, including liver failure and coagulopathy. The other main causes of this clinical scenario are enteroviral infection, bacteremia, and inherited disorders of metabolism. Considering the life-threatening state of patients presenting in this manner, they should be treated

■TAB. 4.1: Comparison of cerebrospinal fluid findings in neonatal HSV encephalitis and enteroviral meningitis.

Reference	No. of leukocytes × 10^6/l		Protein conc. (mg/dl)	
HSV				
Nahmias	0–2500		up to 1000	
Arvin	100–262 (70–95% mononuclear)		63–210	
Gutman	10–315		95–100 (initially)	
Enterovirus				
No. of leukocytes (% of cases in each group)	% neutrophils (% of cases in each group)		Protein conc. (% of cases in each group)	
Rorabaugh	<10	(5)	<50	(66)	<50	(28)
	10–25	(22)	50–75	(19)	50–79	(40)
	26–100	(22)	76–90	(10)	80–119	(23)
	101–500	(31)	>90	(5)	120–170	(7)
	501–1000	(13)			>170	(3)
	>1000	(7)				

with antiviral therapy as well as broad-spectrum antibiotics until a definitive diagnosis can be made. Studies for metabolic diseases should also be performed as part of the initial evaluation.

Enterovirus (Coxsackie and echovirus) infection is common, and enteroviral meningitis usually has a benign course and outcome. Although the infection can occur at any age, most cases are diagnosed within the first few months of life. This is probably due, at least in part, to the frequency with which young febrile infants undergo lumbar puncture. Enterovirus infection in the first few days of life can cause very severe illness. In this case the infection may have been acquired from the mother around the time of delivery or in the nursery, soon after the infant's birth. The infection manifests as a rapidly progressive multiorgan system disease, with myocarditis, hepatitis, pneumonia, and adrenal disease.

What would you like to know?

Considering the large number of diagnostic possibilities in such infants and the rarity of HSV infection, several pieces of information might help in increasing the probability of HSV infection, and thus of favoring initiating empiric antiviral therapy with acyclovir:

History of exposure: (a) genital HSV infection in the mother at the time of delivery (that was the case in this mother); (b) penile lesions in the mother's sexual partner (that had also occurred in this patient's case); HSV infection in close contacts, such as fever blisters.

Examination: The skin should be thoroughly examined, including the scalp. In this case careful examination of the red eye revealed a dendritic ulcer, which is characteristic of HSV keratitis, and, thus clinically confirmed the diagnosis of HSV infection.

What would you like to do?

Management: In suspected cases material from lesions, when available, should be sent to the laboratory for viral culture. In this case the eye culture was positive for HSV. In addition, swabs from the mouth and rectum should also be cultured for HSV. Although laboratories might observe the cultures for up to a week, they are often positive within 48 hours. Cerebrospinal fluid should be tested for HSV by polymerase chain reaction (PCR). Pending the results of tests, empiric therapy should be initiated. This consists of acyclovir administered intravenously at a dosage of 20 mg/kg/dose given every 8 hours. If the diagnosis is confirmed or considered likely this should be continued for a total of 21 days in cases of encephalitis and for 14 days in cases without encephalitis.

Prevention: Intrapartum acquired HSV infection can largely be prevented by performing caesarean sections on mothers in labor with overt genital

HSV infection. If a baby is indeed born vaginally to such a woman, the following should be considered: specimens should be taken about 24 hours after delivery, from the mouth, nose, conjunctiva, and rectum for HSV culture, and the parents be instructed to bring the child for care if there are any signs of illness. If this occurs, or if the cultures are positive, antiviral therapy should be initiated while further evaluation is conducted.

Some infants with neonatal HSV who have been appropriately treated develop recurrences of cutaneous lesions. It is unclear how these patients should be managed.

Reading:

Kimberlin DW: Neonatal herpes simplex infection. Clin Microbiol Rev 2004; 17: 1–13.

References:

Whitley RJ, Corey L, Arvin A et al: Changing presentation of herpes simplex virus infection in neonates. J Infect Dis 1988; 158: 109.

Arvin et al: Neonatal herpes simplex infection in the absence of mucocutaneous lesions. J Pediatr 1982; 100: 715.

Gutman LT, Wilfert CM, Eppes S: Herpes simplex virus encephalitis in children: analysis of cerebrospinal fluid and progressive neurodevelopmental deterioration. J Infect Dis 1986; 154: 415.

Rorabaugh ML, Berlin LE, Heldrich F et al: Aseptic meningitis in infants younger than 2 years of age: acute illness and neurologic complications. Pediatrics 1993; 92: 206.

Nahmias A et al: Herpes simplex. In: Remington J. Klein J (editors): Infections of the fetus and newborn infant. WB Saunders. Philadelphia, 1983, pp. 66–809.

Frenkel LM: Challenges in the diagnosis and management of neonatal herpes simplex virus encephalitis. Pediatrics 2005; 115: 795–797.

Fonseca-Aten M, Messina AF, Jafri HS, Sanchez PJ: Herpes simplex virus encephalitis during suppressive therapy with acyclovir in a premature infant. Pediatrics 2005; 115: 804.

CASE 5. (HYP). A 5-year-old boy presents with a limp. This was preceded by a febrile illness, but there has been no preceding trauma. On examination he has weakness of all muscle groups in his right lower limb. The limb is hypotonic, and deep tendon reflexes cannot be elicited. There is no pain on movement of the joints nor is there tenderness. Sensory examination is normal.

- *What is your differential diagnosis?*
- *What else would you like to know?*
- *What would you do?*

Since there is no pain, trauma or infection of the bones, joints or muscles can be eliminated as causes of the limp. The finding of weakness indicates a muscle or nervous system problem. The main acute disease of muscle is myositis, which is usually associated with pain, and is usually more diffuse. Therefore the disease is most likely one of the nervous system.

Where in the nervous system could a lesion be located that would cause the present illness?

1. *Brain*: If a single lesion, it would have to be localized to the left motor cortex, in the medial aspect of the brain. This would be associated with hypertonia and increased deep tendon reflexes.

The clinical features are those of a lower motor neuron problem. The anatomy of the lower motor neuron is shown in Figure 5.1.

2. *Spinal cord*: If a single lesion, it would have to be located at several levels of the cord on the right side. This would be unlikely in the absence of sensory changes.

However, multiple lesions affecting cells in the anterior horns at several levels could explain this. This is what occurs in poliomyelitis.

3. *Peripheral nerve*: The most common acute peripheral nerve disease of children is the Guillain-Barre syndrome. This presents as an ascending weakness and is symmetrical.

4. *Neuromuscular junction*: Botulism, which presents with a descending, symmetrical paralysis, is the main example of disease affecting this area. One of the important abnormalities in this condition is ptosis.

This child has poliomyelitis. This is an enteroviral infection caused by polio viruses 1, 2, and 3, which are transmitted by the fecal–oral route. It affects motor neurons of the spinal cord and the brain. The infection is characterized by fever, myalgia, and backache, which may resolve completely or may be followed by flaccid weakness. Aseptic meningitis is often present. Although the weakness is usually localized to one limb or muscle group, it

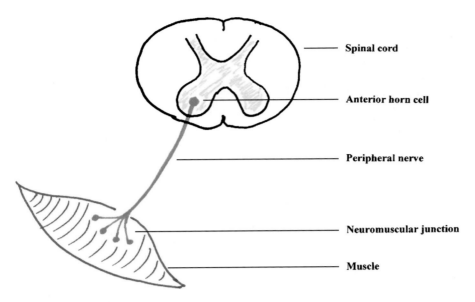

FIG. 5.1.   The different parts of the lower motor neuron unit.

may be generalized. When the brainstem is involved (bulbar poliomyelitis) swallowing and respiration are affected. There may be recovery, but paralysis may persist, with wasting of the affected muscle group (Figure 5.2). Nonpolio enteroviruses and West Nile virus can cause the same clinical syndrome.

A postpolio syndrome, characterized by weakness, muscle atrophy, and generalized fatigue may develop decades after the acute infection.

Poliomyelitis is diagnosed primarily clinically. The diagnosis should be confirmed by culture of the virus from the stool. This makes it possible to examine the viral genome to determine whether the incriminated virus is wild polio virus or oral vaccine virus, which can, rarely, cause paralytic disease. The main exposure questions are (a) has he been adequately immunized against the infection and (b) has he traveled recently to an area where polio is still prevalent (e.g. India)?

Management: In this child the management is concerned with physical therapy. Long-term care will depend on the degree of recovery that occurs. However, in patients with bulbar involvement or involvement of the nerves innervating the muscles of respiration, respiratory support is critical. It is important to notify the case to the local health department because the virus can be spread rapidly in both pharyngeal secretions and by the fecal–oral route. It is important to ensure that his contacts are immunized and that he practices good hygiene. In the United States, polio vaccine is given thrice during the first 18 months of life, and again at the age of 4–6 years. In the

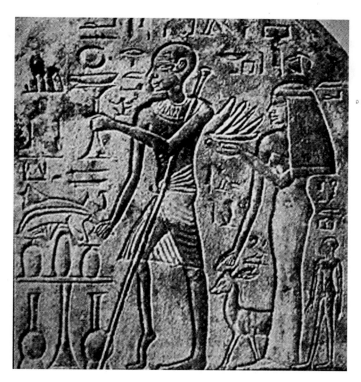

FIG. 5.2.   Unilateral lower limb wasting, typical of the late effect of poliomyelitis. This picture depicts a Pharaoh of the 18th dynasty. (Reprinted from: Loschiavo F: The Lancet. Volume 347, page 628, with permission from Elsevier Publishers).

United States, only the inactivated (Salk) vaccine is used, while in many other parts of the world the oral, live, attenuated (Sabin) vaccine is used. Although significant progress has been made in attempts to eradicate polio from the earth, this has recently been hampered by objection to immunization by some communities in northern Nigeria, resulting in spread of the virus to adjacent countries. Outbreaks can occur in unvaccinated communities within countries with high vaccination rates, as shown by a recent outbreak in the United States.

Reading:

Burk J, Agre J: Characteristics and management of postpolio syndrome. JAMA 2000; 284: 412–414.

Ogra PL: Poliomyelitis as a paradigm for investment in and success of vaccination programs, Pediatr Infect Dis J 1999; 18: 10–15.

Centers for Disease Control and Prevention: Progress toward interruption of wild poliovirus transmission worldwide, January 2004–March 2005. MMWR 2005; 54: 408–412.

Centers for Disease Control and Prevention: Poliovirus infections in four unvaccinated children – Minnesota, August–October 2005. MMWR 2005; 54: 1053–1055.

CASE 6. (COMP). An 18-year-old boy presents with a history of severe sore throat and fever for a few days. On examination he has a temperature of 39°C, very large, red tonsils with exudate, resembling that shown in Figure 6.1, and large cervical lymph nodes.

- *What is your differential diagnosis?*
- *What else would you like to know?*
- *What would you do?*

Differential diagnosis: Infectious mononucleosis, due to Epstein–Barr virus; *Streptococcus pyogenes* tonsillitis; gonococcal tonsillitis; diphtheria; respiratory virus infection.

What would you like to know?

Is he sexually active? If so, does he engage in oro-genital sex, which could expose him to gonococcal tonsillitis?

Is there splenomegaly? This would strongly support the diagnosis of infectious mononucleosis. If he were sexually active, acute HIV infection should also be considered.

Has he traveled to a country where diphtheria is endemic or been in contact with an individual who has come from such a country? Is he immunized against diphtheria?

Management of this patient: Streptococcal tonsillitis should be diagnosed or excluded by performing a streptococcal test on a throat swab. If confirmed

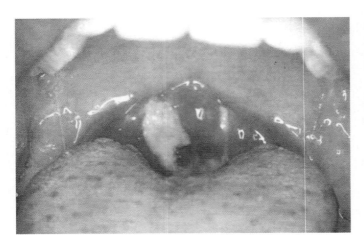

FIG. 6.1. The pharynx of a patient with the same diagnosis as that of the patient described above. (with permission of James H Brien, DO, Texas A and M University College of Medicine)

he should be treated with penicillin. If gonococcal tonsillitis is a consideration, a throat culture, specifically for gonococcus, should be performed. This requires use of a selective medium (Thayer-Martin). The diagnosis of infectious mononucleosis caused by EBV can be confirmed with a heterophile antibody test. In this condition a blood count may show lymphocytosis, and a blood smear may show Downy cells (atypical lymphocytes) (Figure 6.2).

This patient had infectious mononucleosis caused by Epstein–Barr virus.

Epstein–Barr virus (EBV): This gamma herpes virus is spread from one individual (who is usually asymptomatic, but in whom the virus has been reactivated) to another by saliva, but it can be transmitted by blood transfusion. The incubation period is 4–6 weeks.

It becomes latent in oral epithelial cells and B-lymphocytes, where it can become oncogenic. Most individuals are infected in childhood, when the infection is usually asymptomatic or has nonspecific manifestations, such as fever. However, in older children and adults it can cause severe symptomatic disease. It is a cause of severe disease in immunocompromised individuals. Because the virus results in the production of many nonspecific antibodies (heterophile antibodies), infection can be complicated by autoimmune diseases.

Pathogenesis: The virus enters oral epithelial cells and then B-lymphocytes, which proliferate. T-lymphocytes proliferate and attack the infected B-lymphocytes. These T-lymphocytes constitute the primitive-appearing "atypical" lymphocytes on the blood smear described above. The inflammation occurring in the organs is largely the result of the T-lymphocyte response.

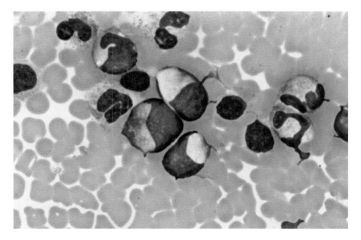

FIG. 6.2. The characteristic "atypical" lymphocytes (Downy cells) in the blood of a 6-year-old child with infectious mononucleosis.

Clinical manifestations of EBV infection

1. Infectious mononucleosis (glandular fever): This affects mainly older children, teenagers, and young adults. It is characterized by:

   (i)   fever, which may persist for a few weeks;

   (ii)   pharyngotonsillitis: this may be very severe, associated with pseudomembrane formation, and may lead to obstruction of the oral pharynx; this form is called "anginose" infectious mononucleosis;

   (iii) cervical lymphadenopathy;

   (iv)   generalized lymphadenopathy;

   (v)   splenomegaly;

   (vi)   hepatitis: chemical evidence of hepatitis (elevated serum transaminase activity) is frequent, but clinical evidence of hepatitis can also occur.

   There may be significant malaise, which can persist for several weeks or months.

2. Several organ systems can be affected as a result of acute EBV infection:

   (i)   blood: autoimmune hemolytic anemia; leucopenia; thrombocytopenia;

   (ii)   nervous system: Guillain-Barre syndrome; transverse myelitis; encephalitis; ataxia; "Alice-in-Wonderland" syndrome (in which objects appear larger or smaller than they should);

   (iii) lungs: pneumonia;

   (iv)   kidneys: glomerulonephritis;

   (v)   heart: myocarditis;

   (vi)   skin: although a rash is unusual in this infection, a macular rash occurs in about 90% of individuals who receive ampicillin or amoxicillin during the infection. This occurs about 10 days after exposure to these drugs.

   (vii) splenic rupture: this a life-threatening complication of EBV infectious mononucleosis. It should be considered in an individual with features of infectious mononucleosis, who develops acute abdominal, flank, or shoulder-tip pain, anemia, or shock. The risk period is up to 1 month after diagnosis.

   The differential diagnosis of infectious mononucleosis caused by EBV includes the similar clinical syndrome caused by other agents, namely cytomegalovirus, toxoplasmosis, and HIV. In sexually active individuals, HIV is the most important consideration. Pharyngotonsillitis due to *Streptococcus pyogenes* and respiratory viruses is associated with the pharyngeal and cervical lymph node manifestations of infectious mononucleosis, but not generalized lymphadenopathy or splenomegaly. The presence of anemia, thrombocytopenia, or leucopenia would also suggest the possibility of leukemia or lymphoma.

3. Fever, with no other manifestations.

4. Diseases in the immunocompromised host:

   (a) X-linked lymphoproliferative disorder (Duncan syndrome): this disorder, affecting males only, is characterized by an immunodeficiency limited to EBV. Affected boys, who cannot contain the infection, develop progressive infection with organ dysfunction, or lymphoma, both of which are fatal.

   (b) posttransplant lymphoproliferative disease (PTLD): this results from the therapeutic immunosuppression used to prevent organ rejection in transplant recipients. It has been a particular risk with cyclosporine therapy. It begins as a focus of polyclonal lymphoproliferation and can progress to a lymphoma. It can affect any area including the transplanted organ or lymph nodes. The diagnosis depends on clinical suspicion, which should lead to biopsy.

   (c) malignancies (see below).

5. Malignancies:

   (a) nasopharyngeal carcinoma

   (b) Burkitt's lymphoma (African type) (Figures 6.3 and 6.4)

   (c) Nasal natural killer-T-cell lymphoma

   (d) Hodgkin's disease

   (e) B-cell lymphoma in immunosuppressed individuals

   (f) leiomyosarcoma in immunosuppressed individuals.

Diagnosis of EBV infection: In most normal children, confirming the diagnosis of infectious mononucleosis caused by EBV is not always necessary. There is value in making a specific diagnosis in the following circumstances:

(i) when a diagnostic work-up for prolonged, unexplained fever, or for lymphadenopathy is planned. Having a specific diagnosis of EBV infection can avert such a work-up.

(ii) advising children against contact sports for 1 month after diagnosis.

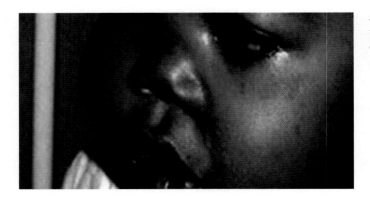

FIG. 6.3.   An African child with Burkitt's lymphoma affecting the right maxilla (external view).

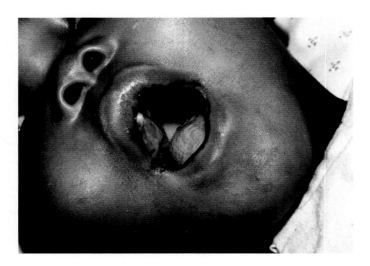

FIG. 6.4.   An African child with Burkitt's lymphoma affecting the right maxilla (internal view).

Diagnostic tests:

(i)   *blood count and smear*: this may show an absolute lymphocytosis and characteristic atypical lymphocytes, described above (Figure 6.2).

(ii) *heterophile antibody*: these are antibodies that are unrelated to the virus and cause agglutination of sheep red cells after absorption with guinea pig kidney cells but not bovine red cells. There are several tests for this such as the "Monospot" test. This test is fairly specific. It is frequently negative in children younger than 4 years.

(iii) *specific EBV antibodies*: antibodies to several different EBV antigens can be detected. Their profile can give an indication of when the infection occurred.

These are shown in Table 6.1. As the table suggests, these tests are frequently difficult to interpret.

■TAB. 6.1: Interpretation of antibody tests to EBV antigens.

Time of infection	Current	Test result Recent (weeks)	Past
Antigen			
Viral capsid antigen (VCA) IgM	+	+/−	−
VCA IgG	+	+	+
Early antigen (EA)	+	+/−	−
Epstein–Barr nuclear antigen (EBNA)	−	+/−	+

(iv)   *PCR:* the detection and quantitation of EBV DNA in the patient's blood has made it possible to examine progression of disease and response to management in immunocompromised patients, such as those who have had transplants, and are suspected of having posttransplant lymphoproliferative disease (PTLD).

(v)   although the virus can be cultured in vitro, this cannot be done in most diagnostic laboratories.

Management: There is currently no drug available that is very active against EBV. Nevertheless acyclovir has some activity against the virus. Treatment of normal hosts is supportive. Treatment of those with PTLD depends on modification of immunosuppression, other forms of immunomodulation, and sometimes chemotherapy, the discussion of which is beyond the scope of this text.

In patients with severe tonsillar swelling and the threat of airway obstruction associated with infectious mononucleosis, administration of corticosteroids is beneficial.

Reading:

Cohen J: Epstein-Barr virus infection. N Engl J Med 2000; 343: 481–492.

Okano M: Epstein-Barr virus infection and its role in the expanding spectrum of human diseases, Acta Paediatr 1998; 87: 11–18.

Thorley-Lawson DA., Gross A: Persistence of Epstein-Barr virus and origins of associated lymphomas. N Engl J Med 2004; 350: 1328–1337.

■CASE 7. (MMWR). A 13-year-old previously healthy boy presents with a history of fever and headache for about 3 days. Now he is generally getting worse. On examination he looks very ill. He has a high fever, is slightly obtunded, and has poor perfusion. During the examination he starts to vomit blood. It is noticed that after blood is drawn, he continues to bleed at the venipuncture site. There are no focal abnormalities.

- *What disturbances are present and what might have caused them?*
- *What else would you like to know?*
- *What would you do?*

The clinical features suggest the presence of an infection that is causing shock, that is systemic, that might be affecting the brain, and that is associated with a coagulopathy. Infections that might do this are:

Viral: hemorrhagic fevers, including those caused by Ebola virus, Marburg virus, Lassa virus, Rift Valley fever virus, Yellow fever virus and dengue virus, and Congo-Crimean hemorrhagic fever;

Bacterial: rickettsioses, sepsis syndrome (in particular meningococcemia), plague, and leptospirosis;

Parasitic: falciparum malaria and African trypanosomiasis.

Therefore it is very important to obtain a history of possible exposures to the above infectious agents.

Additional history of exposures: he has recently returned from a 1-week field trip with his school in a non–malaria-endemic rural part of South Africa. A tick was removed from him. Therefore, with the consideration of a rickettsial infection, when his illness began, he was treated with tetracycline. However, his symptoms progressed.

Management: The most important element of this is supportive care, which should be directed at reversing the shock and the coagulopathy. Treatment for possible treatable infections should be provided at the same time as tests are being performed to make a diagnosis. (All laboratories to which specimens are sent should be informed of the possibility of a viral hemorrhagic fever.) These tests should include blood cultures and, in circumstances in which possible exposure to malaria and trypanosomiasis has occurred, a blood smear, to look for these parasites. Serum should be stored for possible future testing. Blood should be sent to a laboratory with facilities to look for hemorrhagic fever viruses. Appropriate specimens also need to be submitted to the laboratory for evaluation of his physiological derangements (chemistry and hematologic studies). Antimicrobial therapy should be directed at the above-mentioned pathogens (broad-spectrum antibiotic therapy). Although his symptoms suggest the possibility of brain infection, his condition (shock and coagulopathy) contraindicates the performance of a lumbar puncture. Consideration should be given to the administration of ribavirin intravenously, which has activity against some of the hemorrhagic fever viruses, in particular Lassa fever (endemic in West Africa). Strict contact isolation precautions should be employed, in addition to the use of mask and eye protection when procedures are performed that have the potential to cause splashes or aerosols.

The local health department should be notified immediately of a patient with the possibility of a viral hemorrhagic fever, meningococcemia, or plague. In the United States, the Centers for Disease Control and Prevention should also be notified about any case of suspected hemorrhagic fever.

The viruses causing hemorrhagic fevers belong to four main virus families, namely the Arenaviridae (Lassa fever, Argentinian hemorrhagic fever, Bolivian hemorrhagic fever), the Bunyaviridae (Congo-Crimean hemorrhagic fever, Rift Valley fever), the Filoviridae (Ebola and Marburg), and the Flaviviridae (Yellow fever, dengue). Although their clinical manifestations vary, as a group they include the following: fever, headache, sore throat, myalgia, backache, macular rash, hemorrhage, multiorgan dysfunction, and shock.

The diagnosis in this patient was Congo-Crimean hemorrhagic fever (tick-transmitted).

Viral hemorrhagic fever viruses are widespread in Africa and South America. The speed of international air travel facilitates the spread of such viruses. An infected individual can present anywhere in the world. These infections carry a very high fatality rate. Some can be spread from person-to-person and can thus constitute an important nosocomial threat.

Reading:

Androniko S, Hopp M, Thompson PD et al: Congo-Crimean Hemorrhagic Fever – South Africa. MMWR 30: 349–51, July 24, 1981.

Peters CJ: Role of the endothelium in viral hemorrhagic fevers. Crit Care Med 2002; 30: S268–S273.

Borio L, Inglesby T, Peters CJ et al: Hemorrhagic fever viruses as biological weapons. Medical and public health management. JAMA 2002; 287: 2391–2405.

Isaacson M: Viral hemorrhagic fever hazards for travelers in Africa. Clin Infect Dis 2001; 33: 1707–1712.

Geisbert T, Jahrling PB: Exotic emerging viral diseases: progress and challenges. Nat Med. 2004; 10: S110–S121.

Peters CJ: Marburg and Ebola – arming ourselves against the deadly filoviruses, N Engl J Med. 2005; 352: 2571–2573.

CASE 8 (HYP). A 15-year-old boy presents with episodes of agitation and anxiety, and confusion. On examination he has a temperature of 38.2° C and shows slight obtundation and disorientation, but the rest of his examination is normal. A computer tomography (CT) scan is normal and an extended drug-screen is negative. The cerebrospinal fluid reveals 70 leukocytes per microliter of which 95% are lymphocytes, with protein and glucose concentrations of 100 and 50 mg/dl, respectively.

- *What is your differential diagnosis?*
- *What else would you like to know?*
- *What would you do?*

This patient has brain dysfunction and a cerebrospinal fluid (CSF) pleocytosis, suggesting an inflammatory process involving the brain. The following terminology (rightly or wrongly) is often used, according to tradition, to describe disease associated with CSF pleocytosis and brain disease:

(i)   meningitis – CSF pleocytosis with normal brain function. This may be of bacterial or other origin.

■TAB. 8.1:   A list of causes of encephalitis.

Agent	Exposure	Treatment
Viruses		
Herpes simplex	no specific	acyclovir
Enterovirus	no specific	none
Arboviruses	mosquitoes, ticks, flies	none
HIV	human (sexual)	antiretrovirals
Rabies	animal bite	none[a]
Bacteria		
Borrelia burgdorferi	tick	ceftriaxone
Mycoplasma pneumoniae	human	doxycyline
Treponema pallidum	human (sexual)	penicillin
Fungi	OI	amphotericin B, fluconazole
Protozoa		
Toxoplasma gondii	cats, raw meat, OI	pyrimethamine + sulfonamide
Naegleria fowleri	fresh water	amphotericin B + rifampin
Worms		
Baylisascaris procyonis	raccoon feces	
Neurocysticercosis	feces of human who has eaten raw pork	albendazole, praziquantel
Noninfectious disease		
Systemic lupus erythematosus		corticosteroids

[a]Recently a well-documented case of survival from rabies following treatment with ribavirin, interferon, and hypothermia has been reported.

(ii)   meningitis – CSF pleocytosis with brain dysfunction that is thought to be of bacterial, mycobacterial, or fungal origin.

(iii)   encephalitis or meningoencephalitis – CSF pleocytosis with brain dysfunction that is thought to be viral or parasitic in origin (that is not bacterial, mycobacterial, or fungal)

(iv)   cerebritis – focal brain parenchymal inflammation (the equivalent of cellulitis), thought to be of bacterial, fungal, or parasitic origin.

The lymphocytic predominance and normal glucose in the CSF suggest the diagnosis of encephalitis. Although a parameningeal infection such as a brain abscess or subdural empyema can result in this CSF picture, the normal CT scan makes this unlikely. (A CT scan with contrast would be a more sensitive test to detect these conditions.) A wide variety of infectious agents and noninfectious diseases can cause encephalitis. These are shown in Table 8.1.

It is important to obtain an exposure history to determine the possibility of exposure to the above agents. This includes travel, occupational, recreational, and animal exposures.

When appropriate, tests to help to diagnose these infections or conditions should be performed.

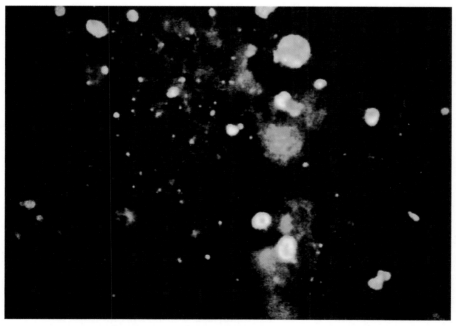

FIG. 8.1.   Immunofluorescence of rabies virus in brain tissue. (Courtesy of Dr Tierkel, Centers for Disease Control and Prevention)

This patient was a spelunker and had frequently entered caves inhabited by bats. This poses a risk of exposure to rabies virus, which could explain his illness.

Tests to diagnose rabies should be performed. These include submission of saliva, CSF, and biopsies of the nape of the neck to a laboratory equipped to perform the tests for rabies (Figure 8.1). In the United States, specimens should be sent to the Centers for Disease Control and Prevention in Atlanta.

Management (a) Supportive; (b) antimicrobial therapy directed against those agents that could cause this clinical picture, and for which therapy is available. Pending the outcome of an epidemiologic enquiry and laboratory tests, I employ the following regimen: (i) acyclovir for its activity against HSV; (ii) cefriaxone for its activity against *Neisseria meningitidis*, *Streptococcus pneumoniae*, and *Borrelia burgdorferi*; (iii) doxycycline for its activity against *Mycoplasma pneumoniae*. (c) contact isolation precautions; (d) if rabies is suspected, the health department should be notified.

Reading:

Hirsch MS, Werner B: Case 17-2003: a 38-year-old woman with fever, headache, and confusion. N Engl J Med 2003; 348: 2239–2247.

Whitley RJ, Gnann JW: Viral encephalitis: familiar infections and emerging pathogens. Lancet 2002; 359: 507–514.

Warrell MJ, Warrell DA: Rabies and other lyssavirus diseases. Lancet 2004; 363: 959–969.

Hemachudha T, Laothamatas J, Rupprecht C: Human rabies: a disease of complex neuropathogenetic mechanisms and diagnostic challenge. Lancet Neurol 2002; 1: 101–109.

Jackson AC: Update on rabies. Curr Opin Neurol. 2002; 15: 327–331.

Willoughby RE Jr, Tieves KS, Hoffman GM et al: Brief report: survival after treatment of rabies with induction of coma. N Engl J Med 2005; 352: 2508–2514.

Romero JR, Newland JG: Diagnosis of viral encephalitides: nonzoonotic-associated viruses. Pediatr Infect Dis J 2006; 25: 739–740.

Romero JR, Newland JG: Diagnosis of viral encephalitides: zoonotic-associated viruses. Pediatr Infect Dis J 2006; 25: 741–742.

CASE 9. A 6-year-old girl presents with a mild fever and a few small blisters on her shoulder and chest (Figure 9.1).

- *What is the diagnosis?*
- *What are the main complications of this infection?*

Observation: Lesions at different stages: tiny papule; vesicle; pustule; crusted lesion.

Diagnosis: varicella (chickenpox).

Varicella is caused by the human herpes virus, varicella zoster virus (VZV). It is a common infection affecting most individuals during childhood (prior to the use of vaccine). It is highly contagious, being transmitted both by direct contact and by the airborne route. The incubation period is 10–21 days. If varicella zoster immune globulin (VZIG) has been administered to an individual in an attempt to prevent infection (see below), the incubation period may be prolonged up to 28 days.

Clinical features: There may be a prodrome of 1 or 2 days during which fever occurs. This is followed by the appearance of skin lesions. These begin as tiny papules, which progress rapidly to clear vesicles, and then, over a few days, to pustules and then scabs. The number of lesions varies from fewer than 10 to several hundred. The course of the illness usually lasts about 7 days. Of importance in differentiating this infection from other infections are:

(i)   different stage lesions are present at the same time (Figure 9.1);

(ii)   the lesions tend to be distributed more centripetally than centrifugally, but they can involve the palms and soles (Figure 9.2);

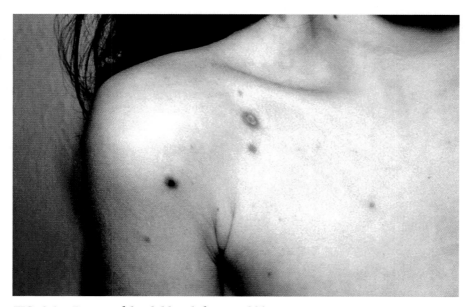

FIG. 9.1.   Picture of the child with fever and blisters.

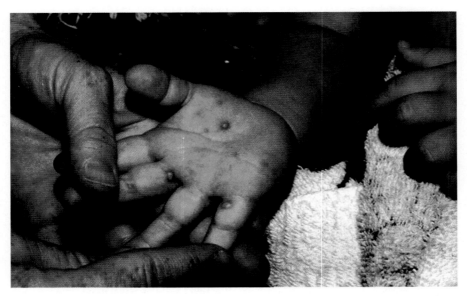

FIG. 9.2.   Varicella in the sibling of child shown in Figure 9.1, showing palmar lesions.

(iii)   they may be present inside the mouth (Figure 9.3); this can be helpful diagnostically.

Fever usually lasts up to about 3 days. If fever persists longer than this time, or if it abates and then recurs, the development of secondary bacterial infection should be suspected. Most children are not very ill with this infection, but adults tend to have more severe systemic illness.

Diagnosis: The diagnosis of chickenpox is made clinically. Although the virus can be cultured, this is difficult and takes several weeks. In situations in which a definitive diagnosis is particularly important, immunofluorescent tests of scrapings from lesions can be used. The differential diagnosis includes:

Smallpox – the lesions are deeper in the skin, are distributed more centrifugally, and all are at a similar stage (Figure 9.4).

Vaccinia – the lesions are usually localized to around the site of inoculation (Figure 9.5).

Bullous impetigo – the lesions start as pustules and do not form a dark red crust. They are generally fewer in number and larger than those in varicella.

Herpes simplex – the lesions appear the same as in chickenpox, but they are localized.

Insect bites – these tend to be papules. Although fire ant (*Solemnopsis invicta*) bites can appear very similar to chickenpox lesions, they are localized, and there is a distinct history of the bite incident (Figure 9.6).

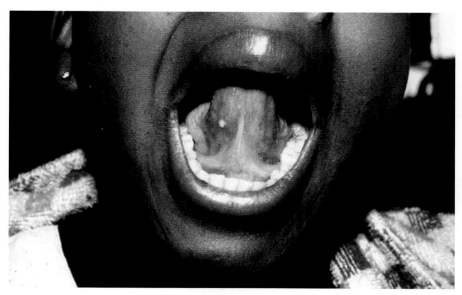

FIG. 9.3.   A woman with the enanthem of varicella.

Management: In most cases symptomatic management is all that is required. This might include an antipyretic (NOT salicylate) and an antipru-
ritic (e.g. diphenhydramine). Cool baths may be soothing. Antiviral therapy
with acyclovir given orally (20 mg/kg/dose every 6 hours) has been shown to
reduce the duration of illness by about 1 day. This is not usually of clinical
significance.

Individuals with impairment of cell-mediated immunity should be treated aggressively, with acyclovir administered intravenously (500 mg/m^2
every 8 hours).

Complications: (i)   The most serous complication is pneumonia. This is very
unusual in normal children, but is important in
adults and immunocompromised children. It is a diffuse
pneumonia that can lead to respiratory failure and death
(Figures 9.7 and 9.8).

It can be followed by pulmonary calcifications. The diagnosis of this complication can usually be made readily. Management entails supportive care
(e.g. oxygen) and antiviral therapy with acyclovir.

(ii)   Secondary bacterial infection of skin lesions (Figures 9.9 and 9.10).
This constitutes the most common complication of varicella. There
may be increasing erythema and induration around the lesion, but
the focus of secondary infection might not always be apparent. The

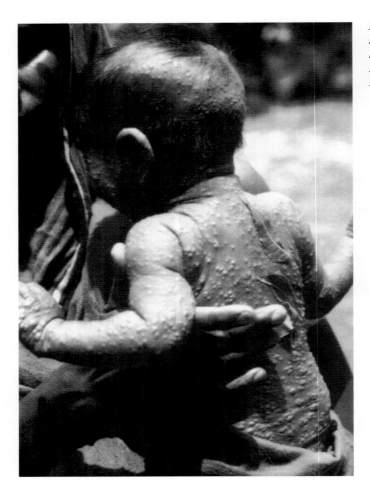

FIG. 9.4.   *A child with smallpox. (Courtesy of James Hicks/Centers for Disease Control and Prevention)*

infecting bacteria are usually *Streptococcus pyogenes* or *Staphylococcus aureus*. These infections can progress to very severe infective complications, including cellulitis, necrotizing fasciitis, bacteremia, osteomyelitis, and staphylococcal toxic shock syndrome or streptococcal toxic shock-like syndrome. This latter complication carries a very high fatality rate.

The diagnosis of secondary bacterial infection is based on clinical suspicion. As alluded to above, fever persisting after 3 days, or recrudescence of fever after it has abated should suggest that this complication has occurred. A very thorough examination of the skin should be made to look for a site of secondary bacterial infection. This is important not only to assist in the diagnosis but also to determine whether there is a focus that requires surgical drainage, or from which infected material can be obtained for culture and

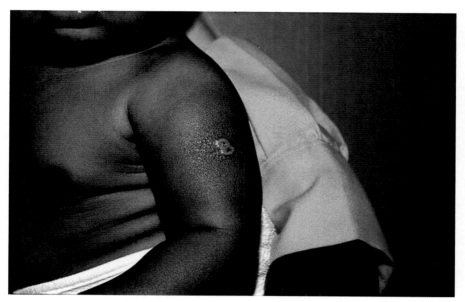

FIG. 9.5.   The appearance of a vaccinia lesion at the site of inoculation.

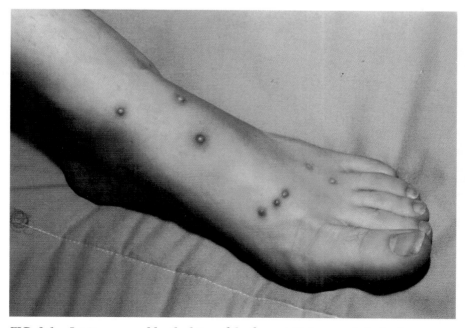

*FIG. 9.6.   Lesions caused by the bites of the fire ant (*Solemnopsis invicta*).*

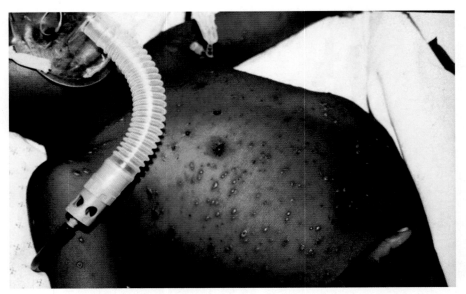

FIG. 9.7.   A child with Hodgkin's disease and a severe case of varicella and varicella pneumonia; note the oxygen mask.

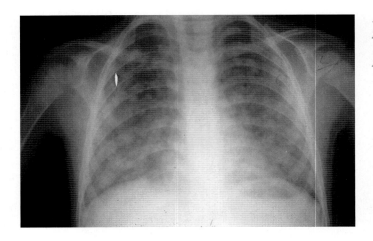

FIG. 9.8.   Chest X ray of patient shown in the Figure 9.7, showing extensive pulmonary infiltrates..

antibiotic susceptibility testing. If there is a suspicion of severe infection, bacteremia, or toxic shock syndrome, a blood culture should be performed, as well as other tests deemed necessary to evaluate physiological functions.

Management: Patients with mild infections can be treated with cephalexin or, where methicillin-resistant *Staphylococcus aureus* (MRSA) is prevalent, clindamycin. Patients with moderately severe or severe infections should

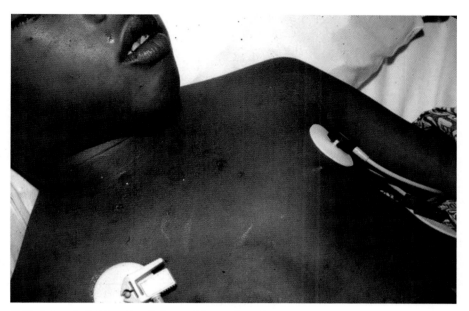

FIG. 9.9.   *A child with cellulitis of the neck and upper chest complicating varicella.*

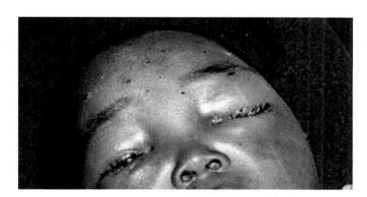

FIG. 9.10.   A child with periorbital cellulitis complicating varicella. Note the swelling of the left upper eyelid and the healed lesions on the forehead.

be hospitalized and receive supportive care as is indicated. Antimicrobial therapy should be directed at the above-mentioned bacteria.

In locales with a low prevalence of MRSA, nafcillin may be used, but where the prevalence of such resistant strains is high, vancomycin should be administered.

(iii)   *Encephalitis*: This can develop during or within a few weeks of chickenpox. In most cases it is probably a parainfectious encephalitis, implying that the virus is not present in the brain.

(iv)   *Acute cerebellar ataxia*: This is a form of encephalopathy characterized by ataxia, suggesting disease of the cerebellum and/or its connections.

The cerebrospinal fluid is generally normal, as are imaging studies. Therefore it may not be an inflammatory disease. It lasts up to a few weeks, but recovery is complete.

(v)   Reye's syndrome.

(vi)   Severe visceral disease (progressive varicella), including hepatitis and myocarditis.

(vii)   *Zoster (shingles)*: Being a herpes virus, VZV becomes latent in sensory or dorsal root ganglia. Zoster represents the recrudescence of the virus. It is characterized by skin disease in a dermatomal distribution. It begins as pain or burning, followed by the appearance of vesicles, which progress to crusting (Figures 9.11 and 9.12).

It can be very painful, and, prior to the appearance of the rash, can be confused with other diseases affecting that location, particularly if it involves the chest or abdomen. Although most patients who develop zoster have no recognized underlying predisposing factor, individuals with defects in cell-mediated immunity are at increased risk of developing this complication. The diagnosis of zoster is made clinically. This is facilitated by the distribution of the rash in one or more dermatomes on one side of the body. A similar appearing rash can be caused by herpes simplex and by allergy to poison ivy.

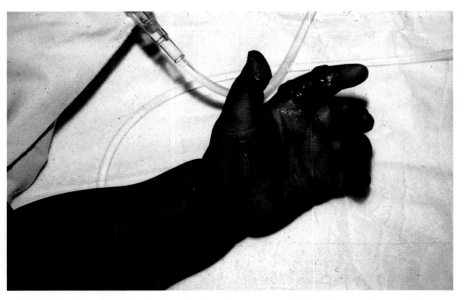

FIG. 9.11.   *Zoster, affecting the skin in dermatome C6 distribution, in a child with leukemia who had had varicella 6 months earlier.*

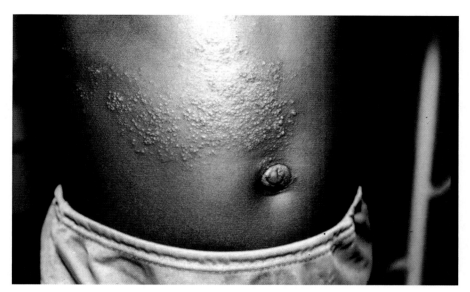

FIG. 9.12. Zoster affecting thoracic dermatomes in a child.

Management: In most cases analgesia is all that is required. The lesion should be covered to prevent spread to individuals who are susceptible to VZV. (Spread is by direct contact.) In individuals with impaired cell-mediated immunity, antiviral therapy should be administered. In severe cases this should be with intravenously administered acyclovir (dosed as for chickenpox, see above), while in mild cases this can be accomplished by the oral route, with acyclovir, valacyclovir, or famcyclovir.

Complications of zoster: (a) *Herpes zoster ophthalmicus*: this is zoster affecting the ophthalmic branch of the trigeminal nerve. This results in disease around the eye, and sometimes of the cornea and uveal tract. If this occurs it should be managed in conjunction with an ophthalmologist, because it can be associated with severe intraocular inflammation and glaucoma. Antiviral therapy (acyclovir or one of its derivatives) should be used. In most cases this can be administered orally. A particularly severe complication of herpes zoster ophthalmicus is contralateral hemiplegia, as a result of infection extending along the sympathetic chain into the carotid artery.

(b) *Postherpetic neuralgia*: This is persistent severe pain following an episode of zoster. Patients with this complication should be managed in conjunction with a neurologist. Carbamazepine can be of value in this circumstance.

(c) *Persistent zoster*: This can occur in individuals with severe cell-mediated immune defects, such as AIDS.

(viii) *Encephalopathy*: There are several possible causes of encephalopathy in patients with varicella. These are listed in Table 9.1.

(ix)   *Congenital varicella*: Although uncommon, maternal varicella can result in fetal infection. This may result in severe scarring of the skin and in brain atrophy (Figure 9.13).

■**TAB. 9.1: Causes of encephalopathy during or following chickenpox.**

Metabolic disease
   Hypoxia due to pneumonia
   Hypoglycemia due to:
      Ketotic hypoglycemia
      Liver failure
      Reye's syndrome
   Reye's syndrome
Infection
   Sepsis syndrome caused by *Streptococcus pyogenes* or *Staphylococcus aureus*
   Toxic shock or toxic shock-like syndromes
   Encephalitis
Intoxication
   Overdosage of diphenhydramine
   Liver failure due to overdosage of acetaminophen

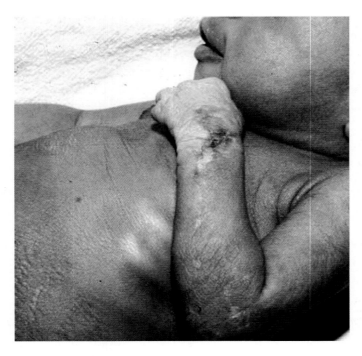

FIG. 9.13.   A newborn baby with left wrist scarring from intrauterine varicella.

Reading:

Nguyen HQ, Jumaan AO, Seward JF: Decline in mortality due to varicella after implementation of varicella vaccination in the United States. N Engl J Med 2005; 352: 450–458.

CASE 10. A 12-year-old girl develops malaise, fever, and rapid breathing 6 weeks after undergoing a renal transplant. On examination she is febrile, tachypneic, and has bilateral crackles on auscultation. Examination of her cardiovascular system is normal, and the rest of her examination is normal other than for the presence of a well-healed abdominal surgical scar, a palpable kidney in the right lower quadrant, and a cushingoid appearance.

- *What is the differential diagnosis?*
- *What would you like to know?*

Differential diagnosis: The clinical features in this child indicate pneumonia. The challenge is to determine its microbial cause. In a renal transplant patient, who is immunocompromised as a result of immunosuppressive therapy, one should consider the following causes of pneumonia:

(a) those causing pneumonia in normal children – *Mycoplasma pneumoniae, Chlamydia pneumoniae,* and *Streptococcus pneumoniae,* respiratory viruses, for example, adenovirus, influenza virus, parainfluenza virus, and respiratory syncytial virus

(b) opportunistic viruses: respiratory syncytial virus, adenovirus, cytomegalovirus (CMV)

(c) opportunistic bacteria: *Legionella pneumophila, Mycobacterium tuberculosis, Staphylococcus aureus, Nocardia asteroides, Rhodococcus equi*

(d) opportunistic fungi: *Histoplasma capsulatum, Cryptococcus neoformans, Pneumocystis jiroveci*

(e) opportunistic parasites: *Toxoplasma gondii, Strongyloides stercoralis.*

The following important questions should be asked to determine possible exposures to unusual pathogens: travel, occupation, recreational activities, exposures to animals and to sick human beings, and blood transfusions.

A very important factor in this patient is the CMV status of the patient before transplantation and of the donor. In this case the patient was CMV seronegative, indicating that she had not ever been infected with the virus, while the donor was CMV positive, indicating prior infection with the virus. This places her at high risk for developing CMV infection, which was ultimately shown to be the case. Considering the number of microorganisms that might cause pneumonia in a transplant patient, and the potential toxicities of antimicrobial therapy directed against them, serious consideration should be given to performing an invasive procedure such as bronchoalveolar lavage or lung biopsy in order to make a microbiological diagnosis. This was not done in this patient. She was treated with ganciclovir intravenously and improved.

CMV infections in the immunocompromised host are discussed below.

Because CMV is markedly cell-associated, cell-mediated immunity is important in controlling viral replication. Therefore individuals with impairment of this defense system are at risk for significant CMV disease. These include patients with AIDS and those who have undergone organ transplantation. The infection manifests with fever, evidence of different organ involvement (see below), leucopenia, and elevated transaminase levels. The organ involvement includes the following:

pneumonia, which is the most serious (Figure 10.1);
retinitis, which is particularly important in patients with AIDS;
encephalitis;
kidney disease, which may lead to graft rejection in renal transplant patients;
hepatitis;
colitis, which may associated with bleeding or intestinal perforation.

Diagnosis: There are currently several types of tests available for diagnosing CMV infection:

(i)   *Serological tests for antibodies*: These are of very limited value. A positive anti-CMV IgG indicates that the patient has had the infection

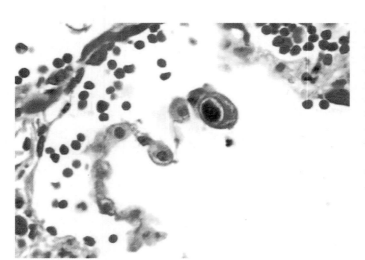

FIG. 10.1. Lung tissue from a patient with AIDS complicated by pneumonia, demonstrating the characteristic large ("megalo") alveolar cell ("cyte") with an intranuclear inclusion, characteristic of cytomegalovirus infection. (Courtesy of the Centers for Disease Control and Prevention/Dr Edwin P Ewing, Jr)

previously or has recently received a blood transfusion. A positive anti-CMV IgM indicates that the patient has recently been infected with the virus or has had a reactivation of the virus. A negative serological test indicates that the patient has not been infected or has been infected but cannot mount an antibody response. The main value of the test lies in determining a patient's susceptibility to the virus prior to transplant, whether a transplant donor has been infected with the virus and whether the patient has seroconverted, implying acquisition of infection.

(ii) *Culture*: Although CMV takes several weeks to produce cytopathic effects in tissue culture, the presence of viral antigens on tissue culture cells can be detected within 48 hours after inoculation. This technique is called the "shell-vial" technique. Body fluids that can be tested in this manner include urine and bronchial fluid.

(iii) *PCR*: This detects viral genome. It is rapid, very sensitive, and can be performed on blood and leukocyte preparations. This test can be used not only for detecting viremia, but also for quantitating viremia ("viral load"), and consequently, for evaluating response to therapy.

(iv) Detection of CMV antigenemia.

(v) Demonstration of virus-infected cells in tissue. Such cells show characteristic inclusions and can be stained with CMV antigen–labeled antibody.

Management: When CMV is diagnosed in an immunocompromised patient, antiviral therapy should be administered, initially with intravenous gancyclovir. Failure of an expected response should suggest the possibility of resistance to the drug. In such a case attempts should be made to culture the virus from urine or blood so that its drug susceptibility can be determined. If resistance is suspected or demonstrated, the antiviral drug foscarnet should be administered.

Various strategies can be considered for patients placed at risk of developing CMV infection through solid organ transplantation. These are as follows: (i) prophylaxis, which involves administering gancyclovir, with or without CMV hyperimmune globulin, to patients at high risk (seronegative recipient, seropositive donor); (ii) pre-emptive therapy, which involves monitoring blood by CMV viral load measurement for the development of infection and, if it occurs, to initiate therapy with ganciclovir; and (iii) therapy for symptomatic disease with ganciclovir. In a situation such as the one described for this patient, in which a seronegative recipient received an organ from a seropositive donor, prophylaxis or pre-emptive therapy with ganciclovir might have prevented her illness.

Reading:

Danziger-Isakov LA, Storch GA: Prevention and treatment of cytomegalovirus infections in solid organ transplant recipients. Pediatr Infect Dis J 2002; 21: 432–434.

Bueno J, Ramil C, Green M: Current management strategies for the prevention and treatment of cytomegalovirus infection in pediatric transplant recipients. Pediatr Drugs 2002; 4: 279–290.

Pereyraa F, Rubin RH: Prevention and treatment of cytomegalovirus infection in solid organ transplant recipients. Curr Opin Infect Dis 2004; 17: 357–361.

CASE 11 (HYP). A 4-year-old boy develops fever 5 weeks after undergoing open-heart surgery for congenital heart disease. On examination he is fairly well appearing and has a temperature of 38.4°C. The surgical wound and sites of previous vascular catheters are well healed. The heart examination reveals a 2/6 short ejection systolic murmur and no pericardial rub. There are no petechiae, splinter hemorrhages, or palmar nodules. He has generalized lymphadenopathy and splenomegaly, but no hepatomegaly, and the rest of his examination is normal.

• *What is the differential diagnosis?*

Differential diagnosis of a febrile illness in a patient who has undergone cardiac surgery:

(a) Infective endocarditis: This is the main concern in a patient with congenital heart disease who has fever following heart surgery. Although splenomegaly is a clinical feature of infective endocarditis, generalized lymphadenopathy is not.

(b) Nosocomial infection complicating use of vascular catheters, a urinary catheter, and ventilation: These usually manifest during hospitalization or soon afterward. Therefore this is unlikely.

(c) Postpericardiotomy syndrome: This is characterized by fever, pericarditis, and pleuritis. It usually develops 1–3 weeks after surgery. This child lacks the clinical features of this condition.

(d) Postperfusion syndrome: This is an infectious mononucleosis syndrome resulting from blood transfusions given during cardiopulmonary bypass. It is usually caused by cytomegalovirus, but can be caused by Epstein–Barr virus, *Toxoplasma gondii*, and human immunodeficiency virus

(HIV). It is characterized by fever, splenomegaly, and lymphadenopathy. Hepatomegaly and a rash may sometimes occur. This is the most likely diagnosis in this patient.

The diagnosis of cytomegalovirus infection can be supported by demonstrating CMV in the blood by PCR, CMV in the urine by culture, seroconversion to CMV, or the presence of CMV IgM antibodies in the blood (see Case 10). Infection with the other causes of infectious mononucleosis can be diagnosed serologically or, in the case of acute HIV infection, by a PCR test.

Many infectious agents can be transmitted in transfused blood. Most of these are present in the blood of the donor at the time of blood collection. These include viruses (hepatitis B and C, cytomegalovirus, Epstein–Barr virus, HIV, and West Nile virus), bacteria that are present in the donor's blood, including *Treponema pallidum*, and especially *Yersinia enterocolitica* and *Listeria monocytogenes*, which can grow during cold storage of the blood, and protozoa, including *Plasmodium* spp., *Toxoplasma gondii*, *Trypanosoma cruzi*, and *Trypanosoma brucei*. The blood can also become contaminated during collection and processing, in which case the infectious agents are usually bacteria. Platelet units are particularly prone to bacterial infection because they are stored at room temperature.

Reading:

Busch MP, Kleinman SH, Nemo GJ: Current and emerging infectious risks of blood transfusions. JAMA 2003; 289: 959–962.

CASE 12. A 6-year-old girl with sickle cell disease is admitted with fever, sore throat, and general malaise. She has no localizing signs of infection. She is treated for the possibility of bacteremia with intravenous cefotaxime, but her fever has persisted. The blood cultures have been negative. On day 3, her hemoglobin concentration has decreased from 7.5 to 5.0 g/dl, and her reticulocyte count has decreased from 10% to 1%.

What do you think has happened?

She has developed worsening anemia in the face of a decreased production of red cells, as demonstrated by a decreasing reticulocyte count. This suggests that the cause of the deterioration is bone marrow failure of red cell production. Possible causes of this are infection, in particular that caused by parvovirus B19, and drugs. Since this illness is associated with fever and she has not received drugs that cause red cell hypoplasia, this is likely caused by parvovirus. This clinical scenario is called an "aplastic crisis." Parvovirus B19 infects many individuals in childhood, sometimes causing an exanthem called erythema infectiosum (fifth disease) characterized by a lacy erythematous rash and red cheeks (Figures 12.1 and 12.2).

The virus infects red cell precursors in the bone marrow, resulting in failure to produce red cells for about 1 week. This does not have a significant effect on individuals with a normal red cell lifespan (about 120 days) but can

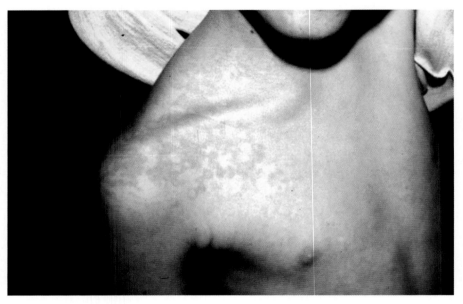

FIG. 12.1.   The lacy rash associated with parvovirus B19 infection.

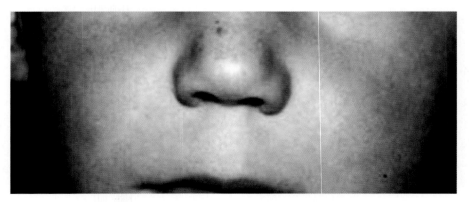

FIG. 12.2.   A boy (sibling of the child in Figure 12.1) with red cheeks ("slapped cheeks") due to parvovirus B19 infection.

cause profound anemia in individuals whose red cell lifespan is short, that is, those with chronic hemolytic anemias such as sickle cell disease and hereditary spherocytosis. This virus also causes severe anemia in the fetus, resulting in hydrops fetalis, and in individuals with immunodeficiencies that limit their ability to eliminate the virus, such as AIDS.

Reading:

Young NS, Brown KE: Parvovirus B19. N Engl J Med 2004; 350: 586–597.

CASE 13. A 5-year-old girl presents with a history that she has difficulty walking and that her speech is becoming difficult to understand. On examination she has generalized increase in muscle tone, her gait is wide-based, and she is dysarthric. Disease of the brain is diagnosed, and a computer tomography scan without contrast is performed (Figure 13.1).

- *What does the scan show?*
- *What is your differential diagnosis?*
- *What would you do?*

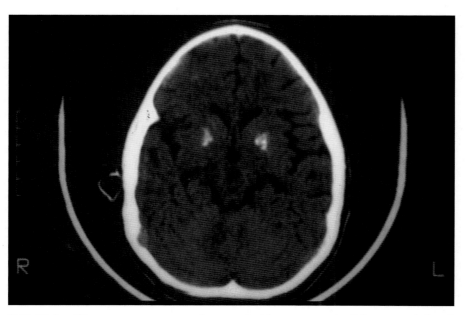

FIG. 13.1.   The computer tomography scan (without contrast) of the patient's head.

The scan shows calcification of the basal ganglia, in addition to cerebral atrophy, as demonstrated by widened sulci. There are several metabolic conditions that can cause this, such as pseudohypoparathyroidism. Intrauterine infections such as toxoplasmosis and cytomegalovirus infection can cause cerebral calcifications, but in such cases the clinical manifestations of cerebral injury are present in infancy. A particular infection that should be considered in such patients is human immunodeficiency virus (HIV) infection, which would likely have been transmitted vertically. Therefore an HIV antibody test should be performed on the child.

She was shown to have HIV infection as was her mother.

Neurological disease is an important complication of HIV infection in children. Most cases are due to direct damage to the brain by the virus, resulting in encephalopathies with varying rates of progression. These can result in failure to attain developmental milestones or loss of intellectual and motor milestones, as in this case. Spasticity is often present, and movement disorders may occur. In my experience, ankle clonus is often present.

Much less common causes of brain disease in HIV-infected children include tumors (primarily lymphoma), stroke resulting from HIV vasculopathy, and opportunistic infections, the most common of which is cytomegalovirus infection.

Other nervous system diseases occurring in HIV-infected children include vacuolar myelopathy and peripheral neuropathy, which is due mainly to antiretroviral therapy.

Reading:

Zuckerman GB, Sanchez JL, Conway EE: Neurologic complications of HIV infections in children. Pediatr Ann 1998, 27: 635–639.

Zeichner SL, Read JS (editors): Handbook of pediatric HIV care. Lippincott Williams and Wilkins, Philadelphia, 1999, pp. 336–351.

Weisberg LA: Neurologic abnormalities in human immunodeficiency virus infection. Southern Med J 2001; 94: 266–275.

Antiretroviral therapy and medical management of pediatric HIV infection and 1997 USPHS/IDSA report on the prevention of opportunistic infections in persons infected with human immunodeficiency virus. Pediatrics 1998; 102 (part 2): S 1005–S 1085.

American Academy of Pediatrics and Canadian Paediatric Society. Evaluation and treatment of the Human Immunodeficiency Virus-exposed infant. Pediatrics 2004; 114: 497–505.

CASE 14. A 6-month-old boy presents (in 1990) with a history of poor feeding, fever, and decreased activity. He weighs 3 kg. He is diagnosed with meningitis due to *Listeria monocytogenes*. He is treated with ampicillin and recovers from this infection. While still in hospital he develops tachypnea and respiratory difficulty. A chest X ray is performed (Figure 14.1).

- *What does the X ray show?*
- *What is the differential diagnosis?*
- *What would you do?*

The clinical scenario is one of an infant with severe failure to thrive and the development of pneumonia while he was recovering from a proven infection (listeriosis) that is opportunistic in individuals with defective cell-mediated immunity. The new respiratory symptoms therefore suggest the possibility of another opportunistic infection. The chest radiograph shows a diffuse alveolar infiltrate. This might be caused by many infectious agents including respiratory viruses (respiratory syncytial virus, human metapneumovirus, adenovirus, parainfluenza virus, and influenza virus) and bacteria (*Streptococcus pneumoniae, Mycoplasma pneumoniae, Chlamydia pneumoniae, Legionella pneumophila*, and *Mycobacterium tuberculosis*). In

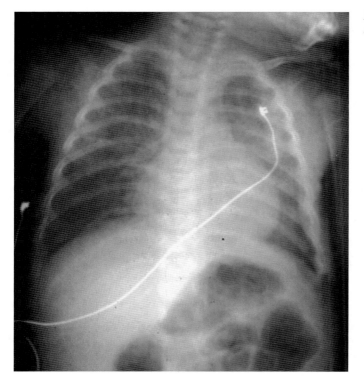

FIG. 14.1.   The infant's chest X ray.

view of the likelihood that he is immunocompromised, an important consideration is infection with *Pneumocystis jiroveci* (formerly called *Pneumocystis carinii*). Considering the long time that it would have taken to demonstrate the presence of the viruses in the pharynx by tissue culture of pharyngeal secretions (rapid diagnostic tests were not readily available at the facility at that time), and the lack of ability to obtain sputum from an infant for examination of bacteria, the dilemma facing the clinicians was the following: should the child be treated empirically for all the treatable diagnostic possibilities or should he undergo an invasive diagnostic procedure such as bronchoalveolar lavage or lung biopsy to obtain pulmonary material for staining of bacteria and *Pneumocystis jiroveci*, culture, and histology?

He underwent open lung biopsy. The histological picture was typical of pneumocystis infection (Figure 14.2), and the silver stain showed cysts of the *Pneumocystis jiroveci* (Figure 14.3).

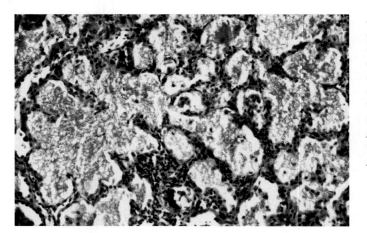

FIG. 14.2. Hematoxylin and eosin stained section of lung tissue from the patient, showing thickening and hypercellularity of the interstitium, and foamy material within the alveoli, characteristic of pneumocystis pneumonia (formerly called interstitial plasma cell pneumonitis).

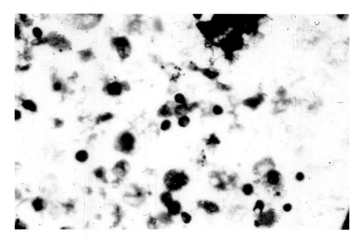

FIG. 14.3. Gomorri methenamine stain of the lung biopsy showing the black-stained cysts of Pneumocystis jiroveci.

The child was treated with trimethoprim/sulfamethoxazole and improved. Further investigation showed that he was infected with HIV, which he had acquired vertically from his mother.

The clinical features of children with HIV infection are discussed below. They can be considered in terms of those due to only the HIV infection itself, those due to the consequences of loss of immune function (mainly opportunistic infections), and those due to management (not discussed here).

Manifestations due to HIV infection itself: Since the virus infection is systemic all parts of the body can be affected.

Growth and nutrition: Failure to thrive and loss of weight; this is due to a combination of increased metabolic demands, in which cytokines play a role, and opportunistic infections.

Reticuloendothelial system: Generalized lymphadenopathy, including epitrochlear lymphadenopathy, hepatomegaly, and splenomegaly.

Blood: Anemia, thrombocytopenia, and leucopenia; the leucopenia can reflect not only lymphopenia, but also neutropenia.

Lung: Lymphocytic interstitial pneumonitis, which is characterized by lymphocytic infiltration of the bronchial walls as well as the alveolar septa. Epstein–Barr virus may play a role in the pathogenesis of this condition. This condition can cause airway obstruction.

Central nervous system: Encephalopathies ranging in manifestations from failure of brain growth and normal acquisition of milestones, to progressive loss of acquired milestones, spasticity, and movement disorders (see Case 13). A vasculopathy predisposing to stroke can also occur.

Heart: Cardiomyopathy.

Skin: Inflammatory lesions resembling atopic or seborrheic dermatitis.

Kidney: Glomerulopathy due to a membranous glomerulonephritis. This is a late manifestation of HIV infection.

Opportunistic infections: Many of these infections are the same as those in normal children, such as frequent episodes of acute otitis media, and caused by infectious agents that infect normal children, in particular *Streptococcus pneumoniae*. However, HIV-infected children may have more severe disease, have these infections more frequently, or be unable to eliminate the infectious agent. Several opportunistic diseases are rare in children compared with adults, probably because of lack of exposure to the organisms. These include toxoplasmosis, cryptococcosis, histoplasmosis, polyoma virus infections, Kaposi sarcoma, and bacilliary angiomatosis.

Virus infections:

The herpes viruses: Herpes simplex virus can cause severe infections of the oral and esophageal mucosae and the skin, while varicella zoster virus can cause severe chickenpox, as well as severe and chronic zoster infections. Cytomegalovirus, which commonly affects many normal children, can cause severe opportunistic infection of the esophagus, intestine, retina, lung, liver, and nervous system. All three herpes viruses can cause a radiculomyelopathy.

Respiratory viruses: Although the clinical diseases are the same as those affecting normal children, pneumonia is common, and viral excretion may be prolonged.

Parvovirus B19: HIV-infected children may not be able to eliminate the virus, which infects red cell precursors in the bone marrow. This can therefore be one of several potential causes of chronic anemia.

Bacterial infections: Although some bacterial infections affecting HIV-infected children do not occur in normal hosts, many of the bacterial infections in such children are the same as those in normal hosts, but they occur significantly more frequently. Otitis media and pneumonia are common. Bacteremia is caused by *Streptococcus pneumoniae, Haemophilus influenzae* type b, and *Pseudomonas aeruginosa*, and occasionally, by *Listeria monocytogenes*. Although tuberculosis occurs as in any exposed individual, the disease is more frequently extrapulmonary than in otherwise normal hosts. *Mycobacterium avium* complex causes both pulmonary and systemic disease, affecting the liver, intestine, and other organs. *Nocardia species* cause opportunistic pneumonia and brain abscess.

Fungal infections: The most important of these by far is *Pneumocystis jiroveci* (formerly *P. carinii*). This causes severe pneumonia, the peak age incidence of which is 4 months. The other important fungal pathogen is *Candida*. This causes oral as well as esophageal disease.

Parasites: In the United States, the most important are those protozoa affecting the intestinal tract, namely *Giardia lamblia, Cryptosporidium parvum*, and *Isospora belli*.

Opportunistic tumors are rare in children. These include B-cell lymphomas and leiomyosarcomas.

Reading:

Zeicher SL, Read JS: Handbook of Pediatric HIV Care. Lippincott Williams and Wilkins, Philadelphia, 1999, pages 336–352.

Domachowske JB: Pediatric human immunodeficiency virus infection. Clin Microbiol Rev 1996; 9: 448–468.

Antiretroviral therapy and medical management of pediatric HIV infection and 1997 USPHS/IDSA report on the prevention of opportunistic infections in persons infected with human immunodeficiency virus. Pediatrics 1998; 102 (part 2); S 1005–S 1085.

American Academy of Pediatrics and Canadian Paediatric Society. Evaluation and treatment of the Human Immunodeficiency Virus-exposed infant. Pediatrics 2004; 114: 497–505.

CASE 15 (COMP). A 2-year-old boy presents with a history of having a cough and fever for 2 days. He has been hospitalized on three previous occasions for a similar problem, and he improved after being treated with antibiotics. On examination he is mildly ill-appearing. His temperature is 38.5°C, heart rate 120/minute, respiratory rate 40/minute, and blood pressure 95/60 mm Hg. He has mild subcostal retractions and decreased breath sounds in the right lower lobe, with crackles in that area. The trachea is central. The ears and pharynx are normal, and the rest of his examination is completely normal.

- *What is your differential diagnosis?*
- *How would you evaluate him?*

This patient has evidence of lobar pneumonia (fever, decreased breath sounds, and crackles). He requires treatment for this episode of illness. However, this is recurrent, and he therefore requires evaluation for an underlying disease predisposing him to this problem.

When evaluating a patient with recurrent pneumonia, one should ask oneself several questions:

(a) Has there indeed been recurrent pneumonia, or have these episodes really represented episodes of asthma or bronchitis? What is the evidence that he has had recurrent pneumonia?

(b) Have these episodes affected the same area of the lung, or different areas?

Answering these two questions requires review of all records and chest X rays available.

If he has indeed suffered from recurrent episodes of pneumonia, and these have affected the same area of the lung each time, this suggests an anatomical abnormality in that area, particularly an abnormality causing obstruction of the bronchus to that area. Causes of this can be considered in terms of abnormalities within the lumen, those affecting the wall, and those causing compression from outside the bronchus. These include the following:

Causes within the lumen:
   Foreign body
   Endobronchial tuberculosis
   Tumor
Causes affecting the wall:
   Asthma
   Bronchomalacia
Causes from external compression:
   Enlarged hilar lymph node due to:
   Tuberculosis
   Lymphoma
   Enlargement of the left atrium compressing the left main bronchus
Other causes of recurrent focal pneumonia:
   Bronchiectasis
   Lung malformations
   Sequestered lobe

If the pneumonias have affected different parts of the lung, a more generalized problem should be considered. The causes should be considered in the following categories:

Heart disease
   heart failure
   left-to-right shunts, for example, ventricular septal defect
Gastrointestinal disease
   Gastroesophageal reflux with aspiration
   H-type tracheoesophageal fistula
Neurological disease
   Lower motor neuron disorders, causing poor lung excursion and clearance
   of secretions, for example, spinal muscular atrophy (Figure 15.1)
Severe spasticity, with pseudobulbar paresis
Systemic diseases affecting the lung:
   Immotile cilia syndromes
   Cystic fibrosis
Immune deficiencies

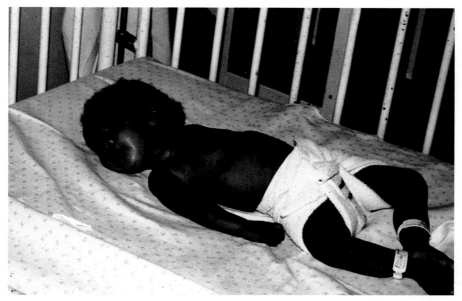

FIG. 15.1. A 10-month-old infant with spinal muscular atrophy (Werdnig-Hoffman type). Note the "frog-leg position" of the lower limbs, and the concavity of the lower chest (Harrison's sulcus), a sign of lung disease beginning at a young age.

Many of these can be diagnosed or suspected clinically. Specific tests may be required for diagnosing others, for example, gastroesophageal reflux, cystic fibrosis, immotile cilia syndromes, and immune defects.

Reading:

Panitch HB: Evaluation of recurrent pneumonia. Pediatr Infect Dis J 2005; 24: 265–266.

CASE 16 (HYP). A baby is born with a rash identical to that seen in the baby shown in Figure 16.1.

Questioning reveals that the mother had a febrile illness during the second trimester of pregnancy.

Examination reveals diffuse raised purple skin lesions. There is no pallor, jaundice, or cyanosis. The eyes are normal externally, the heart has a 3/6 systolic murmur, and there is enlargement of both the liver and the spleen. There is no lymphadenopathy.

- *What is your differential diagnosis?*
- *What would you like to know?*

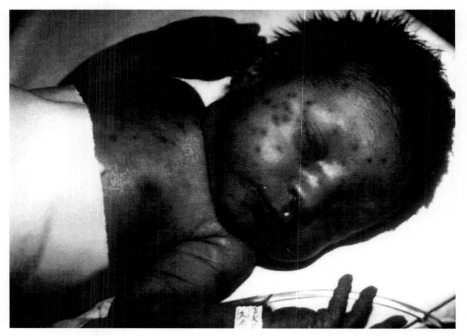

FIG. 16.1.   New born baby with a rash. (Courtesy of the Centers for Disease Control and Prevention).

This child's condition is characterized by a rash, a heart murmur, and enlargement of the liver and spleen.

This rash is generalized and characterized by raised purple lesions.

Several infections may cause rashes that are present in babies at birth. These include the following: congenital rubella, which causes a generalized macular rash or raised purple lesions ("blueberry muffin rash"), which represent areas of extramedullary erythropoiesis; congenital cytomegalovirus (CMV) infection and toxoplasmosis, which can cause the same type of rash as rubella. The rash associated with congenital syphilis is macular or maculopapular, but does not consist of purple lesions; congenital listeriosis, which produces multiple pustules (granulomatosis infantiseptica); candida, which causes macules or generalized erythema; and herpes simplex virus, which produces focal vesicles. The lethal form of epidermolysis bullosa is associated with denudation of areas of skin at birth. Nikolsky sign can be demonstrated in this condition.

Candida and herpes simplex are usually due to ascending infection and are not likely to result from a maternal infection in the second trimester. Congenital listeriosis is usually fatal, so the baby would not likely have survived from the second trimester.

Enlargement of liver and spleen occurs in congenital rubella, CMV infection, toxoplasmosis, and syphilis, as well as in noninfectious conditions, such as hemolytic disease of the newborn (which would be associated with jaundice and pallor). The heart murmur could suggest a congenital heart disease, such as that associated with congenital rubella, but at this age could also represent a flow murmur.

Of the chronic intrauterine infections, congenital CMV infection is, by far, the most common. In considering congenital rubella an important question to be asked is: Was the mother immune to rubella (was she seropositive) before this pregnancy, and is she immune now? Knowledge of immunity only during this pregnancy does not answer the question of whether the infection occurred during this pregnancy (potentially affecting the baby) or previously.

In this case (Figure 16.1) the rash was caused by rubella. The congenital rubella syndrome may be associated with abnormalities affecting many organs: ocular abnormalities, including cataracts (the abnormality that led to the recognition of the entity of congenital rubella infection) (Figure 16.2), microphthalmia, and corneal opacity (Figure 16.3); deafness; congenital heart disease; brain abnormalities, including microcephaly; hepatitis; anemia; thrombocytopenia; and linear lucencies in the long bones ("celery stalk" appearance).

The methods used to diagnose intrauterine infections are shown in Table 16.1.

The development of PCR tests will render diagnosing these infections easier.

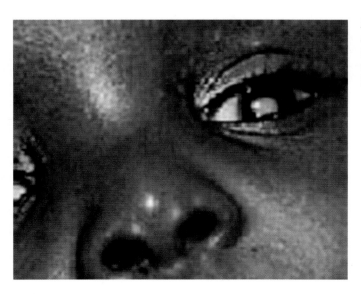

FIG. 16.2.   *A child with a congenital cataract. Note that the opacity can be seen only through the pupil, because the lens is behind the iris.*

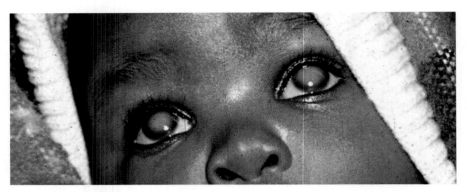

FIG. 16.3.   Corneal opacities. Note that the opacities are in front of the pupil.

■TAB. 16.1:   The usual methods used to diagnose intrauterine infections.

Infection	Method
Rubella	serology (IgM)
Cytomegalovirus infection	urine viral culture, PCR on blood
Human immunodeficiency virus infection	DNA PCR
Lymphocytic choriomeningitis virus	serology
Syphilis	serology (RPR, specific Treponemal test)
Toxoplasmosis	serology (IgM)

Legend: PCR = polymerase chain reaction; RPR = rapid plasma reagin; IgM = immunoglobulin M.

Congenital rubella can be prevented by immunization of all children so that (i) the girls are not susceptible when they become pregnant and (ii) that neither girls nor boys can bring the infection home to their pregnant mothers. In the United States, the rate of congenital rubella syndrome decreased from 10,000 cases per year in 1969 when vaccination was introduced to 1 case per year in 2002.

Reading:

Achievements in public health: elimination of rubella and congenital rubella syndrome – United States, 1969–2004. MMWR 2005;54:1–4.

■CASE 17 (HYP). A 6-year-old girl complains of weakness and muscle pain, and "tightness" in her thighs and legs. About 1 week earlier she had a fever, sore throat, and cough. On examination she cannot stand nor walk due to weakness. Her thighs and calves are tender. Sensation and deep tendon reflexes are normal. Examination of the back and upper limbs is normal.

- *What might be wrong with her?*
- *What would you like to know?*

The differential diagnosis is one of generalized weakness but preserved higher function. This suggests a lower motor neuron lesion affecting her lower limbs. The possible levels of disease should be considered anatomically (Figure 17.1).

It is useful to consider possible etiologies of diseases for each of these sites.

Diseases of the lower motor neuron may be generalized in which case they may affect the muscles of respiration, leading to respiratory failure. They may also be associated with autonomic dysfunction resulting in cardiovascular instability. Therefore cardiorespiratory supportive care is the most important component of management. Secondary infectious problems may complicate the course, such as decubitus ulcers, and the complications of intensive support such as artificial ventilation and intravenous therapy.

The differential diagnosis should include the infectious and noninfectious diseases listed below in Table 17.1.

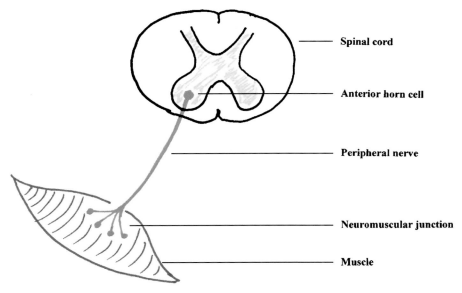

FIG. 17.1.   *The anatomy of the lower motor neuron unit.*

■TAB. 17.1: Causes of acute flaccid weakness.

(A) Spinal cord	Spinal shock (early stage of acute cord disease)
	Transverse myelitis (mixed upper and lower motor)
(B) Anterior horn cell	Poliomyelitis
	Other enterovirus infections
	West Nile virus infection
(C) Peripheral nerve	Guillain-Barre syndrome
	Diphtheria
	Toxins – n-toluene, glue-sniffing
	Acute intermittent porphyria
(D) Neuromuscular junction	Botulism
	Elapid snake bite (cobra, mamba)
(E) Muscle	Myositis
	Electrolyte disturbance
	Hypokalemia
	Extreme hypocalcemia
	Periodic paralysis (several types)
(F) Pseudoparesis (localized)	Skeletal disease
	Traumatic injury
	Osteomyelitis
	Septic arthritis
	Congenital syphilis (osteitis)
(G) Unknown mechanism	Tick paralysis

Management principles:

1. Observe respiratory function. In older individuals this can be done by monitoring inspiratory force. In infants the strength of the cry is helpful. Supporting ventilation may become necessary.
2. Monitor cardiovascular function, in particular heart rate and blood pressure.
3. Make a diagnosis.
4. Provide specific therapy if possible.
5. Prevent decubitus ulcers.
6. Prevent contractures.
7. Ensure adequate nutrition.

The pain and muscle tenderness in this patient indicate muscle inflammation (myositis) as the cause of the weakness.

Muscle disease: Acute muscle disease may be due to injury, inflammation (myositis), or a metabolic disorder, for example, heat stroke. Acute myositis is usually caused by a viral infection such as influenza, enterovirus infection, or acute HIV infection. This is referred to as benign acute childhood myositis, which is to be distinguished from the myositis occurring with dermatomyositis or polymyositis, which have a prolonged course and can result in significant long-term disability. Patients with benign acute myositis present with acute onset of weakness and muscle pain and tenderness, most frequently affecting the calf muscles. The muscles may be swollen and the weakness may be profound. The dangers of myositis are respiratory failure and rhabdomyolysis, which leads to hyperkalemia and to myoglobinuria, which, in turn, can lead to acute tubular necrosis and renal failure. The diagnosis of myositis can be confirmed by the demonstration of elevated creatine phosphokinase (CPK) activity in the serum. Myoglobinuria manifests as red, clear urine (like rosé wine) as opposed to red, cloudy urine that occurs with hematuria. In this clinical circumstance a urine dipstick test that is positive for blood in the absence red cells on microscopy is highly suggestive of myoglobinuria. A microbiological diagnosis of the cause of myositis is not usually helpful, unless HIV infection is suspected.

Treatment is primarily supportive, entailing analgesia and a very high fluid intake. If myoglobinuria is present the urine should be alkalinized to prevent injury to the renal tubules. Monitoring of respiratory function is essential.

Reading:

King BA: Benign acute childhood myositis as a cause of failure to weight bear. J Paediatr Child Health. 2003; 39: 378–380.

Singh U, Scheld WM: Infectious etiologies of rhabdomyolysis: three case reports. Clin Infect Dis 1996; 22: 642–649.

CASE 18 (COMP-MMWR). A previously well 48-year-old man presents with a 4-day history of fever, chills, photophobia, myalgia, arthralgia, nausea, vomiting, constipation, and upper abdominal discomfort. On examination he is ill-appearing and febrile. He is jaundiced and he has upper abdominal tenderness, but has neither enlargement of liver or spleen nor lymphadenopathy. He has several skin papules on his limbs, consistent with insect bites. Laboratory testing reveals marked elevation of transaminases (several thousand IU/dl), serum creatinine, and blood urea, as well as leucopenia and thrombocytopenia.

- *What is your differential diagnosis?*
- *What would you like to know?*

This patient has a systemic infection of very acute onset with liver and renal failure, but without shock. He does not have known underlying disease predisposing him to severe infection. Therefore one should pursue a course looking for exposures to specific infectious agents. We know that he has probably been bitten by "insects."

Arthropod-transmitted infections that cause acute systemic illness are shown in Table 18.1.

Non–arthropod-borne infections that might cause this clinical scenario include arenavirus infections such as Lassa fever, Argentinian hemorrhagic fever and Bolivian hemorrhagic fever, and leptospirosis. The latter is usually acquired from exposure to water into which animals have urinated.

Considering the differential diagnosis, the exposure history is very important.

He had traveled to the jungle in the Amazon region of Brazil. He had not been immunized against yellow fever. He was shown to have this infection, from which he died.

■TAB. 18.1: **Arthropod-borne infections causing acute systemic illness and their vectors.**

Organism	Vector
Viruses	
Flaviviridae – yellow fever, dengue, and others	mosquito
Togaviridae – equine encephalitides	mosquito
Bunyaviridae	
Congo-Crimean hemorrhagic fever	tick
Rift Valley fever and others	mosquito
Reoviridae – Colorado tick fever	tick
Rickettsiae	
Rocky Mountain spotted fever and others	tick
Epidemic typhus	louse
Ehrlichiae	
Ehrlichia chafeensis	tick
Anaplasma phagocytophilum	tick
Spirochetes	
Borrelia – relapsing fever	tick, louse
Gram-negative rods	
Francisella tularensis	tick, fly
Yersinia pestis	flea
Protozoa	
Malaria	mosquito
Babesia	tick
Trypanosoma brucei	fly
Trypanosoma cruzi	reduviid bug

Yellow fever is one of the important global infectious diseases. It is caused by yellow fever virus, which is a flavivirus (the prototypic virus of this group, whence the name "flavi," which is derived from the Latin for yellow). It is transmitted by *Aedes aegypti* mosquitoes, in tropical Africa and tropical South America. There are two epidemiologic patterns, namely the urban pattern in which the virus is transmitted between mosquitoes and human beings, and the sylvatic, in which it is transmitted between mosquitoes and monkeys, and in which human beings are incidental hosts. The virus causes liver and renal failure, and carries a very high case fatality rate. There is a very effective live attenuated vaccine that should be administered to all travelers to endemic areas.

References:

Schwartz F, Drach F, Guroy ME et al: Fatal yellow fever in a traveler returning from Venezuela, 1999. MMWR 49: 303–5, April 14, 1999

Hall P, Fojtasek M, Pettigrove J et al: Fatal yellow fever in a traveler returning from Amazonas, Brazil, 2002. MMWR 2002; 51: 324–325.

Geisbert TW, Jahrling PB: Exotic emerging viral diseases: progress and challenges. Nat Med 2004; 10: S110–S121.

CASE 19. A 6-month-old boy presents with watery diarrhea and a temperature of 38.5°C.

- *What is the most important aspect of the clinical evaluation?*
- *What is the likely clinical diagnosis, and what are its possible causes?*
- *What do you want to do?*

(a) The most important question addresses the physiologic diagnosis, namely: What is his hydration status? The signs of dehydration are:

decreased urine output;
sticky oral mucosa
decreased skin turgor (Figure 19.1)
sunken eyes
sunken fontanelle
tachycardia
poor peripheral perfusion and decreased level of consciousness (shock)

What is the likely diagnosis? This is most likely a case of acute infectious diarrhea (acute gastroenteritis). The possible causes are listed in Table 19.1.

These agents are all spread by the fecal–oral route. In addition, there are several food intoxications (food poisonings) in which bacteria have been

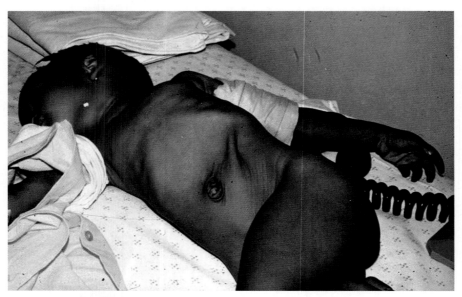

FIG. 19.1. Decreased skin turgor ("tenting") in a dehydrated child.

allowed to grow in food, and produce toxins, which cause vomiting and/or diarrhea. These toxins are produced by *Staphylococcus aureus* and *Bacillus cereus.*

Although these agents have different sources, sites of infection within the intestine, and mechanisms of causing disease, they all cause diarrhea, and hence water loss. Consequently, the most important aspect of evaluation is to determine the state of hydration, and the most important component of treatment is to ensure adequate hydration (see above).

There are risk factors that predispose individuals to acquiring infections with enteropathic organisms:

Poor hygiene in those preparing food

All circumstances leading to poor hygiene

Squalid or crowded living circumstances

Absence of clean water supply and sewage disposal

Eating of uncooked or undercooked meat or seafood or other foods contaminated by these

Lack of refrigeration of foods that have been contaminated

Living or traveling to areas where enteric infections are prevalent (mostly for the above reasons)

■TAB. 19.1: Causes of acute infectious diarrhea.

Agent
Viruses
   Rotavirus
   Enteric adenovirus
   Noroviruses
   Astroviruses
Bacteria
   Salmonella enteritidis
   Shigella species
   Campylobacter jejuni
   Escherichia coli
      Enteropathogenic (EPEC)
      Enterotoxigenic (ETEC)
      Enteroadherent (EAEC)
      Enterohemorrhagic (EHEC)
      Enteroinvasive (EIEC)
   Yersinia enterocolitica
   Vibrio cholerae
   Vibrio parahaemolyticus
   Clostridium difficile
   Clostridium perfringens
Parasites
   Giardia lamblia (intestinalis)
   Cryptosporidium parvum
   Cyclospora cayetanensis
   Isospora belli
   Entamoeba histolytica
   Balantidium coli

Clinical features: The initial symptom is often vomiting followed within a few hours by the development of diarrhea. The viral and invasive bacterial infections are often associated with fever. Abdominal cramps may also occur. In the cases of invasive bacterial infections, blood and pus may appear in the stool after 1 or 2 days. Although most patients with acute enteric infection begin to improve after about 2 days, some take several days to return to normal health. In young children, the stool may remain loose for weeks.

Complications:

1. *Dehydration.* This is the main problem caused by acute diarrheal disease, and the major cause of death from such illnesses. The dehydration leads not only to hypovolemic shock, but also to hemoconcentration. The combination of hypovolemia and hemoconcentration results in a decreased blood flow rate, predisposing the patient to vascular occlusion. This can occur anywhere in the circulation but is most devastating when it affects the brain.

2. *Metabolic and electrolyte disturbances*: As a result of causing diarrhea by different mechanisms, different organisms cause different degrees of salt and other electrolyte losses in the stool. The main electrolyte disturbances that can occur are hyponatremia, hypernatremia, hypokalemia, and acidosis. Abnormalities of blood glucose, both hypoglycemia and hyperglycemia can also occur. These abnormalities should be sought in all children with severe diarrhea in whom neurological disturbances are present, such as changes in level of consciousness, seizures, muscle hypertonia, or hypotonia.

3. *Bacteremia*: This can occur in gut-invasive bacterial infections and is most common in cases of salmonella infection. In countries where water and food hygiene are poor, salmonella enteric infections are very common, and salmonellae are among the most common causes of bacteremia. Salmonellae occasionally cause metastatic infections such as septic arthritis, osteomyelitis, and meningitis. Young infants are at greatest risk of suffering such complications. Individuals with sickle cell disease are also at risk of developing salmonella osteomyelitis. *Yersinia enterocolitica* also causes bacteremia in young infants, as well as in individuals with iron overload.

4. *Hemolytic uremic syndrome*: This is a condition characterized by a vasculopathy, affecting mainly the kidney and the brain, by renal failure and hypertension, and by microangiopathic hemolytic anemia, and thrombocytopenia. Most cases result from infections with enterohemorrhagic *E. coli*, such as serotype O157; H7, but infections with shigella can also cause the disease. It should be suspected in children who have recently suffered from bloody diarrhea, and who develop oliguria, edema, petechiae, pallor, or changes in mental state. The blood smear shows fragmented erythrocytes, "helmet" cells, and schistocytes (Figure 19.2).

5. *Toxic encephalopathy*: This is a frequent complication of shigellosis.

This frequently manifests with seizures but can be associated with a depressed level of consciousness and even coma. Occasionally shigella encephalopathy can be fatal, a condition known in Japan as "ekiri." Causes of altered mental state in children with acute infectious diarrhea are shown in Table 19.2.

6. *Chronic diarrhea*: Previously well children, who suffer an episode of acute infectious diarrhea, may then continue to have diarrhea. By definition diarrhea lasting longer than 2 weeks is considered chronic. The most important cause of chronic diarrhea in this circumstance is villous atrophy, with loss of disaccharidases, especially lactase. The inability of the intestinal mucosa to hydrolyze lactase results in this sugar being presented to the colon, where it causes an osmotic diarrhea. Chronic

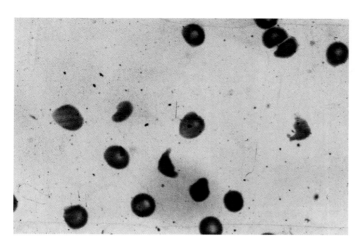

FIG. 19.2.   A blood smear of a child with hemolytic uremic syndrome. Note the large spaces between the erythrocytes, indicating severe anemia (the hemoglobin concentration was 1.8 g/dl) and the schistocytes.

■**TAB. 19.2:   Causes of altered mental status in children who have or have had diarrhea.**

Shock from dehydration
Metabolic and electrolyte disturbance
   Hypoglycemia
   Hyperglycemia
   Hyponatremia
   Hypernatremia
Vascular
   Stroke
   Hemolytic uremic syndrome
Iatrogenic
   Too rapid correction of hypernatremia
   Too rapid correction of hyponatremia (central pontine myelinosis)
   Atropine-containing drugs
   Antiemetic drugs
Complication of bacteremia
   Meningitis
Shigellosis

diarrhea may also result from continued infection. This is most likely to occur with parasitic infections such as giardiasis.

7. *Colonic perforation:* This is a complication of amebiasis and highlights the importance that this infection be considered in individuals who have traveled to high-risk areas and who have bloody diarrhea. It differs from the bacterial causes of bloody diarrhea in that the stool does not have many leukocytes (which are lysed by the parasites) and that the infection may not be self-limited.

8. *Reactive arthritis*: This is a well-recognized, but unusual complication of bacterial enteric infections. Individuals with the HLA B27 haplotype are particularly predisposed to this complication.

9. *Guillain-Barre syndrome*: About one-third of cases of Guillain-Barre syndrome follow infections with *Campylobacter jejuni*.

Management: As mentioned above, the most important element of management is to ensure adequate hydration (Figure 19.3). In most circumstances this can be accomplished by the frequent administration of liquid by mouth.

Diagnosis of enteric infections: There are two components of this. (a) Are the clinical features due to an enteric infection or not? (b) If due to an enteric infection, what is the likely cause?

(a) Noninfectious causes of intestinal symptoms and signs. Vomiting is a common symptom in children. When accompanied by fever, it may be a manifestation of a parenteral infection. Two conditions that should always be considered when vomiting is NOT ACCOMPANIED BY DIARRHEA are raised intracranial pressure, as may occur with meningitis, and intestinal obstruction. Abdominal pain or cramps, WITHOUT DIARRHEA, and with or without the passage of blood per rectum should suggest the possibility of intussusception in children younger

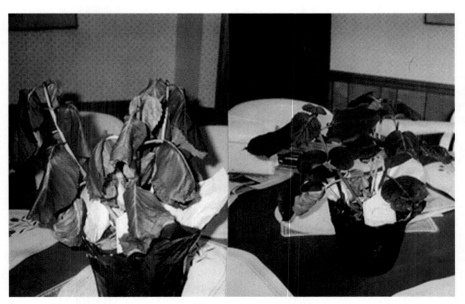

FIG. 19.3. *Dehydration with decreased turgor (left panel), and normal hydration with good turgor (right panel).*

than about 3 years of age. Chronic diarrhea, with obviously bloody stools, or with hematological evidence of blood loss in young infants should suggest the possibility of milk protein allergy. In older children and teenagers, chronic diarrhea, with or without blood, and weight loss, should suggest the possibility of inflammatory bowel disease. The differential diagnosis of enteric infections is listed in Table 19.3.

(b) Differentiating between the different causes of infection is difficult and, in most cases, is unnecessary. Examination of the stool macroscopically is useful. If blood or pus is seen, then further evaluation of the stool is indicated. This should consist of examination of the stool for leukocytes and culture for pathogenic bacteria. Examination of a *fecal smear for leukocytes* can be very useful because it can give an immediate clue as to the type of agent causing the disease. This test is performed as follows: the stool is inspected for blood, mucus, or pus; any areas containing these elements are scraped on to a wooden spatula/tongue depressor, and a thin smear of this is made on a microscope slide and allowed to dry; the slide is stained with methylene blue for about 2 minutes, and examined microscopically (Figure 19.4). The presence of large numbers or sheets of leukocytes suggest that the illness is caused by an invasive bacterium. However, this can also be seen in cases of milk protein allergy.

Culture of stool for bacteria usually takes several days, because various selective processes are needed to eliminate the normal bacteria that are present in feces. Most laboratories routinely culture for *Salmonella* spp., *Shigella* spp., *Yersinia enterocolitica* and *Campylobacter jejuni*. However, they may not culture for enterohemorrhagic *E. coli* or for *Vibrio cholerae*. When

■**TAB. 19.3: Differential diagnosis of intestinal symptoms and signs.**

Vomiting, no diarrhea
  Gastritis
  Acute food poisoning
  Raised intracranial pressure
  Intestinal obstruction, in particular intussusception
  Parenteral infection
Hematochezia, no diarrhea
  Meckel's diverticulum
  Intussusception
  Polyp
  Profound upper intestinal bleeding
Bloody diarrhea
  Milk protein allergy
  Inflammatory bowel disease

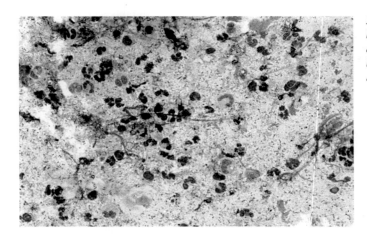

FIG. 19.4.   A methylene blue–stained fecal smear of child with diarrhea caused by *both* Salmonella enteritidis *and* Yersinia enterocolitica.

these organisms are suspected, based on epidemiological, clinical, or stool features, they should be specifically sought. Testing the stool for viruses is not usually very helpful, because no specific therapy is available. However, the results may be of epidemiological value and may restrain one from pursuing other causes of the disease.

The epidemiological, clinical, and stool features associated with different enteric infections are shown in Table 19.4.

Testing the stool for protozoa: In the past this has depended on the observation of the organisms by microscopy of the stool. This is time-consuming and requires significant expertise. *Giardia lamblia* and *Cryptosporidium parvum* can be detected by antigen detection methods. Because giardia forms cysts, it is often the cysts that are seen in the stool rather than the trophozoites. *Cryptosporidium parvum* and *Cyclospora cayetanensis* can be detected, after centrifugation of the stool specimen, by staining with a modified acid-fast stain (see Case 62). *Entamoeba histolytica* should be sought by microscopy. Ideally fresh stool mixed with warm saline is examined under the microscope. Observation of erythrophagocytic trophozoites with ameboid movement confirms that these are invasive amebae. If this test cannot be done immediately, the stool should be submitted in a fixative to the laboratory so that the morphology of the parasite can be observed. However, antigen detection methods are now available for the detection of this organism in stool.

Treatment of patients with enteric infections

1. The most important component of management is rehydration and maintenance of hydration.
2. *Nutrition*: In infants with acute diarrhea, especially those who may have borderline malnutrition, it is very important that adequate nutrition be

■TAB 19.4: Epidemiological, clinical, and stool features associated with different enteric infections, and tests used for their confirmation.

Microorganism	Epidemiology	Clinical	Stool	Test
Rotavirus	winter	acute	no blood	antigen
Enteric adenovirus		acute	no blood	tissue culture
Norovirus	outbreak (human)	acute, vomiting	no blood	RT-PCR[a]
Salmonella	animals, eggs, meat	acute, fever	+/− blood, pus	culture
Shigella	day care, human	acute, fever	+/− blood, pus	culture
Campylobacter	poultry	acute	+/− blood, pus	culture
Yersinia	pork	acute	+/− blood	culture
EHEC	meat	acute	blood	specific culture
Giardia	day care, water	acute-chronic	no blood	micro, antigen
Cryptosporidium	water, outbreak	acute-chronic	no blood	micro, antigen
Cyclospora	outbreak	acute-chronic	no blood	micro
E. histolytica	travel	acute-chronic	blood	micro, antigen

[a]RT-PCR, reverse transcriptase polymerase chain reaction; micro, microscopy.

provided. There is no sound basis for withholding food. Therefore, as soon as the child has been re-hydrated, milk or another appropriate preparation should be administered.

3. *Antimicrobial*: This can be of benefit in selected bacterial and protozoal infections but plays no roll in viral infections. Because the specific etiology is seldom known until a few days after the patient presents, initial treatment should be based on the epidemiological and clinical features, and on the appearance of the stool. The treatment of patients with different enteric infections is shown in Table 19.5. As a generalization, antibacterial therapy is indicated for patients suspected of having shigellosis or bacteremia, or in those with diarrhea associated with foreign travel. Antiparasitic therapy is indicated in those with a demonstrated protozoal infection for which therapy is available.

4. *Antiperistalsis agents*: These have limited value in children, although loperamide has been shown to reduce the volume of stool output in certain circumstances. It should not be used in presumed toxigenic infections.

5. Public health measures: Because these agents are transmitted by the fecal–oral route, attention to hygiene should be emphasized to family members. Those children who are hospitalized should be nursed with

■TAB. 19.5: Antimicrobial therapy of enteric infections.

Microorganism	Antimicrobial agent(s)
Salmonella	None, unless bacteremia suspected Ceftriaxone, TMP/S
Shigella	Ampicillin[a]; TMP/S; cefriaxone; azithromycin, fluoroquinolone[b]
Campylobacter jejuni	Azithromycin, fluoroquinolone [b]
Yersinia enterocolitica	None, unless bacteremia suspected Ceftriaxone, TMP/S; gentamicin
E. coli[c]	
ETEC, EPEC, EIEC	TMP/S; fluoroquinolone [b]
Clostridium difficile	Metronidazole; oral vancomycin
Giardia lamblia	Metronidazole, nitazoxanide
Cryptosporidium parvum	Nitazoxanide
Cyclospora cayetanensis	TMP/S
Entamoeba histolytica	Metronidazole/tinidazole

ETEC = enterotoxigenic Escherichia coli, EPEC = enteropathogenic Escherichia coli; EIEC = enteroinvasive Escherichia coli; TMP/S = trimethoprim/sulfamethoxazole.
[a]Ampicillin-resistant Shigella are widely prevalent.
[b]Fluoroquinolones are very useful, but still not widely used in children. In puppies they have been shown to cause joint disease. This has not been a problem in children.
[c]Rifaximin, a nonabsorbable rifamycin, has been shown to be of value in treating adults with travelers' diarrhea.

contact precautions. Patients with the suspicion of cholera should be reported to the health department.

Reading:

Thielman NM, Guerrant RL: Acute infectious diarrhea. N Engl J Med 2004; 350: 38–47.

Hines J, Nachamkin I: Effective use of the clinical microbiology laboratory for diagnosing diarrheal diseases. Clin Infect Dis 1996; 23: 1292–1301.

Al-Abri SS, Beeching NJ, Nje FJ: Traveller's diarrhea. Lancet Infect Dis 2005; 5: 349–360.

Armon K, Stephenson T, MacFaul R et al: An evidence and consensus based guideline for acute diarrhea management. Arch Dis Child 2001; 85: 132–141.

Glass RI, Parashar UD, Bresee JS et al: Rotavirus vaccines: current prospects and future challenges. Lancet 2006; 368: 323–332.

CASE 20. An 18-month-old girl presents with fever of a few hours duration and a rash that is spreading rapidly. Examination reveals a very ill child with poor perfusion, temperature of 40°C, and a hemorrhagic rash (Figure 20.1).

- *What is the most likely diagnosis?*
- *What would you do?*

This child has septic shock as well as hemorrhagic skin lesions. This scenario is typical of meningococcemia (meningococcal (*Neisseria meningitidis*) septicemia). This is by far the most likely diagnosis, although other infections can cause this clinical appearance, such as pneumococcal bacteremia in an asplenic individual, Gram-negative rod bacteremia, staphylococcal bacteremia or acute staphylococcal endocarditis, and septicemic plague. Rocky Mountain spotted fever, which might be considered, does not have such a short course from onset of symptoms to the appearance of the rash.

Management:

(a) *Institute supportive care immediately*: Intravenous fluids, and, if there is an inadequate response, vasopressor agents.

(b) *Attempt to make a microbiological diagnosis*: Aspirate a skin lesion and culture the aspirate and make a smear for Gram stain (Figure 20.2). Obtain blood for blood culture.

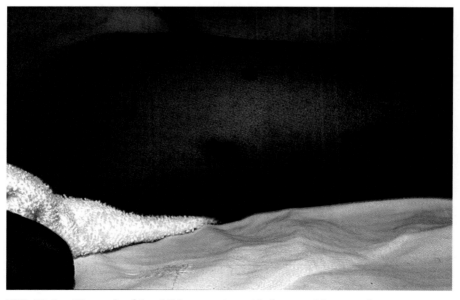

FIG. 20.1.   The rash of the child presenting with fever and hypoperfusion.

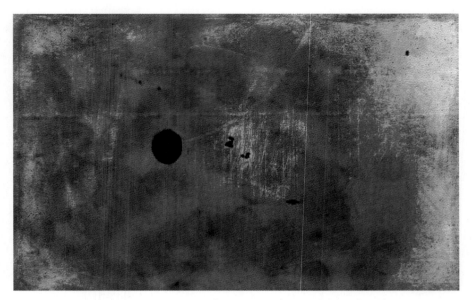

FIG. 20.2.   Gram-negative cocci in a skin aspirate from a child with meningococcemia.

Performance of a lumbar puncture is contraindicated in this child at this time, since she is unstable.

(c) Institute antimicrobial therapy with a third-generation cephalosporin. Although *Neisseria meningitidis* is susceptible to penicillin, the other possible causes of this child's illness may not be. Ceftriaxone has the advantage that it eliminates carriage of meningococcus from the nasopharynx. In considering the recently described syndrome of rapidly progressive systemic infections caused by methicillin-resistant *Staphylococcus aureus*, the addition of vancomycin should also be considered.

(d) Offer antimicrobial prophylaxis to household members and notify the local health department immediately. This prophylaxis should consist of rifampin (consider drug interactions), ciprofloxacin (if >18 years old), or a single injection of ceftriaxone. Any contact who develops fever should be evaluated, even if prophylaxis has been taken.

(e) *Vaccination*: Two vaccines are available in the United States, both against serogroups A, C, Y, and W-135. The older vaccine is a polysaccharide vaccine that is licensed for individuals older than 2 years of age. Its use has been recommended for individuals who are at increased risk of exposure to the organism (military recruits, travelers to high endemicity areas, and college students living in dormitories) and to those at increased risk of disease (asplenic individuals and those with deficiencies in terminal complement pathway components). The new vaccine is a conjugate vaccine that is for use in children older than 11 years. In the United States, it is recommended for all adolescents in addition to the groups mentioned above who are candidates for the polysaccharide vaccine.

Neisseria meningitidis is a Gram-negative coccus. It is often seen in pairs, as shown in the Figure 20.3.

Its carbohydrate capsule is an important virulence factor, enabling it to evade opsonization in the nonimmune host. It colonizes the host's pharynx, whence it may invade the bloodstream. Infection by this organism is highly feared because the bacteremia it causes (meningococcemia) can rapidly develop into a sepsis syndrome with progression to death within a few hours. This syndrome is often associated with petechiae (Figure 20.4), echymoses, and purpura fulminans, characterized by necrotic skin lesions, as shown in this patient, and the patient shown in Figure 20.5.

Occlusion of large vessels can also occur as part of this syndrome, resulting in gangrene of limbs (Figure 20.6).

Gram-stain appearances of Neisseria and Streptococci

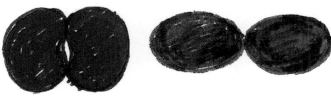

Neisseria   **Streptococcus**

FIG. 20.3.   Contrasting the Gram stain appearances of Neisseria and Streptococci.

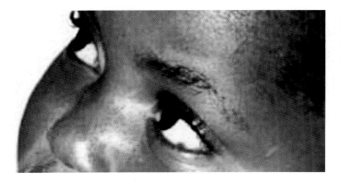

FIG. 20.4.   A subconjunctival hemorrhage in a child with meningococcal meningitis.

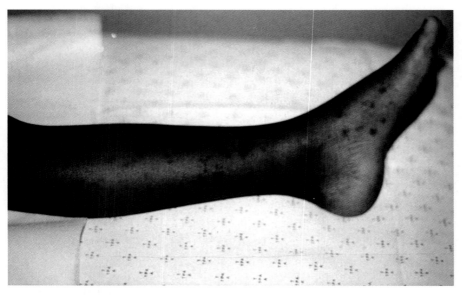

FIG. 20.5. *The hemorrhagic rash and necrotic skin lesions associated with meningococcemia.*

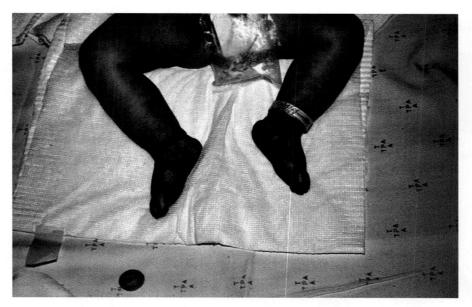

FIG. 20.6. *Peripheral gangrene due to arterial occlusion in meningococcemia.*

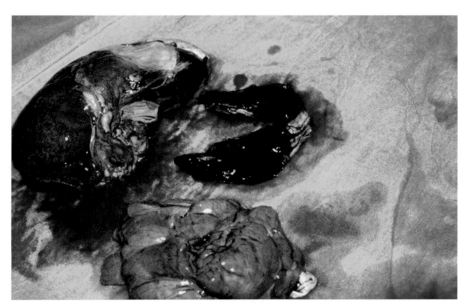

FIG. 20.7.   *The autopsy appearance of adrenal hemorrhage due to the Waterhouse-Friderichsen syndrome.*

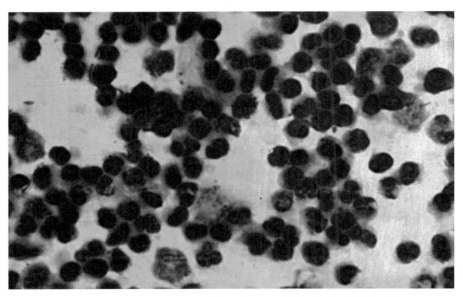

FIG. 20.8.   *Gram-stain appearance of cerebrospinal fluid of a child with meningococcal meningitis, showing numerous polymorphonuclear leukocytes and Gram-negative cocci, many of which are inside polymorphonuclear leukocytes.*

A maculopapular rash may also occur. One of the dramatic clinico-pathological complications of meningococcemia is adrenal hemorrhage, called the Waterhouse-Friderichsen syndrome (Figure 20.7).

These clinical abnormalities are due to activation of inflammatory mediators and of the coagulation and fibrinolytic systems initiated by the large amounts of endotoxin elaborated by the organism. These disturbances result in endothelial cell dysfunction, failure of vascular integrity, and myocardial depression.

The other main disease caused by this organism is meningitis, which gives the organism its name, *N. meningitidis* or meningococcus. The Gram stain appearance of cerebrospinal fluid in this infection is shown in Figure 20.8.

Other clinical syndromes it causes are encephalitis, pneumonia (which is highly contagious), arthritis, which may be septic or reactive, pericarditis, endocarditis, and anterior uveitis.

Reading:

Rosenstein NE, Perkins BA, Steohens DS, Popovic T, Hughes JM: Meningococcal disease. N Engl J Med 2001; 344: 1378–1388.

Jodar L, Feavers IM, Salisbury D, Granoff DM: Development of vaccines against meningococcal disease. Lancet 2002; 359: 1499–1508.

Warren HS, Gonzalez RG, Tian D: A 12-year-old girl with fever and coma. New Engl J Med 2003; 349: 2341–2349.

Kirsch EA, Barton RP, Kitchen L, Giroir BP: Pathophysiology, treatment and outcome of meningococcemia: a review and recent experience. Pediatr Infect Dis J 1996; 15: 967–979.

deKleijn ED, Hazelzet JA, Kornelisse RF, de Groot R: Pathophysiology of meningococcal sepsis in children. Eur J Pediatr 1998; 157: 869–880.

CASE 21. A 5-day infant presents with a 1-day history of a red left eye with a profuse discharge. Examination reveals a well-appearing child with marked swelling and erythema of the left eyelids, a profuse green conjunctival discharge, and marked chemosis (Figures 21.1 and 21.2).

- *What is the likely diagnosis?*
- *What would you do?*

This child has neonatal conjunctivitis. The profuse discharge suggests the possibility of gonococcal infection, but other bacteria can cause this condition, in particular *Staphylococcus aureus*. Chemical conjunctivitis from silver nitrate eyedrops occurs earlier in life and tends not to be very severe.

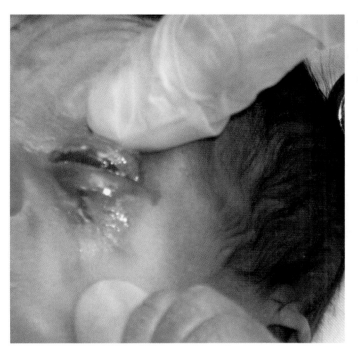

FIG. 21.1.   *The infant's left eye. Note the marked eyelid swelling and yellow discharge. (Courtesy of Dr Timothy Vece, Emory University)*

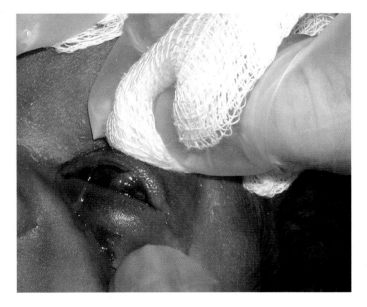

FIG. 21.2.   *The infant's left eye. Note the marked chemosis (conjunctival swelling). (Courtesy of Dr Timothy Vece, Emory University)*

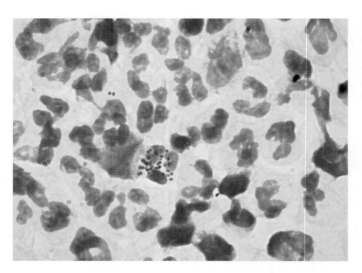

FIG. 21.3.   Gram stain of a conjunctival swab from this child showing Gram-negative cocci, which were confirmed to be Neisseria gonorrhoeae.

This is too early in the child's life for the presentation of chlamydial conjunctivitis.

Management: Make a smear of the discharge for Gram stain (which, in the case of gonococcal conjunctivitis might show Gram-negative diplococci – Figure 21.3) and send a swab to be cultured specifically for *Neisseria gonorrhoeae* (which requires a selective medium).

Infants in whom gonococcal conjunctivitis is suspected should be treated with a single injection of ceftriaxone (125 mg) and frequent instillations of saline eyedrops to rinse out the eyes. They should be re-evaluated the next day. Some authorities recommend performance of blood cultures and lumbar puncture to exclude systemic disease, but I do not do this unless there is evidence of systemic infection. Untreated, this condition can cause severe corneal damage and blindness. Diagnosing this condition implies that the mother is infected with the organism. She and her sexual partner should be treated and the health department should be notified.

This infant's eye swab showed many Gram-negative diplococci and the culture grew out *Neisseria gonorrhoeae*. One day after being treated as described above, the eye was almost normal.

Reading:

Woods CR: Gonococcal infections in neonates and young children. Semin Pediatr Infect Dis 2005; 16: 258–270.

CASE 22 (COMP). A 9-year-old boy presents with a history of pain and swelling of the right knee followed by similar symptoms affecting the left elbow. He also feels tired. On examination he has a temperature of 38.3°C, and a heart rate of 120/min. His apex beat is in the 5th left interspace, anterior axillary line. The first and second heart sounds are normal, and there is a 2/6 holosystolic murmur at the apex. He has swelling of the right knee and left elbow joints with limitation of movement.

- *What is the likely diagnosis?*
- *What would you do?*

This boy has fever, migratory arthritis, tachycardia, and mitral valve insufficiency. These features strongly suggest the diagnosis of acute rheumatic fever. They constitute two of the major Jones criteria for the diagnosis of this condition (arthritis and carditis). The other conditions that might cause these features are infective endocarditis and systemic lupus erythematosus. The other major Jones criteria are Sydenham's chorea, erythema marginatum, and subcutaneous nodules. The diagnosis of acute rheumatic fever depends on two major criteria in addition to evidence of a recent infection with *Streptococcus pyogenes*. There are also minor criteria used for the diagnosis of acute rheumatic fever. These are arthralgia, fever, prolonged PR interval on electrocardiogram, and elevated acute phase reactants. Although one major and two minor criteria may be used for the diagnosis of acute rheumatic fever, the minor criteria are very nonspecific, and one should be wary of using them.

Rheumatic fever is an immunological complication of *Streptococcus pyogenes* (group A streptococcus) pharyngotonsillitis, resulting in inflammation of cardiac valves. It is due to antibodies to streptococcal antigens that cross-react with heart valve antigens. The valves most frequently affected are the mitral and the aortic valves. In the acute phase of the illness, the valve leaflets are swollen. In addition myocarditis or pericarditis may be present. The inflammation may resolve without leaving sequelae, but scarring of the valve can occur resulting in permanent cardiac damage called rheumatic heart disease. Such damage is manifest as valvular insufficiency, and/or stenosis, which, in turn lead to heart failure. Therefore rheumatic fever is a very important cause of acquired heart disease (Figure 22.1).

In individuals who have had an episode of acute rheumatic fever, subsequent episodes of streptococcal tonsillitis may be followed by another episode of rheumatic fever, resulting in further cardiac damage. Treatment of the acute episode entails symptomatic treatment of the arthritis with salicylates or ibuprofen, and treatment of heart failure if this occurs. Prevention of subsequent episodes requires the administration of penicillin until the patient is at least 25 years old. This can be done with oral penicillin twice per day, or with an intramuscular injection of long-acting bicillin every 3–4 weeks. As long as there is any cardiac valvular abnormality, these patients are

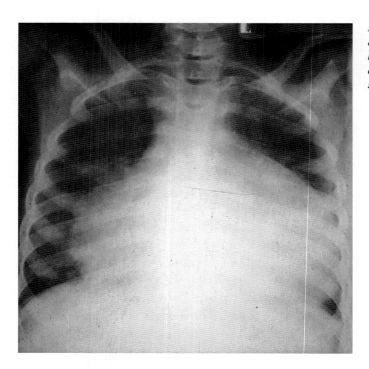

FIG. 22.1. Chest X ray of a child with severe rheumatic heart disease. There is cardiomegaly resulting from severe mitral insufficiency.

susceptible to infective endocarditis. They therefore require *additional* antibiotic prophylaxis for procedures that may cause bacteremia, for example, dental cleaning. The regular penicillin they receive is inadequate for this purpose.

Because rheumatic fever is a potentially devastating albeit rare complication of streptococcal pharyngitis, all patients with streptococcal pharyngitis should be treated with penicillin. Streptococcal pharyngitis cannot be readily differentiated from viral pharyngitis clinically. Therefore throat cultures to detect *Streptococcus pyogenes* should be performed on all patients with pharyngitis to determine who should be treated with penicillin.

Reading:

Stollerman GH: Rheumatic fever. Lancet 1997; 349: 935–942.

Bisno AL, Brito MO, Collins CM: Molecular basis of group A streptococcal virulence. Lancet Infect Dis 2003; 3: 191–200.

Bisno AL: Group A streptococcal infections and acute rheumatic fever. N Engl J Med 1991; 325: 783–793.

Kotloff KL, Dale JB: Progress in Group A streptococcal vaccine development. Pediatr Infect Dis J 2004; 23: 765–766.

Carapetis JR, Steer AC, Mulholland EK et al: The global burden of group A streptococcal diseases. Lancet Infect Dis 2005; 5: 685–694.

CASE 23. A 3-year-old boy presents with swelling of the eyelids on rising in the morning for 2 days. On examination he has swelling of the eyelids and legs, and several healing sores on his legs (Figures 23.1 and 23.2).

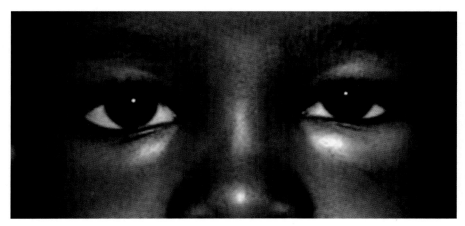

FIG. 23.1.   The eyelid swelling.

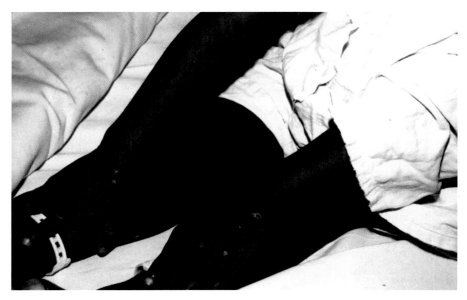

FIG. 23.2.   The skin sores.

- *What else would you like to know?*
- *What is wrong with him?*

Fluid balance between the intravascular space and the interstitial space is dependent on the hydrostatic pressure that tends to force water out of the capillary, the oncotic pressure of the fluid that tends to hold the water within the vascular space, and the integrity of the capillary wall. Edema is the result of one or more of three processes: (a) increased hydrostatic pressure, as occurs in heart failure, or a decreased glomerular filtration rate; (b) decreased oncotic pressure due to hypoalbuminemia, as occurs in the nephrotic syndrome, malnutrition, or liver failure; or (c) increased capillary permeability, as occurs in the sepsis syndrome and in anaphylaxis. Many of these conditions can be diagnosed by history and physical examination alone.

Additional information that should be sought:

Is he short of breath? Is there evidence of pulmonary edema from heart failure or fluid overload from renal failure? Is there elevation of the jugulovenous pressure? What is the blood pressure? Is there evidence of liver disease or malnutrition?

What is the color of the urine? If it is dark reddish brown this suggests hematuria, which, in this case, would suggest the diagnosis of acute glomerulonephritis.

This child has edema, a blood pressure of 150/95 mm Hg, a jugulovenous pressure of about 7 cm water, and a respiratory rate of 30/minute, and the urine is reddish brown and turbid.

These abnormalities are highly suggestive of glomerulonephritis, with fluid overload. An important cause of acute glomerulonephritis is infection with *Streptococcus pyogenes*, either impetigo (of which this patient has evidence) or tonsillitis. The glomeruli are inflamed and swollen, and there is a decrease in the glomerular filtration rate, leading to oliguria and edema. The demonstration of red cell casts in the urine would confirm the diagnosis of glomerulonephritis (although this is a very insensitive test), while the demonstration of *Streptococcus pyogenes* infection in the throat or skin would suggest this as the etiology of the glomerulonephritis. Culture of an infected skin lesion or of a throat swab is the optimal way in which to confirm the presence of *Streptococcus pyogenes* infection. However, serological tests (e.g. antihyaluronidase titer) may be helpful in this regard.

Treatment of acute poststreptococcal glomerulonephritis consists of (a) treatment of pulmonary edema, if present, with oxygen and furosemide; (b) control of hypertension, for example, with nifedipine (furosemide might help in this regard); (c) restriction of fluid intake; (d) penicillin for 10 days to eliminate the streptococcus. Long-term penicillin is not necessary, because, unlike rheumatic fever, this disease does not recur. The long-term prognosis is excellent.

Reading:

Bisno AL, Brito MO, Collins CM: Molecular basis of group A streptococcal virulence. Lancet Infect Dis 2003; 3: 191–200.

Bisno AL: Group A streptococcal infections and acute rheumatic fever. N Engl J Med 1991; 325: 783–793.

Kotloff KL, Dale JB: Progress in group A streptococcal vaccine development. Pediatr Infect Dis J 2004; 23: 765–766.

CASE 24. A 6-year-old boy presents with a sore throat and fever and is found to have large, inflamed tonsils and tender cervical lymphadenopathy, with the appearance of that shown in Figure 24.1 (from a different patient).

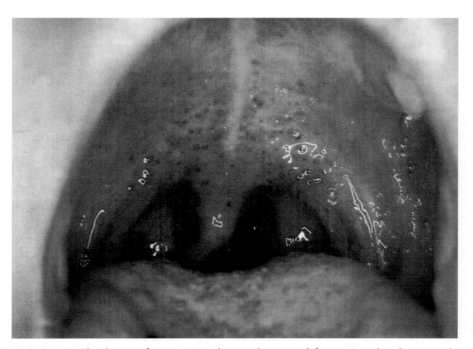

FIG. 24.1.   The throat of a patient with sore throat and fever. Note the pharyngeal erythema and palatal petechiae. (Courtesy of the Center of Disease Control and Prevention/Dr Heinz F Eichenwald)

- *What is the differential diagnosis?*
- *What would you do?*

This child has acute tonsillitis. The differential diagnosis of the cause of acute tonsillitis in this patient is *Streptococcus pyogenes*, infectious mononucleosis due to Epstein–Barr virus, and several respiratory viruses such as adenovirus, respiratory syncytial virus, and parainfluenza virus. Diphtheria should be considered in patients who have traveled to areas where this is endemic. In teenagers and young adults *Arcanobacterium haemolyticum* also causes pharyngotonsillitis and a generalized rash. Of the likely causes antimicrobial therapy is available against only *Streptococcus pyogenes*. Although this infection may spread to cause a peritonsillar abscess, retropharyngeal abscess, otitis media, cervical lymphadenitis, and occasionally spread via the bloodstream to cause metastatic infection such as osteomyelitis, the main reason for confirming the diagnosis of this infection and providing antimicrobial therapy is to prevent the complication of acute rheumatic fever, which can have devastating long-term effects on the heart. *Streptococcus pyogenes* infections may be associated with a rash, characterized by fine sandpaper-like papules and diffuse erythroderma, called scarlet fever. This is mediated by a pyrogenic toxin (Figure 24.2).

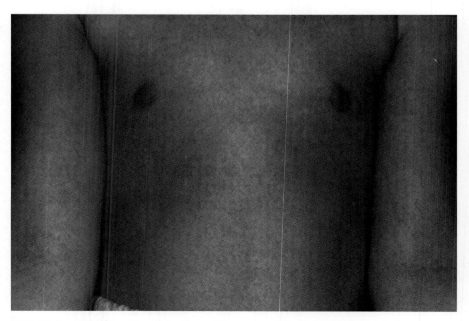

FIG. 24.2. A child with scarlet fever (Courtesy of Dr Michael Radetsky)

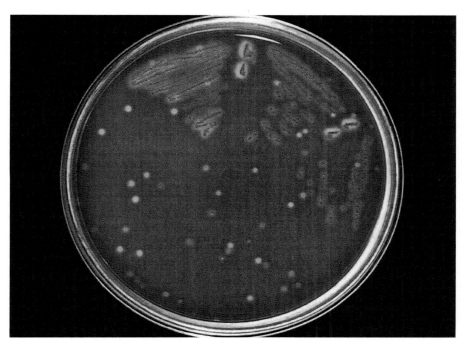

FIG. 24.3.   A culture of Streptococcus pyogenes *on blood agar. Note the β-hemolysis (complete hemolysis) around the colonies. (Courtesy of the Centers for Disease Control and Prevention/Richard R Facklam, PhD)*

The diagnosis of streptococcal tonsillitis can be confirmed with a throat culture (Figure 24.3) or one of the rapid streptococcal antigen detection tests performed on a throat swab.

Treatment consists of penicillin, given as a single dose of long-acting bicillin or as oral phenoxymethyl penicillin administered for 10 days. Other agents such as amoxicillin, cephalosporins, and macrolides may also be used.

Reading:

Bisno AL, Brito MO, Collins CM: Molecular basis of group A streptococcal virulence. Lancet Infect Dis 2003; 3: 191–200.

Bisno AL: Group A streptococcal infections and acute rheumatic fever. N Engl J Med 1991; 325: 783–793.

CASE 25. A premature infant in the neonatal intensive care unit being ventilated for hyaline membrane disease is noted to have temperature instability, dark red spots on the skin, and a swollen red ankle. Further examination reveals a 3/6 ejection systolic heart murmur, heard loudest at the upper sternal border. She has a venous and arterial vascular catheter in place. The abdominal examination is normal.

- *What is the differential diagnosis?*
- *What would you do?*

Dark red spots on the skin suggest the possibility of hemorrhage or infarctions of the skin. The red, swollen ankle suggests a septic arthritis or osteomyelitis. Temperature instability suggests a systemic infection. A unifying diagnosis would be a systemic (bloodstream) bacterial or fungal infection associated with skeletal infection, and causing (a) a hemorrhagic tendency through the mechanisms of thrombocytopenia or disseminated intravascular coagulation or (b) emboli due to infective endocarditis. The heart murmur, which is suggestive of a pathological murmur by its intensity, could be due to a congenital heart disease that could predispose to infective endocarditis, or be due to valvular damage caused by infective endocarditis affecting a previously normal valve. By definition, an infection in this infant is nosocomial. The potential routes of infection are through vascular access sites, through the lungs, especially since the infant is intubated, through the intestine, or through the urinary tract, especially if the infant has a urinary catheter. The likely organisms include staphylococci, *Candida* spp., enterococci, and Gram-negative bacilli.

Specific clinical evaluation should include examination of the optic fundi (to look for Roth spots) and examination of all vascular access sites (past and present) for evidence of infection. The urine should be examined for hematuria. Blood cultures (three) should be performed over a period of 15 minutes, as should a blood count including a platelet count. The ankle and one of the skin lesions should be aspirated and the aspirates should be submitted for culture and Gram stain. A cardiologist should be consulted for both clinical and echocardiographic evaluation of the heart.

Initial (empiric) antimicrobial treatment should be directed at the most likely pathogens, but guided by Gram-stain results, and more definitive treatment should be based on culture and susceptibility results. Initial treatment should be as follows:

(a) If the Gram stain shows Gram-positive cocci in clusters (staphylococci), vancomycin + nafcillin + gentamicin should be used. The reason for using both vancomycin and nafcillin is that for susceptible organisms, nafcillin is superior to vancomycin. However, the vancomycin is necessary in case the organism is resistant to β-lactam antibiotics (methicillin resistant). Gentamicin accelerates the clearance of the staphylococci from the blood.

(b) If the Gram stain shows Gram-negative rods (which could be enteric bacilli or *Pseudomonas aeruginosa*), ceftazidime + amikacin should be used (gentamicin can be used instead of amikacin if the rate of gentamicin resistance among Gram-negative bacilli is very low in the unit);

(c) If the Gram stain shows yeasts, amphotericin B should be used. (In less severely ill patients with intravascular-line–associated fungemia, and without endocarditis, and in whom the vascular line can be removed, fluconazole would be appropriate).

(d) If the Gram stain does not reveal an organism, initial treatment should be directed at staphylococci and Gram-negative rods with vancomycin, nafcillin, gentamicin, or amikacin, and a third-generation cephalosporin.

The Gram stain from a skin aspirate of this patient (Figure 25.1) shows Gram-positive cocci in clusters, the typical appearance of staphylococci.

The skin, blood cultures, and ankle joint fluid grew out *Staphylococcus aureus* susceptible to methicillin. Further evaluation revealed an aortic vegetation, providing additional evidence of infective endocarditis. She was treated successfully with nafcillin.

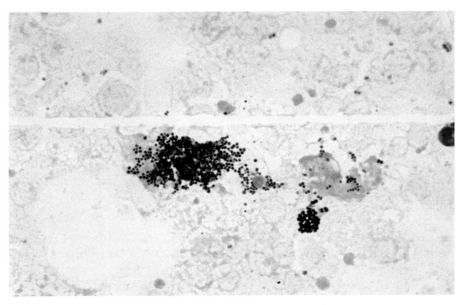

FIG. 25.1. Gram-stained smear of a skin lesion aspirate from the above patient revealing Gram-positive cocci in clusters.

Reading:

Daher AH, Berkowitz FE: Infective endocarditis in neonates. Clin Pediatr 1995; 34: 198–206.

Moreillon P, Que Y: Infective endocarditis. Lancet 2004; 363: 139–149.

CASE 26 (HYP). A 3-year-old boy who broke out with chickenpox 5 days ago seems to be getting worse after initial improvement. He has a high fever, his skin is red all over, and he seems a little confused.

• *What might be the problem?*

The most likely problem is that this boy has developed a complication of chickenpox. The most common complication is secondary bacterial infection of skin lesions with *Streptococcus pyogenes* or *Staphylococcus aureus*. The child's illness is characterized by fever, confusion, and diffuse erythroderma. The confusion could be due merely to delireum associated with the fever, to a more severe problem affecting the brain, including meningitis, a metabolic disturbance such as hypoglycemia or hyponatremia, or to poor brain perfusion. The erythema could be due to scarlet fever, or to streptococcal toxic shock-like syndrome or staphylococcal toxic shock syndrome. Given the apparent severity of the child's condition and the combination of clinical abnormalities, he probably has streptococcal toxic shock-like syndrome, with or without bacteremia, or staphylococcal toxic shock syndrome.

Further clinical evaluation should be directed at determining the adequacy of his perfusion and at finding a septic focus that might be drained. This is very important in toxic shock syndrome.

Management should entail the following: (a) ensuring adequate perfusion with intravenous fluid and vasopressors, if necessary; (b) draining any focus of pus, and sending specimens for Gram stain and culture; a blood culture should also be performed; and (c) antimicrobial therapy – this should consist of antibiotics active against *Streptococcus pyogenes* and *Staphylococcus aureus*, and might consist of the following, depending on the local prevalence of methicillin-resistant *Staphylococcus aureus* (MRSA): vancomycin (for its activity against MRSA) + oxacillin/nafcillin/cephazolin (for its activity against *Streptococcus pyogenes* and methicillin-susceptible *Staphylococcus aureus*) + clindamycin (for its ability to halt protein synthesis by the organisms, and thus halt toxin production).

There is some evidence that intravenous immune globulin (IVIG) is beneficial in patients with streptococcal toxic shock-like syndrome. I would use it in a patient such as this.

Reading:

American Academy of Pediatrics. Committee on Infectious Diseases. Severe invasive group A streptococcal infections: a subject review. Pediatrics 1998; 101: 136– 140.

CASE 27. A 6-month-old previously well girl who attends day care presents with a history of fever, irritability, and decreased activity. On examination she has a temperature of 40°C and is extremely irritable. In addition, she does not interact with her parents as usual. There are no other findings. The cerebrospinal fluid examination reveals 8000 leukocytes per mm^3 with a differential count of 95% neutrophils and 5% lymphocytes. The Gram stain is shown in Figure 27.1.

- *What is the likely diagnosis?*
- *What would you do?*
- *How might this illness have been prevented?*

The Gram stain shows numerous Gram-positive diplococci, resembling streptococci.

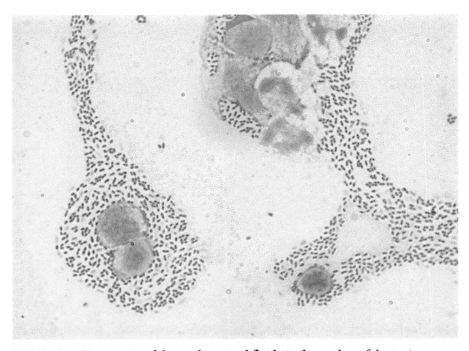

FIG. 27.1. Gram stain of the cerebrospinal fluid similar to that of the patient described.

The likely diagnosis is *Streptococcus pneumoniae* (pneumococcal) meningitis.

Management consists of (a) supportive care, which might entail intravenous fluids if the child is in shock, and ventilation if breathing is impaired and (b) antimicrobial therapy.

The initial empiric antimicrobial therapy is determined by possible resistance of the causative organism to penicillin and third-generation cephalosporins. It should consist of vancomycin 20 mg/kg/dose q 8 hours intravenously plus ceftriaxone 50 mg/kg/dose q 12 hours intravenously (or cefotaxime 75 mg/kg/dose q 6 hours intravenously). Some authors (myself included) recommend the addition of rifampin 10 mg/kg/dose q 12 hours orally.

Once the susceptibilities are known, therapy can be adjusted.

The use of a corticosteroid such as dexamethasone is controversial. I recommend its use.

Acute bacterial meningitis is associated with significant vascular injury, cerebral edema, and raised intracranial pressure. Consequently it can be associated with the following complications:

1. various types of brain injury including hemiplegia, brainstem infarction, and learning disabilities (Figures 27.2–27.4)

2. seizures

3. cranial nerve palsies

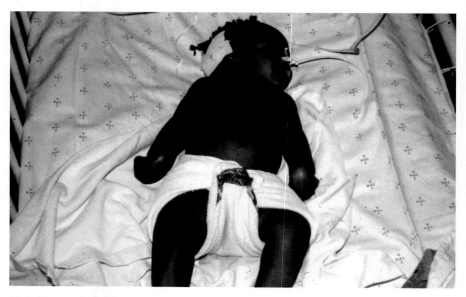

FIG. 27.2.   A child with severe brain damage resulting from pneumococcal meningitis.

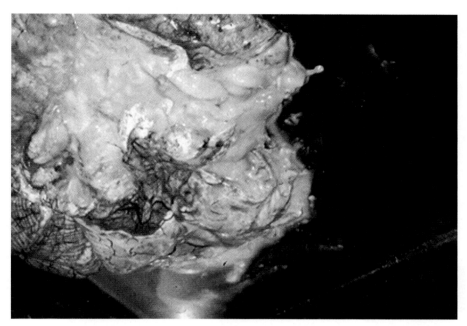

FIG. 27.3.   *The autopsy appearance of the brain of the child shown in figure 27.2. Note the brain liquefaction resulting from ischemia.*

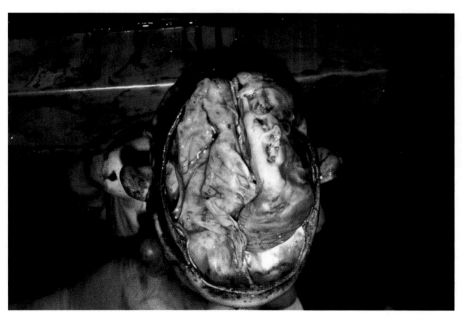

FIG. 27.4.   *Autopsy appearance of the brain of an infant dying from pneumococcal meningitis, showing severe damage.*

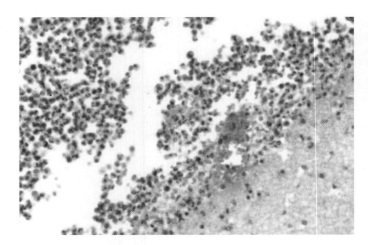

FIG. 27.5.   Histopathology of bacterial meningitis, showing the inflammatory reaction in the subarachnoid space. (Courtesy of Dr Carlos Abramowsky, Emory University).

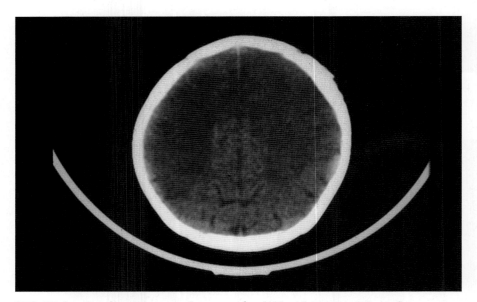

FIG. 27.6.   Computer tomography scan of a child with Haemophilus influenzae *meningitis and profound neurological deficit. The dark (hypodense) areas represent infarctions, which affect both hemispheres.*

4. hydrocephalus

5. subdural fluid collection. This is common and does not usually warrant drainage. However, it may progress to empyema in which case drainage is indicated.

6. brain abscess is rarely a complication of bacterial meningitis, except in the newborn, and particularly in cases caused by *Proteus, Enterobacter,* and *Citrobacter* species.

7. inappropriate secretion of antidiuretic hormone (SIADH)

8. hearing loss. This is due to cochlear damage.

Fever may continue despite treatment in patients with bacterial meningitis. One should consider several causes of fever in such patients.

(A) Those related to the meningitis:

    (a) If the patient is otherwise improving, the fever is probably due to the meningitis itself and may last up to about a week.

    (b) If the patient is not improving as expected, the causative organism may not be susceptible to the antimicrobial therapy; in such a case, a repeat lumbar puncture should be performed to determine whether the cerebrospinal fluid has been sterilized or not.

    (c) Intracranial suppurative complications of the meningitis such as subdural empyema or brain abscess. Brain imaging can help to diagnose these.

(B) Those related to therapy:

    (a) Phlebitis from the intravenous catheter

    (b) Drug fever due to the antibiotic

    (c) Nosocomial infections such as phlebitis, respiratory tract infection

(C) Distant infections resulting from hematogenous spread of the same organism that caused the meningitis, for example, septic arthritis

(D) Immune reactions to the infection, for example, arthritis, which is seen particularly with meningococcal infections.

Evaluation of such patients should be guided by clinical findings.

Reading:

Bedford H, de Louvois J, Halket S et al: Meningitis in infancy in England and Wales: follow up at age 5 years. BMJ 2001; 323: 533–535.

Kaplan SL, Mason EO: Management of infections due to antibiotic-resistant *Streptococcus pneumoniae*. Clin Microbiol Rev 1998; 11: 628–644.

Swartz MN : Bacterial meningitis – a view of the past 90 years. N Engl J Med 2004; 351: 1826–1828.

Kaplan SL, Woods CR: Neurological complications of bacterial meningitis in children. Curr Clin Top Infect Dis 1992; 12: 37–55.

CASE 28. A 1-month-old infant presents with a history of not moving the right arm for 1 day. She is otherwise fine, eating well, and afebrile. On examination the temperature is 36.5°C, and the perfusion is normal. The right upper limb is flaccid and there is mild swelling and marked tenderness around the shoulder joint. The rest of the examination is normal.

- *What is the differential diagnosis?*
- *What would you do?*

The differential diagnosis essentially consists of injury to the limb (accidental or nonaccidental), involving the soft tissue or bone, or infection involving the shoulder joint or bone on either side of the joint, that is, the upper end of the humerus or the scapula, or both. Although an X ray cannot exclude soft tissue injury, it can largely exclude a fracture. Skeletal infections in children of this age typically manifest as failure of the use of the limb, as seen in this patient. The infant usually appears otherwise well, feeds well, and may be afebrile. Osteomyelitis and septic arthritis in children is almost always hematogenous in origin. Osteomyelitis affects the bone metaphysis. In young infants infection can spread through the growth plate into the joint, but in children older than about 18 months the growth plate provides a significant barrier to spread of infection into the joint (Figure 28.1). It can also spread through the periosteum into the muscle and subcutaneous tissue (Figure 28.2).

The common causative organisms of skeletal infection in a 1-month-old infant are *Streptococcus agalactiae* (group B streptococcus), *Staphylococcus*

Anatomy of end of a long bone in infant and older child

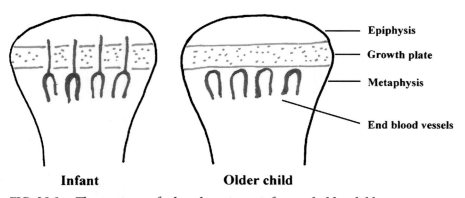

Infant   Older child

FIG. 28.1. *The anatomy of a long bone in an infant and older child.*

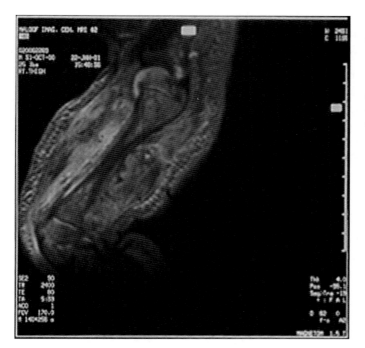

FIG. 28.2.   MRI of the femur of a young infant with osteomyelitis, showing inflammation within the quadriceps muscle, resulting from spread of the infection from the femur through the periosteum.

aureus, and Gram-negative bacilli. It is extremely important to make a microbiological diagnosis in order to provide optimal therapy. This requires obtaining specimens from the joint and the adjacent bone by inserting a needle into the respective area and culturing the aspirated material. Material should be submitted both on a swab or in a sterile tube, as well as inoculated into a blood culture bottle, which can increase the chances of culturing an organism. When the focus of disease is apparent, as in this child, further studies to localize the disease are unnecessary, but when this is not the case, a radionucleide bone scan should be performed to localize a site of osteomyelitis. When the nature of the disease and the specific site are un-clear, an MRI may be helpful. Blood cultures should also be performed. Once appropriate specimens have been obtained, antibiotic therapy directed against the above-mentioned organisms should be initiated. This can be adjusted once an organism is isolated. In areas with a high prevalence of methicillin-resistant *Staphylococcus aureus* (MRSA), vancomycin should be used, in addition to a third-generation cephalosporin for its activity against *Streptococcus agalactiae* and enteric Gram-negative bacilli. In areas with a low prevalence of MRSA, nafcillin or oxacillin can be used instead of vancomycin.

In this child, *Streptococcus agalactiae* was cultured from the shoulder joint. She improved on therapy with ampicillin.

CASE 29. A 6-month-old child, who is 3 weeks post placement of a ventriculoperitoneal (VP) shunt for hydrocephalus, presents with a 3-day history of fever and decreased appetite. On examination she has a temperature of 38.2°C and a large head. The shunt track is not inflamed and the surgical wound is well healed. The rest of the examination is normal. Cerebrospinal fluid taken through the shunt bulb shows 100 leukocytes per mm^3 of which 75% are neutrophils. The Gram stain reveals a few Gram-positive cocci.

- *What is the likely diagnosis and its likely cause?*
- *What should be done?*

The patient has ventriculitis due to a shunt infection. This is probably caused by a staphylococcus, a coagulase-negative staphylococcus more likely than *Staphylococcus aureus*.

Patients with VP shunt infections usually present with fever and evidence of raised intracranial pressure due to shunt malfunction (headache, vomiting, decreased level of consciousness) or abdominal pain caused by infected fluid draining into the peritoneal cavity, causing peritonitis.

Of three different methods of management, namely (i) leaving the shunt in place and using antimicrobial therapy only, (ii) removal of the shunt and immediate replacement with a new shunt, in addition to the administration of antibiotics, and (iii) removal of the shunt, placement of an external drain, in addition to the administration of antibiotics, and replacement of the shunt when the cerebrospinal fluid has become sterile, the last strategy ((iii)) is preferable. The new shunt can usually be replaced within 3–7 days after the infected shunt has been removed and appropriate therapy has been instituted.

References:

Yogev R: Cerebrospinal fluid shunt infections: a personal view. Pediatr Infect Dis J 1985; 4: 113–118.

Schreffler RT, Schreffler AJ, Wittler RR: Treatment of cerebrospinal fluid shunt infections: a decision analysis. Pediatr Infect Dis J 2002; 21: 632–636.

CASE 30. A full-term newborn baby develops respiratory difficulty and shock, and dies within 12 hours of birth, despite vigorous therapy. The Gram stain of the blood culture broth after 12 hours of incubation is shown in Figure 30.1.

- *What is the likely identification of the organism?*

The Gram stain shows Gram-positive cocci in chains.

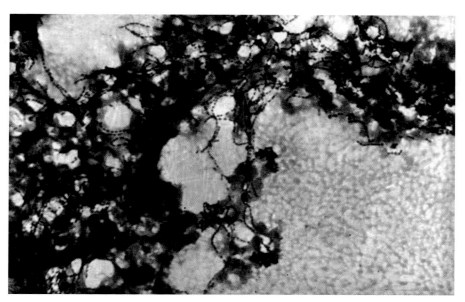

FIG. 30.1.   The Gram stain of the blood culture broth after overnight incubation.

The most likely causative organism is *Streptococcus agalactiae* (group B streptococcus). This organism is the most common cause of neonatal sepsis in the United States at this time. It causes two main types of illness. (a) Early-onset disease (i.e. presenting in babies <1 week, often within a few hours of birth as in this patient), which is characterized by severe pneumonia and septic shock. In this situation, the organism is acquired from the mother's vagina. (b) Late-onset disease (i.e. presenting in babies older than >1 week), which may occur in infants as old as 4 months. Such infants usually present with fever. They usually have bacteremia and/or meningitis. Late-onset disease may also cause skeletal infection (see Case 28).

Several strategies have been used to prevent early-onset infection with this organism. The current strategy recommended by the US Public Health Service entails screening of the mother in late pregnancy and treating colonized mothers with ampicillin during labor. This strategy has been shown to have been associated with a marked decline in the number of cases of early-onset neonatal Group B streptococcal infections but not in that of late-onset infections.

Reading:

Centers for Disease Control and Prevention. Prevention or perinatal group B streptococcal disease. Revised guidelines from CDC. MMWR Recomm. Rep. 2002; 51 (RR 11): 1–22.

CASE 31. An 8-month-old African-American boy presents with a history of fever for several hours. He is found to be in shock. There are no localizing findings. He is treated with fluid resuscitation, pressors, and antibiotics (ceftriaxone and vancomycin intravenously). He dies a few hours later. A blood smear reveals the cause of death (Figure 31.1).

- *What does the blood smear reveal?*
- *What are possible underlying condition predisposing him this disease?*

The blood smear reveals diplococci. When this smear is stained with Gram stain, these can be seen to be Gram-positive diplococci, resembling *Streptococcus pneumoniae* (pneumococcus) (Figure 31.2).

When microorganisms are seen on a blood smear, this indicates at least 10^5 organisms per milliliter of blood and a very poor prognosis for survival. The most likely identity of these organisms is *Streptococcus pneumoniae*. The rapid progression of the illness and the high concentration of organisms in the blood suggests the absence or hypofunction of the spleen. This can occur congenitally (sometimes associated with congenital heart disease), or as a result of sickle cell disease or surgical splenectomy. (The presence of Howell-Jolly bodies (intraerythrocytic inclusions) on a blood smear indicates absence of the spleen (Figure 31.3)). This was indeed a case of pneumococcal bacteremia and the child indeed had sickle cell disease (Figure 31.4), which had not been previously diagnosed. This is the main cause of death in infants and

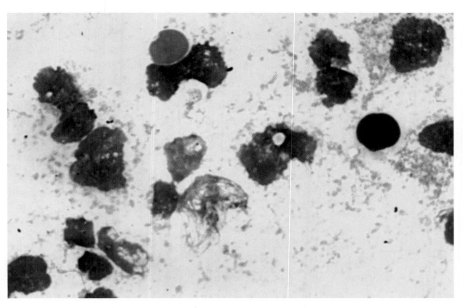

FIG. 31.1. The patient's blood smear stained with Wright's stain.

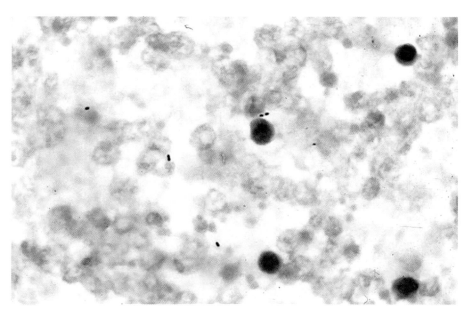

FIG. 31.2.   The blood smear stained with Gram stain, revealing Gram-positive diplococci, resembling Streptococcus pneumoniae.

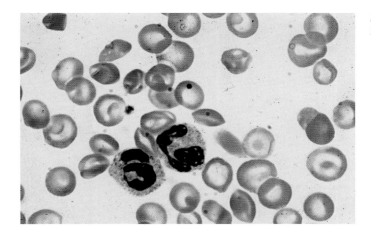

FIG. 31.3.   A Howell-Jolly body inside an erythrocyte.

young children with sickle cell disease. Children at highest risk are those younger than 3 years. The reason for children with sickle cell disease to be susceptible to fulminating pneumococcal sepsis syndrome is hyposplenism resulting from splenic infarcts. This develops progressively during the first year of life.

Pneumococci have a polysaccharide capsule. There are more than 80 different capsular types (serotypes). The host's blood phagocytes (neutrophils,

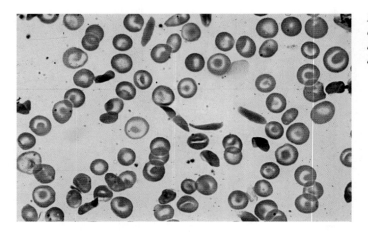

FIG. 31.4.   A blood smear of a child with sickle cell disease. Note the sickle cells and target cells.

The role of phagocytes, antibody, complement, and the spleen in removing pneumococci from the circulation.

FIG. 31.5.   The role of the spleen in removing pneumococci from the circulation.

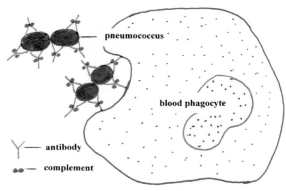

a) presence of antibody

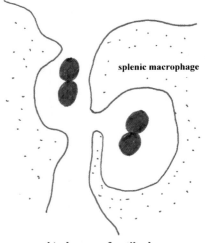

b) absence of antibody

monocytes) depend on complement and capsule-specific antibody to opsonize pneumococci and remove them from the circulation. However, in the absence of antibody, only the splenic macrophages can remove pneumococci from the circulation. In the case of infants and young children, who have not previously encountered the organism and therefore lack antibody, the spleen is therefore very important (Figure 31.5).

Young children with sickle cell disease, who lack both antibody and normal splenic function, cannot prevent pneumococci in the circulation from multiplying rapidly and causing a fulminating sepsis syndrome, as in this case. Penicillin prophylaxis (before the era of significant rates of penicillin resistance) was shown to be very effective in reducing the mortality from this infection. In order to (a) institute penicillin prophylaxis and (b) educate the parents about the importance of bringing such children for evaluation and antibiotic treatment when they have fever, the children must be known to have sickle cell disease. Therefore it is important that children are screened for this hemoglobinopathy as newborns. An additional preventive measure is immunization with the conjugated pneumococcal vaccine beginning at the age of 2 months.

Reading:

American Academy of Pediatrics, Section on Hematology/Oncology, Committee on Genetics: Health supervision for children with sickle cell disease. Pediatrics 2002; 109: 526–535.

Overturf GD and the Committee on Infectious Diseases, American Academy of Pediatrics. Technical report: Prevention of pneumococcal infections, including the use of pneumococcal conjugate and polysaccharide vaccines and antibiotic prophylaxis. Pediatrics 2000; 106: 367–376.

Gaston MH, Verter JI, Woods G et al: Prophylaxis with oral penicillin in children with sickle cell anemia. A randomized trial. N Engl J Med 1986; 314: 1593–1599.

CASE 32.   An infant presents with cough and high fever. On examination she is very ill-appearing; the respiratory rate is 80/minute, and there is dullness to percussion and decreased breath sounds on the left side of the chest. A chest X ray reveals a large left pleural effusion and pneumonia (Figure 32.1).

The effusion is tapped revealing purulent fluid, from which *Staphylococcus aureus* is cultured. A chest tube (intercostal drain) is inserted and she is treated with cloxacillin. She slowly improves. During her convalescence an abnormality, shown in the picture, is noted (Figure 32.2).

- *What is the abnormality, and what is its pathogenesis?*

This picture shows left-sided ptosis. This is part of a Horner's syndrome complicating a pleural empyema. Horner's syndrome, consisting of ptosis, enophthalmos, miosis, and loss of sweating of the forehead, is caused by

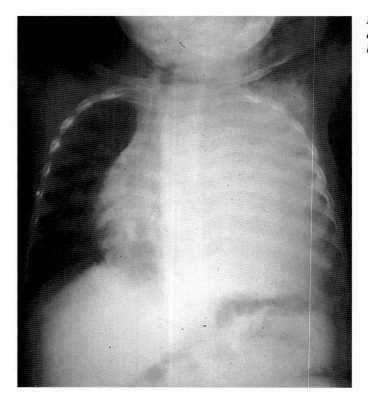

FIG. 32.1.   *The infant's chest X ray showing a left-sided pleural effusion.*

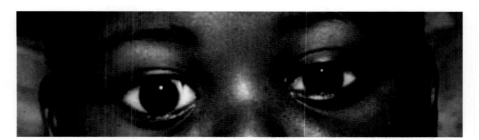

FIG. 32.2.   *Part of the child's face.*

damage to the ipsilateral cervical sympathetic fibers or ganglion. The ganglion is located on the posterior chest wall. This, presumably, was damaged by the empyema.

CASE 33. A 5-day-old infant presents with a history of not being able to breathe properly for a few hours. On examination he appears as shown in the picture (Figure 33.1).

- *What is the diagnosis?*
- *What is the mechanism of disease?*
- *What would you do?*
- *How could this have been prevented?*

This picture demonstrates an infant with stiffness, grimacing, and tightness of the fists. This is characteristic of tetanus. Other diagnostic considerations are: tetany, due to hypocalcemia, and seizures, which, in newborn infants, are not associated with generalized tonic contractions. Tetanus is a major health problem in many parts of the world. Almost all cases of tetanus worldwide occur in newborns, and it accounts for about 7% of neonatal deaths worldwide. The disease is caused by the organism *Clostridium tetani* entering the umbilical stump, which provides an anaerobic environment.

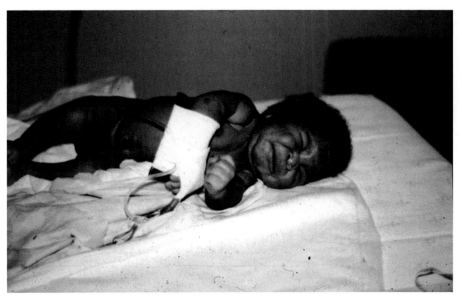

FIG. 33.1.   The infant with inability to breathe properly.

There it elaborates a potent toxin called tetanus toxin (tetanospasmin), which ascends along nerve fibers to the central nervous system. There it causes inhibition of inhibitory neurons, resulting in excitation. This results in the clinical manifestations of muscle spasms. The prolonged contraction of respiratory muscles prevents the victim from inspiring. Infection of the umbilicus occurs as a result of two main factors: (a) the cord is cut with an instrument contaminated with spores of the organism; and (b) the common practice in some cultures of putting dirt or dung, which contain spores of the organism, on the umbilical stump.

Treatment entails sedation, for example, with diazepam, to enable the child to breathe. Artificial ventilation for about 1 month is often necessary. Although tetanus immune globulin (human or animal) and penicillin are used, their value is questionable.

Prevention consists of education regarding cord care and immunization of pregnant women, whose IgG antibodies will enter the fetus and protect it. Later the baby will require active tetanus immunization. Patients who have recovered from tetanus still require active tetanus immunization.

References:

Bryce J, Boschi-Pinto C, Shibuya K et al: WHO estimates of the causes of death in children. Lancet 2005; 365: 1147–1152.

Brook I: Tetanus in children. Pediatr Emerg Care 2004; 20: 48–51.

CASE 34. (HYP). A 10-year-old girl presents with a history of sore throat and difficulty breathing of 1 day's duration. She returned 2 days ago from a trip to Odessa (Ukraine). On examination she is very ill-appearing. She has some inspiratory stridor and thick white-gray material covering her tonsils and faucial pillars, and she has swelling of her neck (Figures 34.1 and 34.2).

- *What is the likely diagnosis and how would you confirm it?*
- *What is the mechanism of disease?*
- *How would you manage her?*

The likely diagnosis is diphtheria, which is caused by *Corynebacterium diphtheriae*. A very large epidemic of diphtheria occurred in the former Soviet Union in the early 1990s. Although other agents can cause a pseudo-membrane on the tonsils, for example, *Streptococcus pyogenes* and Epstein–Barr virus, they do not usually cause stridor. Diphtheria causes stridor

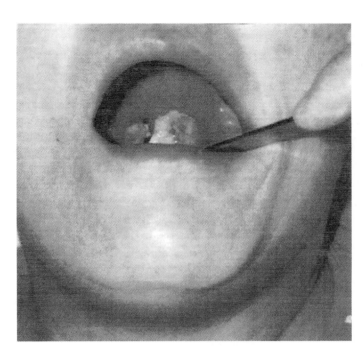

FIG. 34.1. The pharynx of a different patient with the same appearance as that of the child described above. (From Kadirova R, Kartoglu HU, Strebel PM: Clinical characteristics and management of 676 hospitalized diphtheria cases, Kyrgyz Republic, 1995. J Infect Dis 2000; 181 (suppl 1); S110–115, with permission of The University of Chicago Press, © 2000 by the Infectious Diseases Society of America. All rights reserved.)

because the pseudomembrane can descend into the larynx, causing respiratory obstruction, one of the main causes of death in this infection. The organism is not invasive. It elaborates a toxin, diphtheria toxin, which is an ATP ribosylase, which inhibits protein synthesis at the ribosomal site of elongation factor 2. Other clinical effects of the toxin include the following: (i) palatal palsy, which manifests clinically with nasal speech and which may be present in the early stages of the infection; (ii) a toxic myocarditis (cardiomyopathy), which results in atrioventricular block and myocardial failure. This begins 1–2 weeks after onset of the disease; (iii) a peripheral neuropathy resembling that of Guillain-Barre syndrome, which can become manifest 10 days to 3 months after onset of the disease; (iv) renal failure. Fatalities are due to respiratory tract obstruction or cardiac failure.

Diphtheria is confirmed by culture of the causative organism from a throat swab. Culture for *C. diphtheriae* is not routinely performed on throat specimens in the United States. This must be specifically requested, since special media are required.

Management of diphtheria, which highlights the general principles of management of infectious diseases, consists of the following: (a) supportive care – ensuring an adequate airway, which may require endotracheal intubation or tracheostomy; (b) antimicrobial therapy – erythromycin or

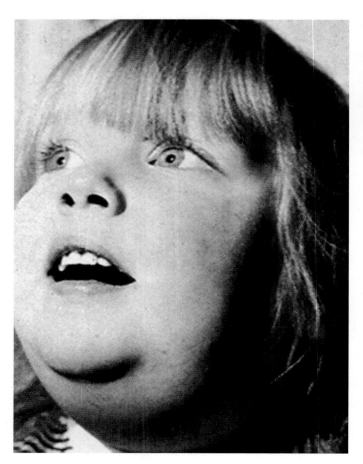

FIG. 34.2.   Appearance of a child with the same diagnosis as the child described. (From Emond RTD: Color Atlas of Infectious Diseases. 1974. Year Book Medical Publishers, Chicago. With permission from Elsevier.)

penicillin, and antidiphtheria globulin, which is made in an animal; (c) sur-gery – tracheostomy (see above); (d) community – notification of the health department; hospital isolation with droplet precautions; contacts should be tested for carriage (by throat culture) and given antimicrobial prophylaxis with erythromycin or penicillin; and (e) prevention – active immunization. Although this infection is very rare in the United States as a result of wide-spread immunization, it is prevalent in many other countries and can be imported into this country.

Reading:

Mattos-Guaraldi AL, Moreira LO, Damasco PV, Junior RH: Diphtheria remains a threat to health in the developing world – an overview. Mem Inst Oswaldo Cruz 2003; 98: 987–993.

Reading:

Kadirova R, Kartoglu HU, Strebel PM: Clinical characteristics and management of 676 hospitalized diphtheria cases, Kyrgyz Republic, 1995. J Infect Dis 2000; 181 (Suppl 1): S 110–115.

CASE 35. A 2-week-old infant presents with a history of fever, poor feeding, and decreased activity over the past 2 days. On examination she looks very ill and is barely responsive. The anterior fontanelle is bulging and tense. The cerebrospinal fluid reveals the following: 1200 leukocytes/mm^3 of which 90% are neutrophils, a protein concentration of 200 mg/dl, and a glucose concentration of 15 mg/dl. The blood glucose concentration is 70 mg/dl. Gram stain reveals Gram-positive rods.

- *What is the likely diagnosis?*
- *What else would you like to know?*
- *How would you manage the child?*

This newborn infant has Gram-positive rod meningitis, which is most likely caused by *Listeria monocytogenes*. This organism is acquired from the mother's vagina, usually during delivery. The mother acquires the organism by ingestion, resulting in intestinal colonization followed by vaginal colonization. Although the organism can be present in many foods including vegetables, an important source is unpasteurized dairy products, including semisolid cheeses, and undercooked meat. Although pregnant women may have transient symptoms such as fever when they become infected, they are often only colonized and asymptomatic. An intrauterine form of listeriosis called granulomatosis infantiseptica, characterized by the presence of multiple abscesses, is usually fatal. *Listeria monocytogenes* is one of the bacteria that can remain within macrophages without being killed, and cell-mediated immunity is therefore necessary for its elimination. (Other bacteria requiring cell-mediated immunity for their elimination include salmonella, brucella, legionella, and mycobacteria.) Therefore individuals with impairment of this arm of immunity due to, for example, AIDS, corticosteroids, and transplantation immunosuppression are at risk for this infection. The elderly are also at risk for this infection.

The treatment of listeriosis consists of ampicillin with or without gentamicin.

Prevention of neonatal listeriosis entails education of pregnant women to avoid the risk factors described above.

Reading:

Braden CR: Listeriosis. Pediatr Infect Dis J 2003; 22: 745–746.

Southwick FS, Purich DL: Intracellular pathogenesis of listeriosis. N Engl J Med 1996; 334: 770–776.

CASE 36. A 5-year-old girl presents with fever, chest pain, and cough and is found to have a pulmonary infiltrate on X ray. She is treated with erythromycin and seems to improve a little. However, her symptoms recur a few weeks later and she is treated with amoxicillin, again with some improvement. She presents a few weeks later with a swelling on the right side of her chest. A chest X ray shows the presence of consolidation in the same place as initially. The swelling is biopsied and the Gram stain has the appearance of that shown in the picture (Figure 36.1).

- *What is the diagnosis?*
- *How should she be treated?*

The biopsy reveals inflammation and a clump of branching Gram-positive bacilli. These are characteristic of actinomyces and nocardia species (both belong to the family Actinomycetales). This patient, who had no known immunodeficiency, is more likely to have had an infection with actinomyces

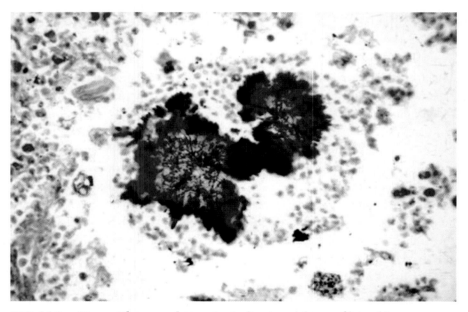

FIG. 36.1.   Biopsy (from another patient) showing a clump of branching, Gram-positive bacilli. (Courtesy of Carlos Abramowsky, MD, Emory University)

than with nocardia. The culture grew out *Actinomyces israelii*, confirming the diagnosis of actinomycosis, which is a bacterial not a fungal infection. There are several species of actinomyces, including *A. israelii* (the most important), *A. naeslundi*, *A. viscosus*, *A. odontolyticus*, and *A. meyeri*. These bacteria, which are considered anaerobes, although they grow best micro-aerophilically, form part of the normal flora of mucosal surfaces. They cause chronic infections, which may spread across tissue plains. Clumps of bacteria become mineralized, resulting in grains called sulfur granules. These infections arise particularly in the mouth (usually as a result of injuries), large bowel, and female genital tract (usually as a complication of intrauterine contraceptive devise usage). However, the organisms can spread to the lung by aspiration and they can spread hematogenously. These organisms require special media for growth in the laboratory, and they are susceptible to many antibiotics. Treatment consists of penicillin for a prolonged period, and sometimes entails surgical drainage. This child improved with penicillin treatment.

Reading:

Mabeza GF, Macfarlane J: Pulmonary actinomycosis. Eur Respir J 2003; 21: 545–551.

CASE 37. An 8-year-old boy, who underwent bone marrow transplantation for leukemia about 1 year ago, presents with cough, chest pain, and fever for a few days. He is currently receiving immunosuppressive therapy. On examination he has evidence of consolidation in his left upper lobe, which is confirmed radiologically.

- ***What is your differential diagnosis?***
- ***What would you do?***

Considering that he is immunosuppressed, there are several possible causes of his lung disease, including the following: (a) bacteria, such as *Streptococcus pneumoniae*, *Staphylococcus aureus*, *Haemophilus influenzae*, and Gram-negative rods, including *Legionella* spp.; (b) bacteria causing more indolent infections such as *Mycobacterium tuberculosis*, *Nocardia* spp., and *Rhodococcus equi*; and (c) fungi, in particular *Aspergillus* species. Pneumonias caused by viruses such as the respiratory viruses and cytomegalovirus, by bacteria such as *Mycoplasma pneumoniae* and *Chlamydia pneumoniae*, and by *Pneumocystis jiroveci* should be considered, but they tend to be diffuse more than focal.

Considering the wide microbiologic differential diagnosis, the lack of practicability of providing antimicrobial therapy directed at all the possible causes of pneumonia, and the high probability of significant adverse effects if such broad spectrum therapy were instituted, it is important to make a microbiological diagnosis in such a patient.

The methods for making a microbiological diagnosis are staining, antigen detection, nucleic acid detection, and culture of potentially infected material for the wide variety of pathogens described above. The major problem is in obtaining appropriate specimens. The specimens used are (i) sputum – this is difficult to obtain in children, and is, by its nature, contaminated with saliva; (ii) bronchoalveolar lavage fluid; and (iii) lung biopsy material, which requires the most invasive procedure. The latter may become necessary if the other procedures fail to provide a diagnostic answer.

This patient underwent bronchoalveolar lavage. Gram stain of the fluid revealed fine, beady, branching Gram-positive rods, with the same appearance as those, from a different patient, shown in Figure 37.1.

Now what is the most likely diagnosis?

This picture reveals beaded, branching, Gram-positive rods, which are highly suggestive of *Nocardia* spp. The genus *Nocardia* includes *N. asteroides,*

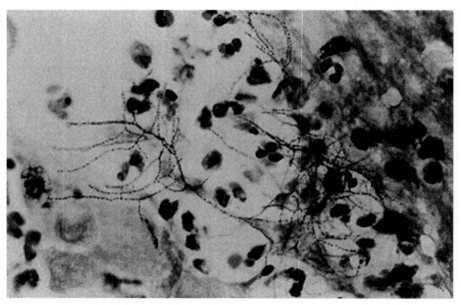

FIG. 37.1. *Gram-stained preparation of bronchoalveolar lavage fluid, from another patient with the appearance of that seen in the fluid from this patient. (From Smilock JD: Pulmonary and disseminated nocardiosis. N Engl J Med 1999; 341: 885. Copyright © 1999 Massachusetts Medical Society. All rights reserved, with permission.)*

N. farcinica, *N. nova*, *N. otitidiscaviarum*, *N. brasiliensis*, and *N. transvalensis*. They may stain with Kinyoun's modified acid-fast stain, which can help to differentiate them from *Actinomyces* spp., which are also branching Gram-positive rods, but do not stain with this stain. *Nocardia* spp. grow on regular media such as blood agar. They are present in the environment, and they cause infection mainly in immunocompromised hosts. They enter the host via the lung but may spread hematogenously, particularly to the brain. However, *N. brasiliensis* causes cutaneous infections in normal hosts following skin inoculation. Although *Nocardia* spp. are usually susceptible to trimethoprim/sulfamethoxazole, their antimicrobial susceptibilities are very variable, so it is very important to have isolates tested for their antimicrobial susceptibilities. They are sometimes susceptible to cephalosporins, minocycline, imipenem, fluoroquinolones, and amikacin. Treatment should be initiated with trimethoprim/sulfamethoxazole, with or without amikacin, pending results of susceptibility tests, which may take several weeks. All patients with pulmonary nocardiosis should undergo brain imaging to look for evidence of spread there.

This patient was treated with trimethoprim/sulfamethoxazole and improved.

Reading:

Lerner PI: Nocardiosis. Clin Infect Dis 1996; 22: 891–903.

Choucino C, Goodman SA, Greer JP et al: Nocardial infection in bone marrow transplant recipients. Clin Infect Dis 1996; 23: 1012–1019.

CASE 38. A 4-month-old breast-feeding infant presents with a history of constipation for a few days. Now she does not move much and seems floppy. On examination she is indeed hypotonic and very weak. She does not open her eyes, but when you open them, she seems to look at you. Her cry is very weak. She has the appearance of the infant shown in Figure 38.1.

- *What is your differential diagnosis?*
- *What would you do?*

This child has an acute diffuse lower motor neuron problem. Although infants with acute cerebral disease, such as bacterial meningitis or hemorrhage, can be hypotonic, in such circumstances they are encephalopathic and do not "look at you." The differential diagnosis of acute lower motor diseases should be considered anatomically (Figure 38.2).

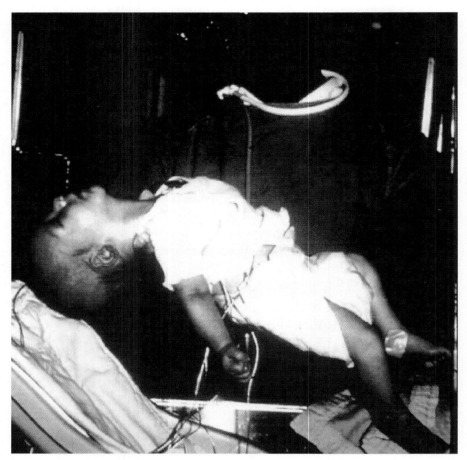

FIG. 38.1.   *A hypotonic infant. (Courtesy of the Centers for Disease Control and Prevention)*

(a) anterior horn cell:

poliomyelitis – in this infection the weakness is usually focal and asymmetric, but may be generalized;

spinal muscular atrophy – although this is a disease of the anterior horn cell, it does not manifest acutely.

(b) peripheral nerve:

Guillain-Barre syndrome and toxic peripheral neuropathies.

(c) neuromuscular junction

botulism, which, in infants, can present exactly as this child has presented.

myasthenia gravis – which does not usually present acutely.

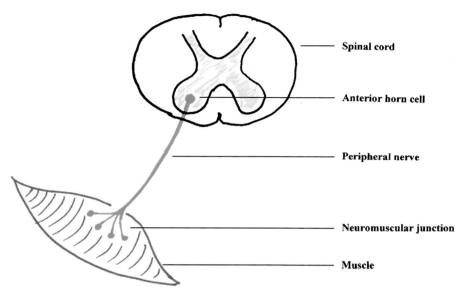

Spinal cord

Anterior horn cell

Peripheral nerve

Neuromuscular junction

Muscle

FIG. 38.2.   Diagram showing the lower motor neuron unit.

(d) muscle:

   acute muscle disease, such as myositis, is usually associated with muscle tenderness.

   Considering this infant's age, the most likely diagnosis is infant botulism. Infant botulism is an *infection* caused by *Clostridium botulinum*. Spores of the causative organism are ingested by the infant. In the gut they germinate producing botulinum toxin, which is absorbed. The toxin, which, like many bacterial exotoxins, has a light (toxic) component and a heavy (attachment) component, prevents release of acetylcholine from the presynaptic end of the neuromuscular junction, resulting in weakness. Clinically, infant botulism presents with constipation and hypotonia, as in this case. Classic botulism typically presents with descending paralysis. Ptosis is a notable feature. The diagnosis is confirmed by the demonstration of toxin in the stool (performed at reference laboratories). Honey fed to the infant is an identified risk factor and should therefore not be given to infants, but specific risk factors are identified in few cases.

   Management: This is mainly supportive, consisting of ensuring adequate ventilation and nutrition. Antibiotics are not indicated. Botulinum immune globulin, obtainable from the California State Health Department, has been shown to ameliorate the condition.

   Classic botulism is an *intoxication* in which the toxin, produced by the organism in contaminated food, such as home canned vegetables, is ingested.

Wound botulism, in which the organism is inoculated into a wound where it produces toxin, is an infection, like infant botulism.

Botulinum toxin is used therapeutically in conditions associated with muscle spasm and for cosmetic purposes to remove wrinkles. It also has the potential to be used as a biological weapon.

Reading:

Arnon SS, Schechter R, Inglesby T et al: Botulinum toxin as a biological weapon. Medical and public health management. JAMA 2001; 285: 1059–1070.

Arnon SS, Schechter R, Maslanka SE et al: Human botulism immune globulin for the treatment of infant botulism. N Engl J Med 2006; 354: 462–471.

CASE 39 (HYP). A 15-year-old Turkish shepherd develops a sore on his forearm. This progressively enlarges and appears as shown in Figure 39.1 (from a different patient).

This sore is characterized by an ulcer with a black center.

- *What might have caused this?*
- *What would you do?*

Sores on the arm can be caused by many microorganisms as a result of minor trauma, for example, *Staphylococcus aureus*. These do not usually have black centers. Specific diseases for which this individual may be at risk due to his place of residence and his occupation are rickettsial infection, cutaneous

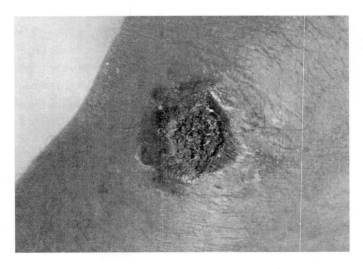

FIG. 39.1.   A sore that has the appearance of that noted in the patient described. (Courtesy of the Center for Disease Control and Prevention/James H Steele)

leishmaniasis, and cutaneous anthrax. (In central Africa, African trypanoso-miasis would also be a consideration.) Being a shepherd is a specific risk factor for acquiring anthrax, the diagnosis in this case.

Anthrax is caused by the spore-forming Gram-positive rod *Bacillus anthracis*, which may be present in soil and on the hides of animals. It causes three clinical forms of disease. (a) Cutaneous, which is the most common. The organism is inoculated into the skin by a mild abrasion, and causes a painless sore that develops into a black eschar associated with significant swelling. (The term "anthrax" is derived from the Greek word for black). (b) Inhalation anthrax, which is characterized by a rapidly progressive mediastinitis that is usually fatal. This form is difficult to diagnose and is frequently complicated by bacteremia and meningitis. (c) Ingestion anthrax, caused by ingestion of contaminated meat. *Bacillus anthracis* has several virulence factors including a polygluconate capsule and three exotoxins which act synergistically.

The diagnosis is confirmed by culture of the organism. Laboratory staff should be informed of the clinical suspicion, because aerosolized organisms pose a significant risk to them. Management is antimicrobial, with cipro-floxacin or doxycycline. Public health authorities must be informed imme-diately about the suspicion of anthrax, especially in light of its use as an agent of bioterrorism.

Reading:

Dixon TC, Meselson M, Guillemin J, Hanna PC: Anthrax. N Engl J Med 1999; 341: 815–826.

Swartz MN : Recognition and management of anthrax – an update. N Engl J Med 2001; 345: 1621–1626.

Mock M, Fouet A: Anthrax. Annu Rev Microbiol 2001; 55: 647–671.

CASE 40. A 10-year-old girl presents with a history of pain and swelling of her calf for a few hours. Her history is significant for several severe bacterial infections, including meningitis, leading to the assumption that she has an immunodeficiency. A specific immune defect has not been dem-onstrated despite very extensive testing. On examination the swelling of the leg is confirmed, in addition to which purple discoloration is also noted. She is diagnosed with a deep venous thrombosis, hospitalized, and treated with heparin intravenously. Over the ensuing few hours the swelling and pain progress to the thigh and she develops brownish cutaneous bullae. An aspirate of a bulla reveals, on Gram stain, what is shown in the Figure 40.1.

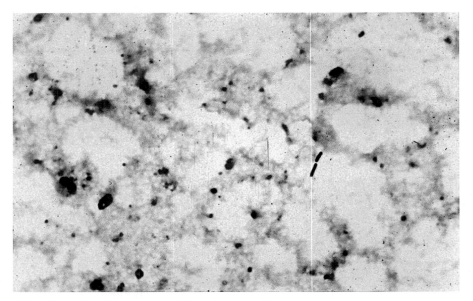

FIG. 40.1.   The Gram stain of fluid from a bulla.

- *What is the diagnosis?*
- *What would you do?*

The picture shows Gram-positive rods and the absence of leukocytes. The clinical and Gram-stain appearance of the organism are characteristic of clostridial gas gangrene (myonecrosis).

Clostridial myonecrosis is caused by histotoxic clostridia, the most important of which is C. *perfringens*. This organism elaborates an exotoxin, which is a lecithinase and lyses cellular membranes, including those of erythrocytes. It thus causes tissue necrosis and intravascular hemolysis. The causative organism in this case was C. *septicum*, which is recognized to cause infections in immunocompromised individuals.

Management consists of antimicrobial therapy and aggressive surgical debridement. Although several drugs, including penicillin, clindamycin, metronidazole, and carbapenems are active against the histotoxic clostridia, a combination of penicillin and clindamycin is considered preferable. Hyperbaric oxygen therapy is also sometimes used. This patient was treated with penicillin, underwent a hindquarter amputation and hyperbaric oxygen therapy, and survived.

Reading:

Stevens DL, Musher DM, Watson DA: Spontaneous, nontraumatic gangrene due to *Clostridium septicum*. Rev Infect Dis 1990; 12: 286–296.

Brook I: Microbiology and management if infectious gangrene in children. J Pediatr Orthop 2004; 24: 587–592.

■CASE 41. Infants between the ages of 0 and 3 months present as shown in the pictures.

• *What is the diagnosis, and what would you do?*

These are all features of congenital syphilis, which is a form of secondary syphilis acquired transplacentally from the mother, and which manifests during the first few months of life. These represent the following:

1. *Snuffles:* this is rhinorrhea caused by mucosal ulcers;
2. *Peeling soles:* this is one of several cutaneous manifestations of congenital syphilis. Macular rashes are also a feature of congenital syphilis;
3. Condylomata lata;
4. *Pitting edema:* this is caused by the nephrotic syndrome due to syphilitic glomerulonephritis.

Other manifestations or sites of infection in congenital syphilis are the following:

meningitis;
pneumonia alba – this is a severe form of pneumonia that is frequently fatal;
enlargement of the liver and spleen, and hepatitis;
anemia and thrombocytopenia;
generalized lymphadenopathy, including involvement of the epitrochlear nodes; chorioretinitis;
osteitis, which may manifest with pseudoparesis (Figure 41.5).

Syphilis is caused by the spirochete *Treponema pallidum*, which is spread sexually and vertically. It can also be spread through blood transfusion.

Other congenital infections, notably cytomegalovirus infection, toxoplasmosis, rubella, and human immunodeficiency virus (HIV) infection may manifest with some of these abnormalities, including chorioretinitis, hepatosplenomegaly, hepatitis, anemia, thrombocytopenia, and cerebrospinal fluid pleocytosis, but they do not cause mucosal disease, nephrotic syndrome, or symptomatic bone disease. In addition, in these infections (with the exception of HIV infection), the abnormalities are present at birth, and their cutaneous manifestations are characterized by purple raised lesions ("blueberry muffin" lesions) caused by extramedullary hematopoiesis.

Late manifestations of congenital syphilis, in untreated individuals, include interstitial keratitis, joint effusions (Charcot's joints), Hutchinson's

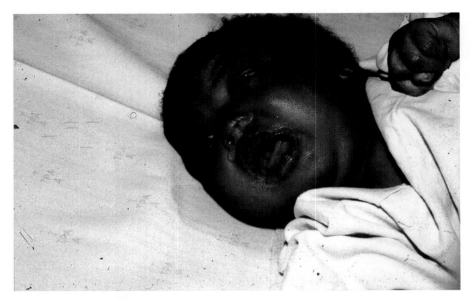

FIG. 41.1. *Cracked lips; runny nose.*

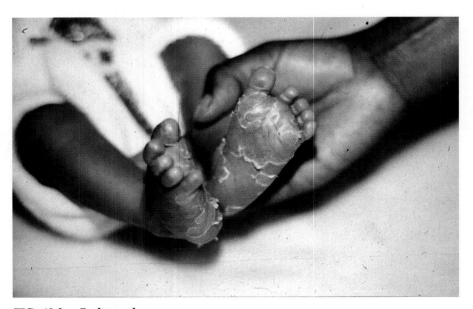

FIG. 41.2. *Peeling soles.*

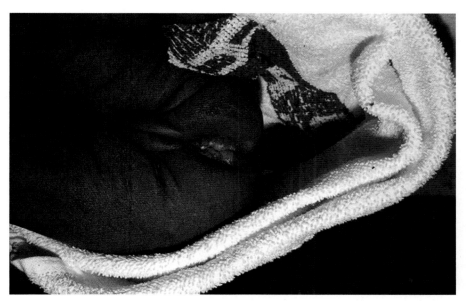

FIG. 41.3.   Perianal swellings.

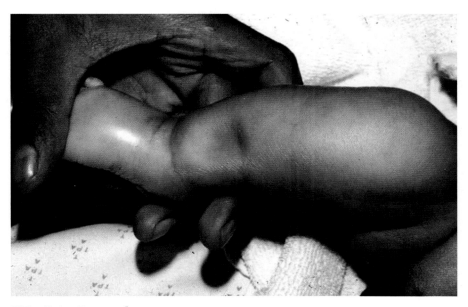

FIG. 41.4.   Pitting edema.

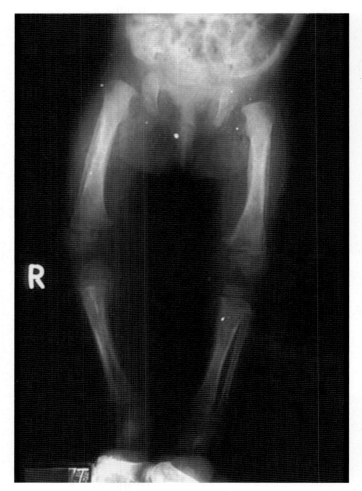

FIG. 41.5.   X ray of the lower limbs showing marked periosteal reactions of the femora and tibias, and metaphysitis of the upper ends of the tibias, caused by congenital syphilis. The lytic lesions of the proximal tibial metaphyses are called "Wimberger's sign."

teeth (which are peg-shaped permanent incisors), sensory deafness, and manifestations of tertiary syphilis, namely brain disease and aortitis of the ascending aorta.

The diagnosis of congenital syphilis is confirmed by (a) dark-field micros-copy of specimens from mucous membrane lesions to detect spirochetes (seldom available) and (b) serology – positive nonspecific serological tests in the mother (e.g. rapid plasma reagin (RPR)) should be confirmed with a specific antibody test (e.g. microhemagglutination test or fluorescent trep-onemal antibody-absorption test (FTA-ABS)). The nonspecific test titers return to negative over time after treatment, but the specific antibody tests do not. Because the mother's specific IgG will be present in the infant, even if she has been adequately treated, the serological confirmation of infection in the infant requires demonstration of a nonspecific antibody (RPR) titer fourfold or greater than in the mother. In suspected cases the cerebrospinal fluid should also be examined for evidence of meningitis (with measurements of cell count, and glucose and protein concentrations) and of antibody production within the central nervous system using the Venereal Disease Research Laboratory (VDRL) test. The presumptive diagnosis and the decision to treat the infant should be guided by the serological test results of the mother and infant, the mother's treatment status (adequate treatment requires parenteral penicillin at least 4 weeks before delivery), and the clinical and laboratory findings in the infant.

Treatment of congenital syphilis consists of parenteral penicillin administered for 10 days.

Reading:

Stoll BJ: Congenital syphilis: evaluation and management of neonates born to mothers with reactive serologic tests for syphilis. Pediatr Infect Dis J 1994; 13: 845–853.

Fiumara NJ, Lessell S: Manifestations of late congenital syphilis. An analysis of 271 patients. Arch Derm 1970; 102: 78–83.

Woods CR: Syphilis in children: congenital and acquired. Semin Pediatr Infect Dis 2005; 16: 245–257.

American Academy of Pediatrics. Syphilis. In: Pickering LK (editor). Red Book: 2006 Report of the Committee on Infectious Diseases. 27th edition. American Academy of Pediatrics, Elk Grove Village, IL, 2006, pp. 631–644.

CASE 42. (HYP). A 13-year previously healthy boy presents with fever, headache, myalgia, and general malaise lasting about 3 days. There has not been a sore throat or other respiratory tract symptoms. He improves, but after a week the fever returns. On examination he has a temperature of 39°C and enlargement of the liver and spleen. The rest of the examination is normal.

- *What would you like to know?*
- *What would you do?*

The main cause of fever and hepatosplenomegaly in a teenager is infectious mononucleosis, caused by Epstein–Barr virus (EBV). This illness is also associated with a sore throat and cervical lymphadenopathy.

Acute human immunodeficiency virus (HIV) infection, as well as cytomegalovirus infection and toxoplasmosis can cause a similar syndrome.

What is unusual about this presentation is fever that remits for a few days and then relapses. This suggests the possibility that this patient has an infection that is associated with a cycle of waxing and waning in the number of organisms in the host or of clinical manifestations being caused by an immune response to the organism. Such infections include malaria, babesiosis, relapsing fever, and leptospirosis. Therefore a history of exposure to such pathogens should be sought, including a history about travel and recreational activities.

Exposure history: This boy was staying in a cabin in the Colorado Rocky Mountains a few days before his symptoms began. This environment is not endemic for malaria or babesiosis but is for borrelial relapsing fever.

The type of relapsing fever occurring in the United States, as in this case, is caused by several species of borrelia, including *B. hermsii*, *B. parkeri*, and *B. turicatae*. These are transmitted by soft ticks of the genus *Ornithodoros* between rodents and human beings. Two types of relapsing fever carry a high fatality rate. These are caused by *B. recurrentis*, which is louse-borne, and has a worldwide distribution, being most prevalent in Africa, and *B. duttoni*, which is tick-borne and occurs in East Africa. Both of these borrelia are transmitted between humans beings and their respective arthropod vectors. The reason for the relapsing nature of the infection is the phenomenon of antigenic variation. The organism has the genetic ability to change an

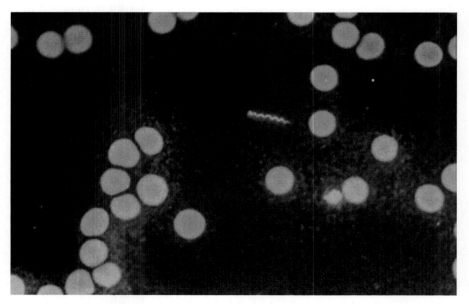

FIG. 42.1.   A positive fluorescent antibody test for Borrelia. (From: Cooper RI, Neuhauser T: Images in clinical medicine. Borreliosis. N Engl J Med 1998; 338: 231. Copyright © 1998. Massachusetts Medical Society. All rights reserved, with permission.)

antigenic coat protein, called variant major protein, so that, as the host makes antibodies to the organism and the clinical illness remits, the antigenic surface of the organism changes and its numbers rise, causing a relapse of clinical symptoms. Each successive relapse becomes milder.

The diagnosis can be made by examination of a Giemsa-stained blood smear on which spirochetes can be seen. The sensitivity of this test is, however, only about 50%. This is increased by the use of fluorescent antibody staining of the blood smear (Figure 42.1).

Serological tests can also be performed. Several drugs can be used to treat such patients, including penicillin, macrolides, and tetracyclines. It is important to note that patients may experience the Jarisch-Herxheimer reaction, characterized by high fever, chills, and hypotension, after initiation of therapy. They should therefore be monitored for about 12 hours after initiation of therapy.

Reading:

Dworkin MS, Schwan TG: Anderson DE: Tick-borne relapsing fever in North America. Med Clin N Am 2002; 86: 417–433.

CASE 43 (HYP, based on two reports in the MMWR). Soon after returning from a competition in Borneo, a 20-year-old triathlon athlete presents with a history of fever, myalgia, and abdominal pain. He improves after about 3 days, and he concludes that he has had a "virus." However, the illness returns with a vengeance 5 days later, causing very severe headache and photophobia. On examination he is ill-appearing with neck stiffness, abdominal tenderness, muscle tenderness, and a macular rash.

- *What is your differential diagnosis?*
- *What would you do?*

In patients with simultaneous potential exposures to multiple infectious agents, such as living in the tropics and exposure to unclean fresh water, as is the case in this patient, one should consider the possibility that the patient has more than one illness, with one illness not necessarily explaining all the clinical features. Although he has evidence of a systemic disease, there is evidence of focal infection in the meninges. The differential diagnosis should include arbovirus infection, in particular dengue, enterovirus infection, meningococcal meningitis and bacteremia, typhoid fever, leptospirosis, malaria, the early stage of schistosomiasis, acute human immunodeficiency virus (HIV) infection, and rickettsial infection. Of these, enterovirus infections and leptospirosis may have a biphasic pattern of fever, while malaria has a multiphasic pattern. Schistosomiasis is not endemic in Borneo.

The following tests should be performed, in order of their priority in contributing to the management of the patient:

Lumbar puncture with Gram stain and culture of the cerebrospinal fluid;

Blood smears for malaria;

Blood culture for *Salmonella typhi* and *Neisseria meningitidis*;

Serology for dengue (Culture of blood for the virus can be performed but is rarely available.). Serology for *Leptospira interrogans* (Blood can be cultured in the early phase of infection and urine in the later phase; however, special medium is required.).

Treatment should be directed at the likely causes of illness after the initial test results have become available. This should consist of a combination of doxycycline, for its activity against *Leptospira interrogans* and rickettsiae, and a third-generation cephalosporin, such as ceftriaxone or cefotaxime, for its activity against *Neisseria meningitidis* and *Salmonella typhi*. Once culture results have become available, therapy can be adjusted. Serological test results may not be available for days or weeks.

This patient had leptospirosis. This is often a biphasic illness, affecting many organ systems. The illness is characterized initially by fever, myalgia, headache, abdominal pain, vomiting and diarrhea and conjunctival injection. In the later stage meningitis, kidney, liver, and pulmonary disease may occur. The causative organism is a spirochete, *Leptospira interrogans*, of which there are many serovars, that causing the most severe disease being serovar *L. icterohaemorrhagiae*. Leptospira organisms are excreted in the urine of animals, such as dogs and rodents. Bodies of water are often the sites of urinary contamination, and thus frequently the source of infection. In athletic events such as the one described many individuals are often infected. Penicillin or doxycycline are the preferred treatments.

Readings:

Katz AR, Ansdell VE, Effler PV et al: Assessment of the clinical presentation and treatment of 353 cases of laboratory-confirmed leptospirosis in Hawaii, 1974–1998. Clin Infect Dis 2001; 33: 1834–1840.

Kaul DR, Flanders SA, Saint S: Clear as mud. N Engl J Med 2005; 352: 1914–1918.

CDC: Public health dispatch: outbreak of acute febrile illness among participants in EcoChallenge Sabah 2000 Malaysia, 2000. MMWR 2000; 49: 816–817.

CDC: Update: outbreak of acute febrile illness among participants in Eco-Challenge-Sabah 2000-Borneo, Malaysia, 2000. MMWR 2001; 50: 21–24.

CDC: Update: leptospirosis and unexplained acute febrile illness among athletes participating in triathlons – Illinois and Wisconsin, 1998. MMWR 1998; 47: 673– 676.

CASE 44 (HYP). A 13-year-old boy presents with a history of a painful left knee. On examination he has a swollen, tender left knee with slight limitation of movement. He is afebrile. The rest of his examination is normal.

- *What is your differential diagnosis?*
- *What else would you like to know?*
- *What would you like to do?*

This boy has acute arthritis. The differential diagnosis includes:

traumatic hemarthrosis – there is no history of trauma;

septic arthritis – unlikely in view of the lack of fever;

acute rheumatic fever;

rheumatoid arthritis;

reactive arthritis following an enteric infection – there is no history of a recent infection, except that there is a history of a large red area on his skin about 2 months ago;

Lyme disease – he lives in Connecticut, where he walks in the woods frequently. This exposure history and the history of a skin lesion makes Lyme disease very likely, likely enough to provide treatment with doxycycline or amoxicillin for 1 month. The diagnosis can be confirmed serologically.

Lyme disease is caused by the spirochete *Borrelia burgdorferi*. It is transmitted to human beings by ticks of the genus *Ixodes*. (*I. scapularis* in the eastern US, and *I. pacificus* in the western US.) Reservoir hosts are mainly rodents and deer. The clinical illness occurs in two overlapping phases:

(a) Early stage (<8 weeks after exposure): the most characteristic clinical feature and that most useful in the diagnosis is erythema chronicum migrans. This is a skin lesion characterized by an area of erythema without elevation extending for several centimeters from the site of the tick bite. It may develop central clearing (Figure 44.1). There may be associated itching or a burning sensation in the area. Mild constitutional symptoms may occur.

Disseminated disease is manifested by the following:

(i)   Multiple skin lesions of erythema chronicum migrans;

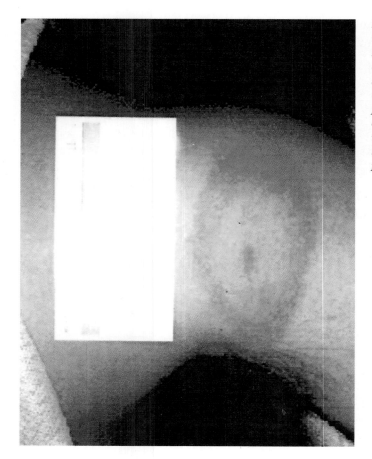

FIG. 44.1. *Erythema chronicum migrans. (From: Smith RP, Schoen RT, Rahn DW et al: Clinical characteristics and treatment outcome of early Lyme disease in patients with microbiologically confirmed erythema migrans. Ann Intern Med 2002; 136: 421–428, with permission.)*

(ii)　Neurological disease manifesting with cranial nerve palsies, especially of the facial nerve, other neuropathies, aseptic meningitis, optic neuritis, and encephalitis;

(iii)　Heart disease, usually manifesting with conduction abnormalities such as heart block. This constitutes the only potential cause of death in cases of Lyme disease.

(b) Late stage (> 8 weeks after exposure):

(i)　*Arthritis*: this may occur during the early stage. It presents acutely, but may become chronic or have a waxing and waning course. It affects mainly large joints, especially the knee.

(ii)　*Late neurological disease*: the manifestations are cognitive deficits, peripheral neuropathies, and low-grade encephalopathy. This is rare in children and difficult to diagnose.

The diagnosis of Lyme disease is based on a history of exposure, clinical manifestations (arthritis following a history highly suggestive of erythema chronicum migrans is sufficient to make the diagnosis), and sometimes serological tests. Although the organism can be detected by culture and polymerase chain reaction (PCR), this testing is not widely available. Therefore testing largely depends on serology. Serological tests can be very misleading and should not be undertaken for "screening," because in situations in which the pretest probability of infection is low, a positive test is very likely to be a false-positive. Positive ELISA tests must be followed by a Western blot test, which is more specific.

The recommended treatment of Lyme disease depends on the stage and the type of involvement. In most situations children should be treated with amoxicillin (or doxycycline in those older than 8 years). In those with neurological disease (other than isolated facial nerve palsy) ceftriaxone should be used.

Prevention depends on avoidance of tick bites and removal of ticks from the skin (transmission occurs only after about 24 hours of tick attachment).

Reading:

Sood SK: Lyme disease. Pediatr Infect Dis J 1999; 18: 913–925.

CASE 45. A 12-year-old girl presents with a history of severe abdominal pain and fever for 2 days. On examination she is in significant pain and febrile. There is no specific area of abdominal tenderness, but the liver and spleen are enlarged. There is also marked enlargement and tenderness of a left axillary lymph node, and a healed sore on the dorsum of her left hand.

- *What is your differential diagnosis?*
- *What more would you like to know?*
- *What would you do?*

This patient clearly has a systemic disease, based on the enlargement of the liver and spleen. Fever, abdominal pain, and hepatosplenomegaly should suggest the diagnostic possibilities of typhoid fever, infectious mononucleosis, and leukemia or lymphoma. However, neither typhoid fever nor infectious mononucleosis is associated with localized lymphadenopathy. Localized lymphadenopathy, which is tender indicates lymphadenitis, which suggests an infection occurring in the areas drained by the node. These are the upper limb and chest wall in the case of an axillary node. The sore on the left hand might well have been the site of inoculation of an infectious agent.

The most common infections causing this are staphylococcal and streptococcal infections of the skin. Systemic infections associated with these organisms would imply bacteremia, with or without infective endocarditis, in which case the patient would appear very ill. Infective endocarditis may be associated with splenomegaly but not hepatomegaly, unless heart failure is present. Infections associated with localized lymphadenopathy and evidence of systemic infection include cat-scratch disease, tularemia, and plague. Plague is associated with marked toxicity and not associated with enlargement of the liver and spleen. The bacteremic ("typhoidal") form of tularemia may be associated with such visceromegaly. Cat-scratch disease, which is caused by *Bartonella henselae*, usually manifests with localized lymphadenopathy and, in cases with the hepatosplenic form, is associated with enlargement of liver or spleen. This form may be associated with severe abdominal pain.

Considering the above differential diagnosis, obtaining a history of possible risk factors for these infections is very important. The questions should address the following: Has there been exposure to any animals (asking whether the family has pets may not adequately address this question), and what has been the nature of the exposure? Has the patient been exposed to arthropods (fleas, ticks)? Has she traveled to areas where plague is endemic (southwestern United States, Africa, Asia, South America)?

Further history from this patient revealed that she has several cats and has been scratched frequently. This illness was preceded by the presence of a pustule on the left hand. A clinical diagnosis of cat-scratch disease with hepatosplenic involvement was therefore made.

The diagnosis of cat-scratch disease can be confirmed by the demonstration of antibodies against the causative organism, *Bartonella henselae*. In cases with hepatosplenic involvement focal lesions can often be demonstrated in these organs by ultrasound or computer tomography (CT), as was the case in this patient. The CT appearance of the liver in hepatosplenic cat-scratch disease in such a patient is shown in Figure 45.1.

Cat-scratch disease is usually self-limited, but it can be associated with severe complications, including an encephalopathy (associated with seizures), retinitis (Figure 45.2), and osteomyelitis. It is an important cause of prolonged unexplained fever in children. In such cases treatment is worth trying, although it may not prove successful. Antimicrobial agents that are sometimes effective include gentamicin, trimethoprim/sulfamethoxazole plus rifampin, a fluoroquinolone, and azithromycin. The only controlled trial for the treatment of patients with cat-scratch disease has demonstrated that lymphadenitis improves more rapidly in patients treated with azithromycin than in those treated with a placebo.

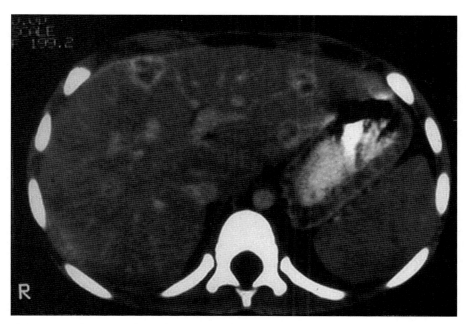

FIG. 45.1.   *CT scan of another patient showing multiple microabscesses in the liver due to cat-scratch disease. (Courtesy of Dr Gillian Sherbourne)*

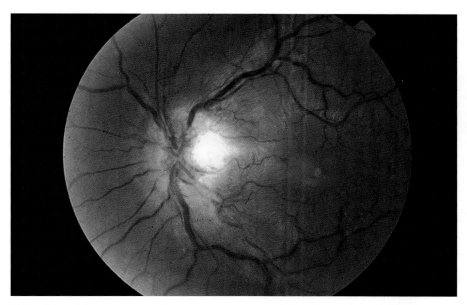

FIG. 45.2.   *The retinitis and optic neuritis associated with cat-scratch disease. Note the blurring of the disc margin and the radial streaking around the macula. (Courtesy of Hans Grossniklaus, MD, Emory University)*

Bartonella henselae also causes bacillary angiomatosis, which is characterized by wart-like vascular lesions, in immunocompromised individuals, such as those with AIDS. The possibility of the elaboration of an angiogenic substance by this organism is particularly interesting. *Bartonella bacilliformis*, the first recognized bartonella species, is transmitted by flies and infects erythrocytes causing Oroya fever (Carrion's disease), which is endemic in parts of the Andes Mountain range. This infection is characterized by a hemolytic anemia, followed by the development of hemangioma-like lesions, called verruga peruana.

Reading:

Bass JW, Vincent JM, Person DA: The expanding spectrum of *Bartonella* infections: II. Cat-scratch disease. Pediatr Infect Dis J 1997; 16: 163–179.

Loutit JS: Bartonella infections. Curr Clin Topics Infect Dis 1997; 17: 269–290.

CASE 46. An 18-month-old boy presents with a history of rash and fever for about 1 week. He was seen by his primary care doctor during this illness and diagnosed with a viral exanthem. His general condition has deteriorated. On examination he is febrile, ill-appearing, extremely irritable, and he has a generalized petechial rash as shown in the pictures (Figures 46.1 and 46.2). The rest of his examination is normal.

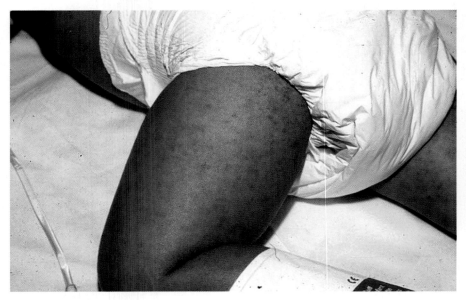

FIG. 46.1.   The child's rash.

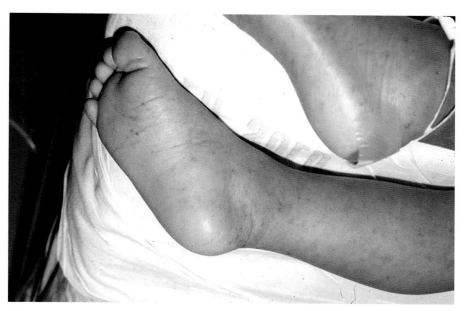

FIG. 46.2.   *The child's rash and an echymosis, partially covered by a bandage, on the left heel.*

- *What might be wrong with him?*
- *What would you do?*

Differential diagnosis:

(a) The most imminently life-threatening condition that this might be is meningococcal bacteremia and meningitis. This diagnosis is unlikely, however, because the history of a week is a long period for this child to have had this infection without his condition having significantly deteriorated.

(b) Rocky Mountain spotted fever (infection with *Rickettsia rickettsii*): Although this disease usually begins with a fever and severe headache, followed a few days later by the appearance of a rash, typically beginning around the wrists and ankles, the progression of this child's illness, especially considering the evidence of brain disease (extreme irritability), strongly suggests this diagnosis.

(c) *Ehrlichiosis:* These are tick-transmitted infections, caused by *Ehrlichia chaffeensis, Anaplasma phagocytophilum,* and *Ehrlichia ewingii,* which cause systemic disease febrile illness, often associated with leukopenia, thrombocytopenia, and elevated hepatic transaminases. Treatment is the same as for rickettsial disease (see below).

(d) Viral exanthems, including rubella, parvovirus infection, and human herpes virus 6 and human herpes virus 7 infections are possible but unlikely given the progressive nature of this child's illness. Furthermore, the rashes in these conditions are macular (blanching), except for the petechial rash occurring in a "glove and stocking" distribution sometimes associated with parvovirus infection. Measles does not cause a petechial rash and is associated with very prominent respiratory tract symptoms.

Management: After blood cultures have been drawn, treatment with both ceftriaxone (for its activity against *Neisseria meningitidis*) and doxycycline (for its activity against *Rickettsia rickettsii*) should be initiated immediately.

This child was treated with ceftriaxone and doxycycline. He developed seizures within a few hours of admission to hospital and a hemiplegia, but he survived. The diagnosis of Rocky Mountain spotted fever was later confirmed.

Rickettsiae are small Gram-negative bacilli that can multiple only intracellularly. They are transmitted by arthropods, in most cases by ticks. There are three groups of rickettsial diseases:

(a) Typhus group consisting of *R. prowazekii*, the cause of epidemic typhus, which is louse-borne, and *R. mooseri (typhi)*, the cause of endemic typhus, which is flea-borne.

(b) *Spotted fever group:* Most areas of the world have their peculiar spotted fever rickettsia, for example *R. rickettsii* (Rocky Mountain spotted fever – the Americas), *R. conori* (Mediterranean spotted fever), *R. africae* (African tick bite fever), *R. sibirica* (northern Asia), and *R . australis* (Australia).

(c) Rickettsialpox (*R. akari*)

R. rickettsii is present in Canada, the United States, Mexico, Central America, and South America. In the United States, it is most prevalent in the southeastern and southern states, where it is transmitted by species of *Dermacentor*, the dog tick.

The diagnosis of Rocky Mountain spotted fever is, for management purposes, a clinical one. There is currently no readily available, rapid, and sensitive laboratory test that is useful for diagnosing this infection, or, more importantly, for excluding this diagnosis. Laboratory tests such as serum sodium concentration and platelet count can be misleading and their value lies only in evaluating the patient for physiological disturbances. Untreated patients have a case fatality rate of about 10%. Only a minority of patients have a known history of a tick bite. Therefore, when Rocky Mountain spotted fever is suspected, treatment with a *tetracycline MUST* be instituted immediately. Doxycycline is usually used. Although there may be concern

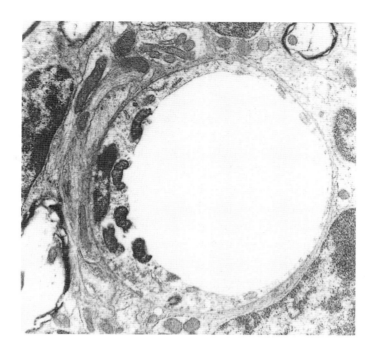

FIG. 46.3.   An electron micrograph of a cross section of a capillary with rickettsiae (in this case Orientia tsutsugamushi)*. (Courtesy of the Centers for Disease Control and Prevention/Dr Edwin P Ewing, Jr)*

about staining of the teeth in children younger than 9 years, this is a minor concern with a 5–7 day course, and *should NOT* deter one from prescribing this agent in children of *any age*. Rickettsiae invade endothelial cells, and therefore the infection can affect every organ, including the brain, heart, lungs, liver, and kidneys (Figure 46.3).

The diagnosis can be confirmed serologically in retrospect, using acute and convalescent sera. This information is only of epidemiological value, and of no value to the patient.

Reading:

Sexton DJ, Kaye KS: Rocky Mountain spotted fever. Med Clin N Am 2002; 86: 351–359.

Dumler JS, Walker DH: Rocky Mountain spotted fever – changing ecology and persisting virulence. N Engl J Med 2005; 353: 551–553.

CASE 47. (Adapted from the patient's account) A 24-year-old man presents with a history of severe headache, fever, myalgia, and abdominal pain, followed after about 5 days by the development of a rash, which started on his upper trunk and then spread to his limbs. Examination confirms these findings. The rash is maculopapular, petechial in areas, and widespread, sparing his face, palms, and soles.

- *What is your differential diagnosis?*
- *What would you like to know?*

The differential diagnosis includes meningococcal disease, rickettsial infection, a systemic viral infection such as West Nile virus infection and dengue, acute human immunodeficiency virus (HIV) infection, leptospirosis, and syphilis.

Young, presumably healthy, adults are not at great risk for the development of infectious diseases unless they have had specific exposures such as animal, arthropod, geographic, environmental, occupational, and recreational, including sexual. The exposure history is therefore very important. This patient's history is that one of his coworkers had developed a similar illness a few days earlier. Their *occupations* were working in a microbiology laboratory, making vaccine against *Rickettsia prowazekii*, the cause of epidemic typhus.

The diagnosis in this patient was laboratory-acquired epidemic typhus. He recovered without antimicrobial therapy, which was not available at the time (about 1943).

Epidemic typhus is a disease that has had a significant impact on human history. It is transmitted by the body louse, *Pediculus humanus corporis* (Figure 47.1), the infestation of which is associated with crowded living conditions, particularly during wars. The louse lives and lays its eggs (nits) in clothing (Figure 47.2).

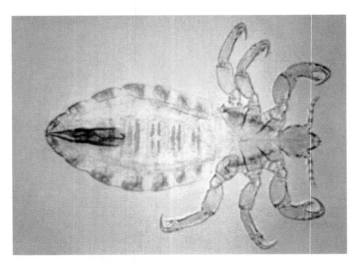

FIG. 47.1. A body louse (Pediculus humanus corporis). (Courtesy of the Centers for Disease Control and Prevention)

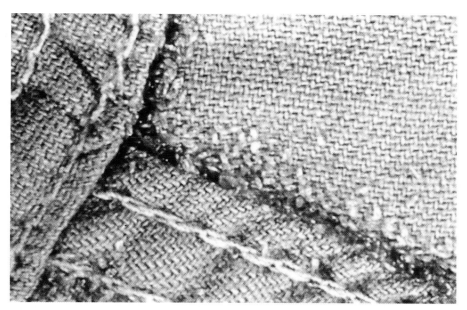

FIG. 47.2. *Nits of the body louse in clothing. (Courtesy of Reed and Carnrick Pharmaceuticals)*

It depends on blood meals from the human host and transmits the infection through its feces. The infection is characterized, as in this case, by fever, headache, myalgia, conjunctival injection, rash, which may be petechial, and mental status changes, which accounts for the name (from the Greek for stupor). The rickettsial organism can remain dormant in the human host for many years after he or she has recovered from the infection and cause a recrudescence, called Brill-Zinsser disease. If such a host is infested with body lice, an outbreak can be initiated. The diagnosis is generally made clinically, and the treatment is doxycycline. Even a single dose of this drug can be effective.

Reading:

Raoult D, Woodward T, Dumler JS: The history of epidemic typhus. Infect Dis Clin N Am 2004; 18: 127–140.

Raoult D, Roux V: The body louse as a vector of reemerging human diseases. Clin Infect Dis 1999; 29: 888–911.

CASE 48. A 13-year-old girl presents with a history of a painful left eye. There is no history of trauma or foreign body entering the eye. There is no significant past medical history. On examination she has photophobia, marked conjunctival injection, and some corneal clouding on the left. Her visual acuity is markedly decreased on the left and slightly decreased on the right. She is also noted to have a swollen left knee, which contains fluid, but which is not painful, and which does not have limitation of movement. Her teeth have an unusual shape (Figure 48.1).

- *What is your differential diagnosis?*
- *How would you manage this patient?*

The combination of a painful, red eye and photophobia suggests corneal inflammation (keratitis) and/or anterior uveitis (iridocyclitis), not merely conjunctivitis. Keratitis is confirmed by the presence of corneal clouding. Keratitis can cause significant visual impairment, and such patients should be referred to an ophthalmologist immediately. In the absence of trauma or a foreign body, it is usually due to a virus infection, in particular herpes simplex virus. Herpes simplex keratitis may have a suggestive appearance, with the corneal ulcer having a serpiginous outline (dendritic ulcer). The joint effusion might have been caused by trauma or reaction to an infection, such as parvovirus or an enteric infection. There was no history to suggest that one of these preceding events had occurred.

Examination by the ophthalmologist revealed bilateral *interstitial* keratitis. This can be caused by untreated congenital syphilis. Therefore a Rapid Plasma Reagin (RPR) test was performed, which was strongly positive, suggesting the diagnosis of syphilis. The diagnosis of syphilis was confirmed by a positive treponemal test. The joint effusion probably represented a "Clutton's joint," also a manifestation of late, untreated congenital syphilis.

She was treated with corticosteroid eyedrops and intravenous penicillin for 10 days, and her mother was referred to the health department for management and contact tracing. Her eyes improved markedly. Her notched upper incisors are called "Hutchinson's teeth," also a manifestation of late congenital syphilis. The molars may have multiple cusps, giving rise to the name "mulberry molars." The combination of interstitial keratitis,

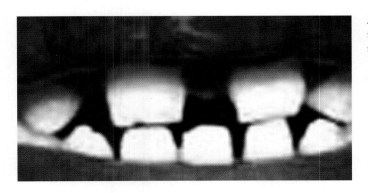

FIG. 48.1.   The small teeth, with notching of the upper central incisors.

Hutchinson's teeth, and sensorineural deafness (which she did not have) constitutes "Hutchinson's triad" of manifestations of late congenital syphilis.

Patients with congenital syphilis may progress to develop tertiary syphilis, the manifestations of which are cardiovascular (aortitis of the ascending aorta) and cerebral (tabes dorsalis and dementia).

Other manifestations of late congenital syphilis include frontal bossing of Parrot and saber shins, due to localized periostitis; rhagades, which are linear scars radiating from the corners of the eyes and mouth; and consequences of nasal inflammation, including saddle nose and short maxilla.

Reading:

Fiumara NJ, Lessell S: Manifestations of late congenital syphilis. An analysis of 271 patients. Arch Derm 1970; 102: 78–83.

CASE 49. An 18-month-old boy presents with a limp and fever for 1 day. He has had no previous significant illnesses. He is fully immunized with oral polio, diphtheria, tetanus and pertussis, Haemophilus influenzae type b, measles, mumps and rubella, and hepatitis B vaccines. On examination there is fever and a swollen, slightly red knee joint with markedly limited range of movement. A diagnostic knee tap is performed, which reveals turbid fluid. The fluid has 5×10^4 leukocytes per microliter and a negative Gram stain. The child is treated with antibiotics. After 2 days a Gram-negative rod is grown from the knee fluid.

What is the diagnosis and the likely causative organism?

This child has septic arthritis of the knee. Prior to the advent of the vaccine against *Haemophilus influenzae* type b, this organism, a small, pleomorphic Gram-negative rod, was a common cause of septic arthritis in young children. In communities in which the children have received this vaccine, this infection has become very rare. Therefore, in this child, although *H. influenzae* should be considered (which would render this a case of vaccine failure), one should consider other Gram-negative rods, including enteric rods, particularly *Salmonella* spp. An organism that has become prominent as a cause of both septic arthritis and osteomyelitis in young children is *Kingella kingae*. This organism is one of the "HACEK" group of organisms, which constitute part of the normal oral flora and which should be considered as causes of infective endocarditis. They are

Haemophilus aphrophilus
Actinobacillus actinomycetemcomitans

Cardiobacterium hominis
Eikenella corrodens
Kingella kingae

Kingella kingae is usually susceptible to all β-lactam antibiotics, although some strains have been shown to elaborate a β-lactamase. The treatment of children with skeletal infections caused by this organism should consist of amoxicillin/clavulanic acid, or a third-generation cephalosporin.

This child had septic arthritis caused by *Kingella kingae*, and he responded well to therapy with amoxicillin.

Reading:

Moylett EH, Rossmann SN, Epps HR, Demmler GJ: Importance of *Kingella kingae* as a pediatric pathogen in the United States. Pediatr Infect Dis J 2000; 19: 262–265

Lundy DW, Kehl DK: Increasing prevalence of *Kingella kingae* in osteoarticular infections in young children. J Pediatr Orthop 1998; 18: 262–267.

CASE 50. A 3-year-old boy presents with a 1-week history of fever and headache. These symptoms started 1 week after he had returned from a visit to a rural part of South Africa with an altitude of about 5000 feet. On examination he is febrile, he has enlargement of the liver and spleen, and he has a few blanching pink spots on his abdomen and chest (Figure 50.1). There is no lymphadenopathy, and the rest of his examination is normal.

- *What is the differential diagnosis?*
- *What would you do?*

Fever and enlargement of the liver and spleen in the absence of jaundice are features of the following:

(A) Infectious diseases:

(i) *viral:* infectious mononucleosis caused by Epstein–Barr virus, cytomegalovirus, and acute human immunodeficiency virus (HIV) infection, (which would likely imply sexual molestation in this child);

(ii) *bacterial:* subacute systemic bacterial infections such as typhoid fever and infective endocarditis (in which case the hepatomegaly would be due to heart failure) and chronic systemic bacterial infections such as tuberculosis (miliary) and brucellosis;

(iii) *parasitic infections:* malaria, toxoplasmosis, and the early egg-laying stage of schistosomiasis;

(iv) *fungal:* systemic fungal infections such as histoplasmosis.

A rash can occur in patients with infectious mononucleosis, especially if they have received ampicillin or amoxicillin; however, it is not a feature of tuberculosis, brucellosis or malaria. The spots occurring in infective endocarditis are nonblanching and are most marked peripherally. The high altitude where this patient has visited would be an unlikely area for malaria transmission. The migrating stage of schistosomiasis is associated with a marked blood eosinophilia, which can readily be demonstrated.

(B) Noninfective conditions, including leukemia, lymphoma, and juvenile rheumatoid disease.

Appropriate tests would be a blood count with differential count, blood culture, and a chest X ray. Depending on their findings, serological tests might be indicated.

This patient's blood culture grew out a Gram-negative bacillus, which was identified as *Salmonella typhi*, the cause of typhoid fever.

Typhoid fever is a common food and water-borne infection in many parts of the world. It is spread by the fecal–oral route. After the organism is ingested, it multiplies in the lymphoid tissue of the small bowel, then spreads, via the mesenteric nodes, to the reticuloendothelial system, where its numbers are amplified. It continues to multiply in the lymphoid tissue of the small bowel eventually causing ileal ulcers. Clinical symptoms begin when the organism, having multiplied in the reticuloendothelial system, spills into the bloodstream (secondary bacteremia). Clinical features include fever, abdominal pain and diffuse abdominal tenderness, enlargement of the liver (particularly in children) and spleen, and slight clouding of consciousness. At the time of acquisition of the infection diarrhea may occur, and after 2–3 weeks this becomes a prominent feature. The main complications of typhoid fever are related to ulceration of the bowel, namely bowel hemorrhage and perforation.

Other complications include encephalopathy (the origin of the term typhoid is from the Greek for stupor), pneumonia, myocarditis, and Zenker's degeneration of muscle.

This diagnosis should always be considered in febrile patients from Latin America, Asia, or Africa. The diagnosis is best confirmed by blood culture. Stool culture becomes positive after 2–3 weeks of illness. Serology (Widal test) can be helpful but is less so in individuals who have lived in endemic areas.

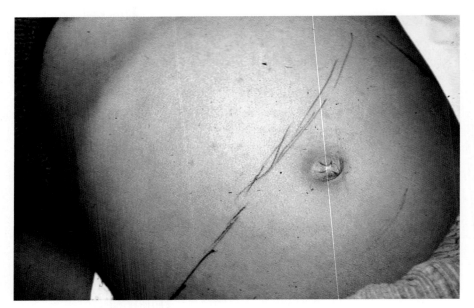

FIG. 50.1. ***The spots and markings of the liver and spleen edges.***

In the past, antibiotic therapy consisted of amoxicillin, trimethoprim/ sulfamethoxazole, or chloramphenicol. However, due to the high rates of resistance to these drugs, a fluoroquinolone or ceftriaxone should be used until antibiotic susceptibilities are known. Despite appropriate therapy relapse of illness can occur.

The diagnosis of typhoid fever carries important public health implications. The causative organism is strictly a human pathogen. Therefore cases should be notified to the health department, so that a source can be identified. Such a source may be an asymptomatic intestinal carrier. Long-term excretion is due to colonization of the liver or gallbladder. This occurs more frequently in adults than in children.

Hospitalized patients should be nursed with contact precautions.

Reading:

Parry CM, Hien TT, Dougan G et al: Medical progress: typhoid fever. N Engl J Med 2002; 347: 1770–1782.

Bhan MK, Bahl R, Bhatnagar S: Typhoid and paratyphoid fever. Lancet 2005; 366: 749–762.

Basnaya B, Maskey AP, Zimmerman MD, Murdoch DR: Enteric (typhoid) fever in travelers. Clin Infect Dis 2005; 41: 1467–1472.

CASE 51. A 1-month-old infant presents with a history of poor feeding and generally appearing ill to the parents. They think he looks a little yellow and his urine is darker than usual. On examination he is ill-appearing, and afebrile. His sclerae are yellowish-green in color. There is enlargement of the liver, but not of the spleen. There is no pallor. The rest of his examination is normal. The urine is indeed dark.

What is the most imminently life-threatening diagnosis?

This infant has evidence of biliary tract obstruction based on "greenish" jaundice and dark urine. The differential diagnosis includes the following:

(A) Hepatitis caused by:

Infections:

  (a) *intrauterine infections:* cytomegalovirus infection; rubella; toxoplasmosis; syphilis;

  (b) *hepatitis viruses:* these do not usually cause clinical hepatitis in infants of this age, and the incubation period is too short for post-natally acquired hepatitis B or C;

  (c) sepsis syndrome, in particular urosepsis caused by enteric bacilli such as *Escherichia coli*;

  (d) "neonatal hepatitis" of unknown etiology;

(B) *Metabolic diseases:* galactosemia, tyrosinemia, α-1-antitrypsin deficiency, hypothyroidism

(C) Biliary atresia

(D) Choledochal cyst

Among these conditions, the only one that is imminently life threatening is urosepsis due to *Escherichia coli*. Therefore the investigation of such cases must include blood and urine cultures to exclude this condition. Urinalysis and urine microscopy and Gram stain are rapid diagnostic tests that can be used to guide decisions about therapy. The fact that this child is ill-appearing suggests that he might have the sepsis syndrome and that empiric antimicrobial therapy should be initiated immediately with an agent such as a third-generation cephalosporin. Meningitis should also be considered.

Reading:

Seeler RA, Hahn K: Jaundice in urinary tract infection in infancy. Am J Dis Child 1969; 118: 553–558.

CASE 52.   A 12-year-old girl has had fever for 1 week. About 1 month ago she had severe abdominal pain and fever, which improved after she had been treated with amoxicillin/clavulanic acid for a few days. On examination she has fever and looks mildly ill. She has some central abdominal tenderness, but no other abnormal physical findings. Blood cultures, performed because of the prolonged fever, have grown a Gram-negative rod and Gram-positive cocci in pairs.

- *What organ is the likely source of the bacteremia?*
- *What is the likely diagnosis?*
- *What are the likely identities of the isolates?*

The isolation of two organisms from the blood (polymicrobial bacteremia) suggests that the bacteremia arose from a mucosal surface. The morphology of these isolates suggests the likelihood of an enteric rod and a streptococcus. This suggests, in turn, that the source of infection is the intestine. In a child with no history given of underlying disease, but a history

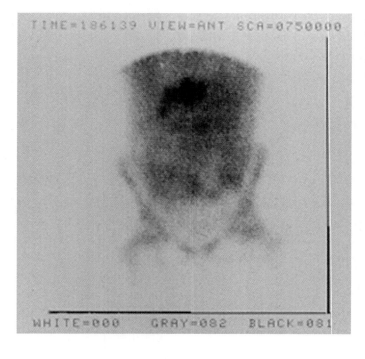

FIG. 52.1.   Gallium scan showing increased intra-abdominal uptake due to an appendix abscess. (Courtesy of Dr Andrew Wiesenthal)

of severe abdominal pain recently, the most likely diagnosis is a perforated appendix, leading to a focal abscess. This child underwent a Gallium-scan study, which showed an area of increased uptake in the abdomen (Figure 52.1).

An appendix abscess was confirmed at surgery. The antimicrobial therapy that she received initially (amoxicillin/clavulanic acid) has broad-spectrum activity, including activity against *E. coli* and enterococci (which were the identities of the organisms isolated from the blood cultures), and anaerobes. Therefore it is likely that the initial infection following the appendiceal perforation had been suppressed by amoxicillin/clavulanic acid and had flared up after the antimicrobial effects of this agent had waned.

Reading:

Solemkin JS, Mazuski JF, Baron EJ et al: Guidelines for the selection of anti-infective agents for complicated intra-abdominal infections. Clin Infect Dis 2003; 37: 999–1005.

CASE 53. A 16-year-old boy presents with an annoying cough, which he has had for about 3 weeks. The illness started with a runny nose. On examination he is completely normal, but he exhibits several episodes of severe coughing.

- *What is the differential diagnosis?*
- *What would you do?*

Differential diagnosis:
Respiratory tract infection:
    Virus:
        Adenovirus
        Other respiratory viruses
    Bacteria:
        Mycoplasma pneumoniae
        Chlamydia pneumoniae
        Bordetella pertussis
        Mycobacterium tuberculosis
    Fungal:
        Histoplasma capsulatum
        Other dimorphic fungi
        Noninfectious diseases:
        Asthma
        Foreign body inhalation

The course of this child's illness, beginning with a runny nose, followed by episodes of severe coughing, suggests a respiratory tract infection. This clinical picture, in particular the 3-week duration of the cough, is highly suggestive of pertussis (whooping cough). Pertussis is a severe, contagious infection that causes significant morbidity and mortality worldwide. It is caused by the small Gram-negative bacillus, *Bordetella pertussis*. This organism becomes attached to the columnar epithelium of the respiratory tract causing effacement of the brush border and necrosis of epithelial cells, resulting in the accumulation of debris within the airway. Pertussis causes mainly bronchitis, but pneumonia may also occur. Classic pertussis has three clinical stages: (a) the catarrhal stage, characterized by a runny nose, which is indistinguishable from that of the common cold. This is followed after about a week by (b) the paroxysmal stage, characterized by paroxysms of

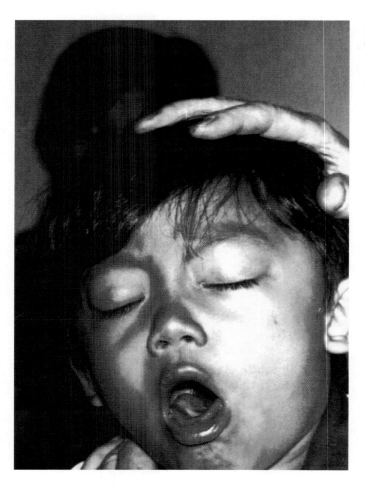

FIG. 53.1.   A child with a paroxysm of coughing caused by pertussis. (Courtesy of the Centers of Disease Control and Prevention)

prolonged cough during which the patient cannot catch his/her breath. At the end of the paroxysm, air is inspired through a partially closed glottis resulting in the characteristic whoop. During the paroxysm the patient may become hypoxic and lose consciousness. Such an attack is frightening to experience or to witness (Figure 53.1). Young infants may not experience the coughing paroxysm, but may just become apneic. The paroxysmal stage lasts for several weeks. This stage is followed by (c) the convalescent stage, during which the paroxysms become less frequent. If the patient develops a viral upper respiratory infection during this time paroxysms may recur. This stage lasts for several weeks.

Complications of pertussis
   hypoxia, with hypoxic brain injury;
   pneumonia;
   bronchiectasis;
   death. Most deaths occur in infants younger than 6 months of age and are due to pneumonia or apnea.

Teenagers and young adults with pertussis often present with a prolonged cough, as in this case. Although such individuals are not at high risk for significant morbidity, they pose an important source of spread of the organism.

Diagnosis: This should be suspected clinically in cases demonstrating the classic whooping cough. A blood count may reveal an absolute lymphocytosis, which can be very marked. The diagnosis is confirmed by culture specifically for the causative organism. A nasopharyngeal swab should be inoculated at the bedside on to a specific selective medium or appropriate transport medium. A direct fluorescent antibody test can be used. This is more rapid than culture, but not as specific nor as sensitive as culture. Polymerase chain reaction tests of respiratory specimens are also available in some laboratories.

Treatment: There is no proven treatment for paroxysms, other than artificial ventilation, which is occasionally necessary. Antimicrobial therapy consisting of erythromycin, given for 14 days, or azithromycin given for 5 days, is used with the following aims: (a) to abort infection if diagnosed in the catarrhal stage; (b) to eliminate carriage and thus infectivity in a patient with the disease; (c) to prevent the development of disease in close contacts.

Prevention: The most important health intervention regarding pertussis is active immunization. Pertussis vaccine has had a significantly beneficial impact on the incidence of this disease. This has been highlighted by the rise in incidence when vaccination rates have dropped, and the decrease in rates associated with its widespread use. In the United States, the rates of this infection prior to vaccination were 450/100,000, while current rates are 1–2/100,000. The older vaccine is the killed whole cell vaccine. The newer vaccine, currently used in the United States, is an acellular vaccine composed of several purified pertussis antigens. This has fewer adverse effects than the whole cell vaccine. It is combined with tetanus and diphtheria vaccines, the combination being referred to as DTaP. In the United States, it is administered at ages 2, 4, 6, and 12–18 months, and at 4–6 years. Because teenagers and adults play a major role in the spread of the infection, they should also receive a vaccine booster, in the form of Tdap (tetanus, diphtheria, and acellular pertussis vaccine).

All cases of pertussis should be reported to the health department, and close contacts should be treated with a course of a macrolide antibiotic. Individuals who are hospitalized should be nursed with droplet precautions.

Reading:

Hewlett E, Edwards KM: Pertussis – not just for kids. N Engl J Med 2005; 352: 1215–1222.

Greenberg DP: Pertussis in adolescents. Increasing incidence brings attention to the need for booster immunization of adolescents. Pediatr Infect Dis J 2005; 24: 721–728.

Halperin SA: Pertussis – a disease and vaccine for all ages. N Engl J Med 2005; 353: 1615–1617.

Crowcroft NS, Pebody RG: Recent developments in pertussis. Lancet 2006; 367: 1926–1936.

CASE 54 (HYP). A 10-year-old boy develops a tender swelling in his right armpit, and fever. On examination he is toxic-appearing and has a large, red, tender lymph node in his right axilla. The rest of the examination is normal.

- *What is the differential diagnosis?*
- *What questions would you like to ask?*
- *What would you do?*

The clinical diagnosis is one of a suppurative lymphadenitis. The differential diagnosis relates to its microbial cause. Most cases of suppurative lymphadenitis are caused by *Staphylococcus aureus* and *Streptococcus pyogenes*, complicating an infected skin lesion or wound drained by the affected node, in this case on the upper limb or chest wall. The other causes require specific exposures. These are: *Francisella tularensis*, the cause of tularemia, *Yersinia pestis*, the cause of plague, and *Bartonella henselae*, the cause of cat-scratch disease. Since they are all transmitted by animals or arthropod vectors, obtaining a history of possible exposures to animals is of the utmost importance. Other questions about exposure are related to travel, occupation, and recreational activities.

This boy had been hunting in Colorado. He had shot and skinned a hare.

This information strongly suggests the diagnosis of tularemia. *Francisella tularensis* is acquired by direct inoculation from infected material as in this case, by the bite of an infected tick or fly, by inhalation, or by ingestion of infected food. There are several clinical syndromes associated with infection with this organism: glandular or ulceroglandular, as in this patient; oculoglandular (Parinaud's syndrome); oropharyngeal, characterized by pharyngitis; typhoidal; and pneumonic. The diagnosis of glandular disease can be confirmed by Gram stain and culture of material from an aspirate of the lymph node. In this case the laboratory personnel should be made aware of the suspicion of tularemia, which poses a laboratory hazard, so that appropriate precautions can be taken. Serology can also be used. Antimicrobial therapy should consist of streptomycin or gentamicin.

Reading:

Dennis DT, Inglesby TV, Henderson DA et al: Tularemia as a biological weapon. Medical and public health management. JAMA 2001; 285: 2763–2773.

CASE 55. A 6-month-old infant presents with a high fever and irritability. On examination she looks toxic, is very irritable, and has a bulging anterior fontanelle. The cerebrospinal fluid reveals the following: leukocytes 1200/µl (95% neutrophils), protein 150 mg/dl, and glucose 24 mg/dl; the Gram stain is shown in Figure 55.1.

• *What is the likely diagnosis?*

This child has bacterial meningitis. The Gram stain shows pleomorphic Gram-negative rods, most likely *Haemophilus influenzae* type b. Prior to the advent of a vaccine against this organism, this was the most common cause of

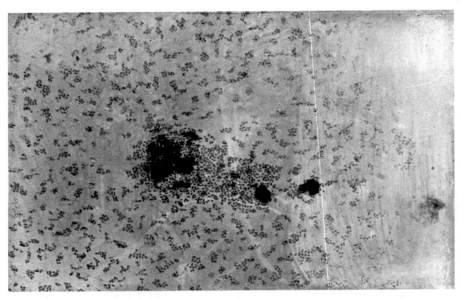

FIG. 55.1.   A Gram stain of the cerebrospinal fluid.

bacterial meningitis in children in the United States. This serotype of *Haemophilus influenzae* is considered contagious and not part of the normal pharyngeal flora. It is spread by droplets from one child to another. It colonizes the pharynx whence it enters the bloodstream. From the bloodstream it can spread to the meninges, joints, pericardium, and other foci. Buccal cellulitis and periorbital cellulitis are focal infections that may also be caused by this organism. These invasive infections affect mainly children younger than 3 years. Acute epiglottitis, a life-threatening disease of the airway, caused by this organism, affects older children, mainly those 4–6 years old. Antimicrobial therapy for patients with haemophilus meningitis consists of a third-generation cephalosporin. Dexamethasone, preferably started 15 minutes before the first dose of antibiotic, reduces the frequency of neurological sequelae, especially of hearing loss.

Because *Haemophilus influenzae* type b is contagious, when a case of invasive disease is diagnosed, the local health department should be notified. Members of families with a case of invasive haemophilus infection and in which a child younger than 5 years lives should be offered chemoprophylaxis with rifampin.

This infection has been largely eliminated in areas where the vaccine is widely used. The vaccine is a conjugate of the polysaccharide capsule, a very important virulence factor for the organism, and a protein such as

meningococcal outer membrane protein, a mutant diphtheria toxin or tetanus toxoid. It is administered in the first and second years of life.

For further discussion of bacterial meningitis, see Case 27.

Reading:

Peltola H: Worldwide *Haemophilus influenzae* type b disease are the beginning of the 21st century: global analysis of the disease burden 25 years after
the use of the polysaccharide vaccine and a decade after the advent of
conjugates. Clin Microbiol Rev 2000; 13: 302–317.

CASE 56. (COMP). A 12-year-old child is in the pediatric intensive care
unit for multiple injuries following a motor vehicle accident. She has been
improving, but on the 8th hospital day she develops a high fever and
becomes hypotensive. On examination she is on a ventilator and receiving
vasopressors. She has an arterial catheter, several venous catheters, and
a urinary catheter in place. There is a red line with swelling extending
proximally from one of the venous catheters.

- *What is the likely diagnosis?*
- *How would you confirm the diagnosis?*
- *What would you do?*

The clinical features of high fever and hypotension suggest septic shock.
This child has many risk factors predisposing her to different nosocomial
infections: (a) vascular catheters, (b) ventilator,; (c) a urinary catheter. This
type of patient is shown in Figure 56.1.

Many such patients have tubes in every natural orifice (mouth, nose,
urethra) except the anus, and tubes in man-made holes. Each of these constitutes a breach in the patient's defenses against infection. The examination
of this patient demonstrates a focus of inflammation, namely phlebitis,
which is the likely cause of the child's infection, and which may well have
led to a bloodstream infection. The most common organisms to cause vascular catheter infection are staphylococci (*S. aureus* and coagulase-negative
staphylococci). In patients who have received antibiotics, *Enterococcus* spp.
and *Candida* spp. are also important, as are Gram-negative rods, including
enteric bacilli and *Pseudomonas* spp.

Management should consist of the following:

(a) Supportive care – correct hypotension;

(b) *Making a microbiological diagnosis*: (i) Culture the blood and urine;
   (ii) remove the catheter and culture its tip; milk the vein toward the

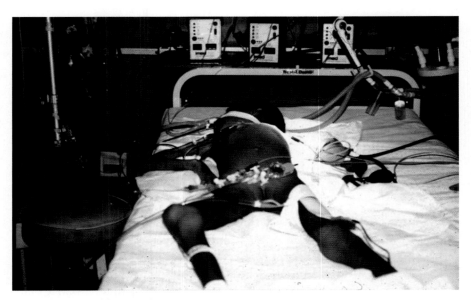

FIG. 56.1.   A patient such as the one described above.

exit site of the catheter and collect any fluid (blood or pus) that emerges. If no material can be obtained in this manner, insert a hypodermic needle percutaneously into the affected area, as if you were drawing blood, and aspirate. Perform a Gram stain and culture of this material.

(c) Initiate antimicrobial therapy with agents active against the likely pathogens. The results of the Gram stain can be very helpful in narrowing the spectrum of such therapy. If no organism is seen, then initial therapy should be directed against methicillin-resistant staphylococci (with vancomycin) and hospital-acquired multiresistant Gram-negative rods (e.g. amikacin). Once culture results are available the therapy may be adjusted. If a yeast is seen, amphotericin B or fluconazole should be administered.

(d) *Surgery*: If pus is expressed from the vein, a diagnosis of suppurative (septic) thrombophlebitis should be made and the affected part of the vein should be excised.

Although infection of intravascular catheters cannot be totally prevented, the rate of infection can be reduced by meticulous cleanliness at the time of catheter insertion and adequate immobilization of the catheter.

CASE 57 (HYP). A 10-year-old child who has had many admissions for episodes of pneumonia in different parts of the lungs, from which she does

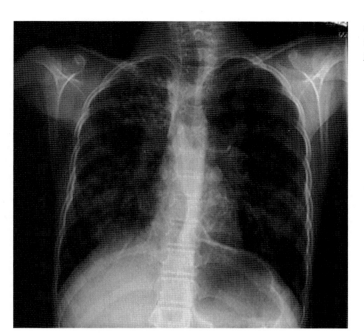

FIG. 57.1.   A chest X ray of a patient similar to the one presented.

not completely recover, presents yet again with a fever and worsening cough. On examination she is thin, cyanosed without supplemental oxygen, tachypneic with intercostal retractions, and she has digital clubbing. Her lungs are hyperinflated, and she has diffuse pulmonary crackles. Her sputum grows very mucoid colonies of a Gram-negative rod. A chest X ray of such a patient is shown in Figure 57.1.

- *What is the likely diagnosis?*
- *What is the likely identity of the isolate?*

This history suggests that she has a generalized disease of the lungs associated with bronchiectasis. The most likely causes are cystic fibrosis and an immunodeficiency. Bronchiectasis may also complicate other conditions such as pertussis, measles, adenoviral infections, and tuberculosis. The presence of very mucoid colonies of a Gram-negative rod suggests mucoid strains of *Pseudomonas aeruginosa* that are characteristic of isolates from patients with cystic fibrosis. Such strains form microcolonies within the lung of such individuals, rendering the organism impossible to eliminate. Children with cystic fibrosis initially acquire pneumonia with *Haemophilus influenzae* and *Staphylococcus aureus*, and later develop infections with *Pseudomonas aeruginosa*. Other pathogens that infect such patients are *Burkholderia cepacia*, which portends imminent deterioration of the patient's condition, and *Stenotrophomonas maltophilia*.

Management of patients with cystic fibrosis must address several issues, including the following: malabsorption and malnutrition due to pancreatic exocrine failure; bronchial obstruction and chronic and recurrent pneumonia, leading to bronchiectasis and cor pulmonale; and living with a severe chronic illness that results in shortened longevity. Of particular relevance to this case is the management of a patient with recurrent pneumonia caused by *Pseudomonas aeruginosa*. Therapeutic strategies include: treatment of acute exacerbations (which manifest with increased respiratory symptoms and crackles on lung examination) with parenteral antipseudomonal antimicrobial agents, such as a combination of ceftazidime and tobramycin. With recurrent use of these agents, resistance often develops. Other suitable agents are fluoroquinolones and carbapenems. Tobramycin administered by inhalation is useful in suppressing the growth of the organism. Azithromycin is useful in suppressing the chronic inflammation that results in lung damage. DNAse administered by inhalation is also of value. It lyses the DNA derived from the cells involved in the inflammation, which contributes toward the high viscosity of the sputum and which, in turn, contributes toward the airway obstruction.

Reading:

Davis PB: Cystic fibrosis. Pediatr Rev 2001; 22: 257–264.

Orenstein DM, Winnie GB, Altman H: Cystic fibrosis: a 2002 update. J Pediatr 2002; 140: 156–164.

Lyczak JB, Cannon CL, Pier GB: Lung infections associated with cystic fibrosis. Clin Microbial Rev 2002; 15: 194–222.

Miller MB, Gilligan PH: Laboratory aspects of management of chronic pulmonary infections in patients with cystic fibrosis. J Clin Microbiol 2003; 41: 4009–4915.

CASE 58. A 4-year-old boy presents with a history of diarrhea, abdominal cramps, and fever starting a few days after he acquired a turtle for a pet.

What is the likely cause of the diarrhea?

This child has acute gastroenteritis (acute infectious diarrhea). The diagnostic challenge lies in determining its microbiologic cause. Many

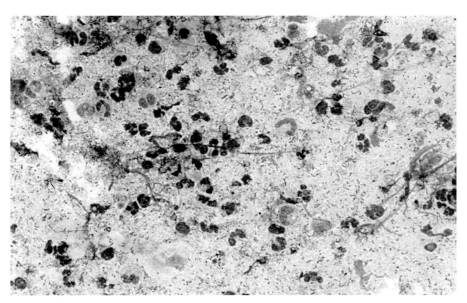

FIG. 58.1. A methylene blue–stained fecal smear showing large numbers of polymorphonuclear leukocytes. This was from a child with enteric infection caused by both Salmonella enteritidis *and* Yersinia enterocolitica.

different organisms (viral, bacterial, and protozoal) could have caused this child's illness. In most circumstances making a microbiological diagnosis is not very important to the patient. Ensuring adequate hydration is the most important component of management (see Case 19). The exposure history suggests very strongly that he has become infected with salmonella, which is excreted by most reptiles.

A rapid diagnostic test that can help to limit the microbiological differential diagnosis is the fecal smear stained with methylene blue. If it reveals many leukocytes (Figure 58.1), an invasive bacterial cause such as *Salmonella* spp., *Shigella* spp., *Campylobacter jejuni*, or *Yersinia enterocolitica* is likely. In such cases the stool should be cultured for these bacteria. The method of performing the fecal smear test is important. The part of the stool containing mucus, pus, or blood should be smeared thinly on a microscope slide and allowed to dry. After the methylene blue stain has been applied for 1–2 minutes, the slide should be rinsed with water, allowed to dry, and examined.

Nontyphoid salmonellae are excreted by many different animals. Human beings become infected by ingesting undercooked meat, eggs, unpasteurized dairy products, and contaminated water. There are over 2500 different serotypes of these organisms, many having interesting names, including those of

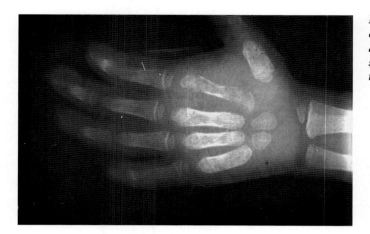

FIG. 58.2.   The hand X ray of a child with sickle cell disease and chronic salmonella osteomyelitis of the second metacarpal.

animals (such as *S. gallinarum* and *S. pullorum*), of diseases they cause in animals (such as *S. typhimurium* and *S. choleraesuis*), and of cities (such as *S. kaapstad* and *S. montevideo*). Most salmonella infections are characterized by acute gastroenteritis. Although salmonella bacteremia is not unusual, metastatic infection is unusual. When it occurs it affects mostly young infants. Such infections include meningitis, septic arthritis, and osteomyelitis. Patients with sickle cell disease are at particular risk of developing salmonella osteomyelitis (Figure 58.2). In parts of the world where a clean water supply is lacking, intestinal and systemic salmonella infections are very common.

Antimicrobial therapy of patients with salmonella gastroenteritis does not hasten recovery but may prolong the duration of excretion of the pathogen. Therefore it is not usually indicated. However, if systemic infection is suspected, antimicrobial therapy should be used. Because of widespread antimicrobial resistance, empiric therapy in children should usually consist of a third-generation cephalosporin. If the isolate is susceptible, amoxicillin or trimethoprim/sulfamethoxazole should be used. In adults a fluoroquinolone can be used.

Salmonellae can live within macrophages. They therefore require cell-mediated immunity for their elimination. Therefore individuals with defects in this arm of immunity, such as those with AIDS, are at risk for persistent salmonella infections. Chronic salmonella bacteremia can occur in individuals with schistosomiasis, in which the worm, which lives within venous plexuses, serves as an infected intravascular foreign body.

Salmonella typhi, which is solely a human pathogen, causes typhoid fever (see Case 50).

Reading:

Stam F, Romkens THE, Hekker TAM et al: Turtle-associated human salmonellosis. Clin Infect Dis 2003; 37: e167–169.

CASE 59. A 2-year-old boy presents with fever and skin lesions of 1-day duration. On examination he is febrile and toxic-appearing but not in shock. There are no localizing findings, except for the skin lesions shown in the picture (Figure 59.1).

- *What are these lesions called?*
- *What do they represent?*
- *What organisms should be considered in the microbiological differential diagnosis?*

These skin lesions are called *ecthyma gangrenosum*. They are metastatic skin infections complicating bacteremia caused by Gram-negative bacilli, in particular *Pseudomonas aeruginosa*, which was the case in this patient. They are caused by infection of the adventitia of subcutaneous blood vessels. They resemble the lesions seen in meningococcemia and acute staphylococcal endocarditis. It is important to aspirate the lesion to get material for Gram stain and culture, the former of which can give immediate information as to

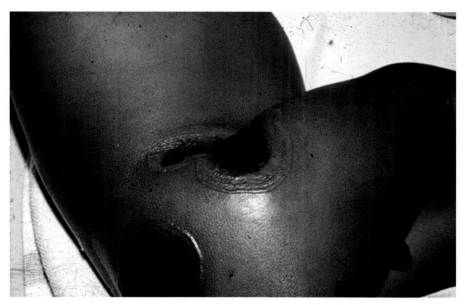

FIG. 59.1. The child's skin lesions. (Reprinted from: Anderson MG: Pseudomonas septicaemia and ecthyma gangrenosum. S Afr Med J 1979; 55: 504, with permission.)

whether this is likely caused by a Gram-negative rod, meningococcal, or staphylococcal infection.

Aspiration is performed as follows: (i) a few drops of nonbacteriostatic, sterile saline is aspirated into a 10 or 20 ml syringe, using a 21- or 22-gauge needle (this is to provide enough volume of aspirate to perform the Gram stain and culture); (ii) the needle is inserted into the lesion and as much suction as possible is applied for about 30 seconds; usually a drop or two of blood-stained fluid will be aspirated into the syringe; this fluid is mixed with the saline, and then a drop is used to prepare a slide for Gram stain, and the remainder is injected onto a culture swab or into a blood culture bottle.

Antimicrobial treatment should include an aminoglycoside and a beta-lactam active against *Pseudomonas aeruginosa*, for example, ceftazidime, and, if staphylococcal infection is suspected, vancomycin.

Reference

Anderson MG: Pseudomonas septicaemia and ecthyma gangrenosum. S Afr Med J 1979; 55: 504–508.

CASE 60. A 13-year-old boy with β-thalassemia major, for which he has received many blood transfusions, presents with a high fever and malaise, of 1 day's duration. He had a mild diarrheal illness a few days earlier. On examination he is ill-appearing, with a temperature of 38.7°C, heart rate of 140/minute, and blood pressure of 80/40. He is pale, mildly jaundiced (his usual color), and his face has a slightly greyish color (also his usual color). His heart is enlarged, and both his liver and spleen are markedly enlarged (all usual for him).

- *What is the likely cause of his acute problem?*
- *What is the likely underlying abnormality predisposing him to this problem?*
- *What would you do?*

This patient's clinical picture suggests that he is in septic shock and that he might also be significantly anemic.

The immediate management should address ensuring adequate perfusion, with intravenous fluids and adequate hemoglobinization with a blood transfusion. (A hemoglobin concentration measurement can rapidly determine whether this is necessary.) The second issue to address is the likely cause of his septic shock and, based on this, optimal empiric antimicrobial management.

This patient has three particular risk factors for infections:

(a) Previous intravenous catheters for blood transfusion. A long-term central venous catheter would be a very likely focus of infection. The most likely causes of infection of such sites are staphylococci.

(b) *Blood transfusion:* Many infectious agents can be transmitted in blood, including the following:

(i) Viruses such as hepatitis B and C viruses, human immunodeficiency virus (HIV), Epstein–Barr virus, cytomegalovirus, and West Nile virus.

(ii) Bacteria, either from the donor's blood, for example, *Treponema pallidum*, or contaminating the blood during collection from the donor. Since a well or mildly ill bacteremic donor would likely have a very low concentration of bacteria in the blood, these would likely not grow to large numbers during refrigeration of the blood. Exceptions are *Listeria monocytogenes* and *Yersinia enterocolitica*, which can multiply in the cold (this is in fact one of the methods used to selectively culture *Yersinia enterocolitica* from feces).

(iii) Protozoa, such as *Plasmodium* spp., *Babesia microti*, *Trypanosoma cruzi*, *Trypanosoma brucei*, and *Toxoplasma gondii*.

(c) *Iron overload:* This patient is at risk for iron overload, and his greyish complexion suggests that he indeed has this complication of repeated blood transfusions. Iron overload predisposes to bacterial infections, in particular that due to *Yersinia enterocolitica*. The preceding diarrheal illness might have been a bacterial enteric infection caused by *Salmonella* spp., *Yersinia enterocolitica*, *Shigella* spp., or *Campylobacter jejuni*.

Therefore this child's blood should be examined for protozoal parasites (by blood smear) and cultured for bacteria. Antimicrobial therapy against Gram-negative bacilli, such as *Salmonella* spp. and *Y. enterocolitica* should be instituted, with, for example, a third-generation cephalosporin and gentamicin, or with a fluoroquinolone. If a long-term central venous catheter is in place, vancomycin should also be administered.

Reading:

Berkowitz FE : Hemolysis and infection: categories and mechanisms of their interrelationship. Rev Infect Dis 1991; 13: 1151–1162.

Busch MP, Kleinman SH, Nemo GJ: Current and emerging infectious risks of blood transfusions. JAMA 2003; 289: 959–962.

CASE 61. Musa Noormohamed, a 3-year-old boy, who has no previous medical history, presents to a hospital in Colorado, USA, with a history of fever for approximately 1 month's duration. He has undergone many diagnostic tests, including blood counts, blood cultures, urine cultures, and intravenous pyelography, but a diagnosis has not been made. On examination he has a temperature of 38.5°C and a slightly tender, enlarged liver. There is no jaundice, pallor, splenomegaly, or lymphadenopathy, and the rest of the examination is normal.

- *What is the differential diagnosis?*
- *How would you make a diagnosis?*

The clinical features suggest disease in the liver or gallbladder, most likely an infection, although cancer, such as hepatoblastoma or lymphoma, would also be a consideration. Infections of the gallbladder tend to be more acute than this child's illness suggests and is unlikely in a 3-year-old previously well boy. Although hepatitis is a consideration, one would expect some jaundice or a history of jaundice in the presence of an enlarged tender liver. A hepatic abscess should be considered. This is not usually associated with jaundice. There are four types of hepatic abscess: (a) pyogenic abscess, which usually results from hematogenous spread of bacteria either from the systemic circulation (as in staphylococcal bacteremia) or from the portal circulation, arising, for example, from appendicitis; (b) amebic abscess, resulting from trophozoites of *Entamoeba histolytica*, present in the colon, being carried to the liver in the portal circulation; (c) an abscess forming in a site of hematoma within the liver; (d) an abscess complicating ascending cholangitis. The patient's name should suggest the possibility of travel outside the United States and such a history should be sought. He visited Libya, his native country, about 1 month before the onset of symptoms. This travel history increases the probability of an amebic liver abscess. The easiest and least invasive test to look for this possibility is an abdominal ultrasound of the liver. The result is shown in Figure 61.1.

This showed a hepatic abscess. Considering his travel history, this was presumed to be amebic. He was treated with metronidazole and made a rapid recovery.

Amebiasis is a very important infection with a worldwide distribution. It is caused by the ameba *Entamoeba histolytica*. This parasite is transmitted by the fecal–oral route. The infectious form is the cyst, which is formed in the colon or in the stool of an infected individual. After ingestion in stool-contaminated food or water, it excysts, and invades the colonic mucosa, producing ulcers. This is associated with diarrhea, which may be bloody

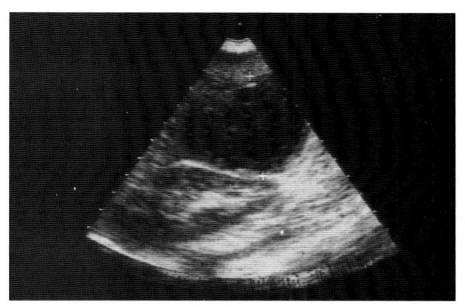

FIG. 61.1.   Ultrasound showing an abscess within the liver.

(amebic dysentery). These ulcers can extend through the colonic wall, resulting in colonic perforation, which carries an extremely high fatality rate. The clinical features of colitis include abdominal tenderness, distension, and, on rectal examination, a rough mucosa, which feels like sandpaper or cobblestones. Other manifestations of colonic disease are toxic megacolon and ameboma, which is a focal annular area of granulation tissue. The organism can enter the portal venous blood and spread systemically. This spread is primarily to the liver, resulting in a liver abscess, as in this patient. Such abscesses can extend to the surface of the liver and rupture into the peritoneal cavity, or they may extend through the diaphragm into the pleural space or the pericardium (Figure 61.2).

The abscess is a collection of liquefied tissue, rather than a pus-filled cavity. Most cases of amebic liver abscess respond to medical therapy only. Surgical drainage is indicated only if rupture appears imminent. The diagnosis of amebiasis can be confirmed by the detection of erythrophagocytic amebae in a fresh stool specimen. Because this is difficult to accomplish, a fresh stool specimen should be placed in a container with a fixative and sent thus to the laboratory (Figure 61.3).

Antigen and PCR techniques have been developed for detecting the organism in the stool or liver abscess fluid. Serological tests are useful in confirming the diagnosis of invasive disease. Therapy consists of metronidazole

Spread of Entamoeba histolytica

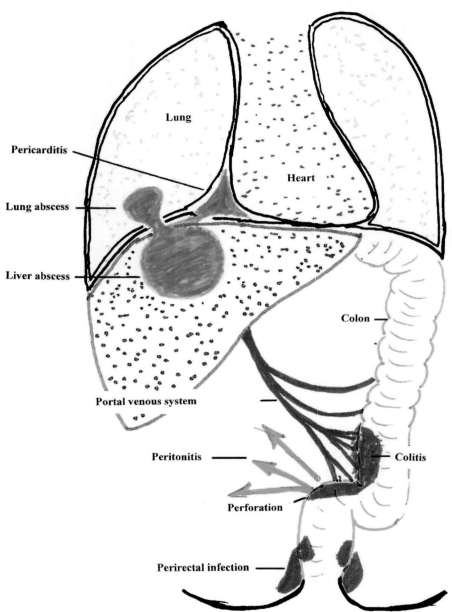

FIG. 61.2.   *The pathogenesis of amebiasis and its complications.*

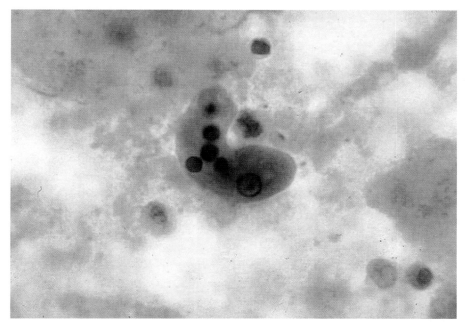

FIG. 61.3. *A fecal specimen showing a trophozoite of* Entamoeba histolytica *with ingested erythrocytes. (Courtesy of Dr NJ Wheeler, Jr/Centers for Disease Control and Prevention)*

or tinidazole for tissue invasion and iodoquinol for eliminating luminal parasites.

Reading:

Stanley SL: Amoebiasis. Lancet 2003; 361: 1025–1034.

Haque R, Huston CD, Hughes M et al: Amebiasis. N Engl J Med 2003; 348: 1565–1573.

CASE 62. A 35-year-old physician with three young children, living in the United States, presents with a history of acute onset of upper abdominal discomfort and nonbloody diarrhea, which began 1 week earlier and has persisted. On examination he appears well, is afebrile, and well-hydrated. The abdominal examination shows very mild distension, but no tenderness, and the rest of the examination is normal.

- *What might be the cause of his illness?*
- *How would you make a diagnosis?*

Many viruses, bacteria, and protozoa cause diarrhea in human beings. A physician is potentially exposed to these more than the general population as a result of his/her occupation. In addition, this patient has the potential exposures from his own children, who might attend day care, an important site for spread of infections. Intestinal pathogens of particular importance in day-care centers are rotavirus and other enteric viruses, *Shigella* spp., *Giardia lamblia*, a flagellated protozoan, and *Cryptosporidium parvum*, a sporozoan. Other possible exposures to diarrheal agents, such as travel to another country, should be sought. The patient's well appearance and mild symptoms suggests that this is probably not a bacterial infection. In a normal adult, one would not expect a viral intestinal infection to have persisted for 1 week without signs of abatement. Therefore protozoal infections become more likely. Specific antimicrobial therapy is available for treating patients with some of them; so diagnostic tests should be directed toward these pathogens. They are *Giardia lamblia (intestinalis)*, *Cryptosporidium parvum*, and *Cyclospora cayetanensis*, which all affect the small intestine. *Entamoeba histolytica*, which affects the colon, is not frequently transmitted in the United States and is often associated with bloody stools. *Giardia lamblia* trophozoites or cysts can be visualized in fresh or preserved stool specimens (Figures 62.1

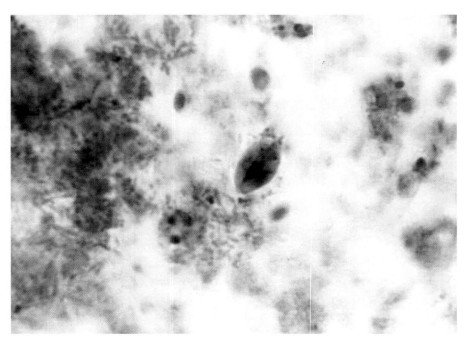

FIG. 62.1.   *Fixed, stained fecal specimen showing a trophozoite of* Giardia lamblia. *(Courtesy of Dr Mae Melvin/the Centers for Disease Control and Prevention)*

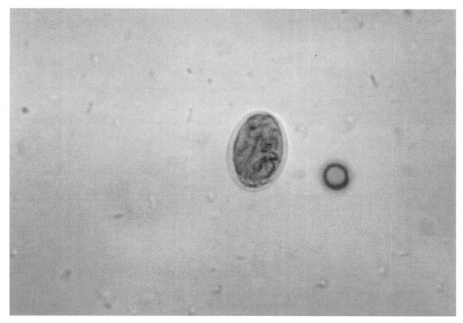

FIG. 62.2.   Unstained fecal specimen showing a cyst of Giardia lamblia. (Courtesy of the centers for Disease Control and Prevention)

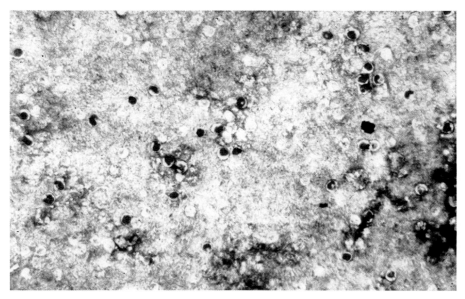

FIG. 62.3.   Acid-fast stain of a stool specimen showing cysts of Cryptosporidium parvum.

■TAB. 62.1:　Enteric protozoal infections causing diarrhea.

Family	Treatment
Ameba	
Entamoeba histolytica	metronidazole or tinidazole
Flagellate	
Giardia lamblia	metronidazole, nitazoxanide, tinadazole, paromomycin, furazolidone, quinacrine
Sporozoa	
Cryptosporidium parvum	nitazoxanide
Cyclospora cayetanensis	trimethoprim/sulfamethoxazole
Isospora belli	trimethoprim/sulfamethoxazole
Microsporidia	
Enterocytozoon bieneusi	fumagillin
Encephalitozoon intestinalis	albendazole
Ciliate	
Balantidium coli	tetracycline, iodoquinol, metronidazole

and 62.2). However, antigen detection methods are more sensitive than microscopy.

Cryptosporidium parvum and *Cyclospora cayetanensis* can be seen after staining the specimen with an acid-fast stain (Figure 62.3). Antigen detection and PCR tests for detecting cryptosporidium have also been developed.

Therapy for patients with giardiasis is metronidazole or tinidazole and for those with cyclospora is trimethoprim/sulfamethoxazole. A newly available treatment for patients with cryptosporidium infection is nitazoxanide, which can also be used for treating patients with giardiasis.

Examination of this patient's stool revealed cysts of *Giardia lamblia*. He was treated with metronidazole. His children, one of whom had diarrhea, were treated with furazolidone.

The different protozoa that can cause diarrhea and treatment of affected patients are listed in Table 62.1.

Reading:

Schuster H, Chiodini PL: Parasitic infections of the intestine. Curr Opin Infect Dis 2001; 14: 587–591.

The Medical Letter. Drugs for parasitic infections. The Medical Letter. August 2004.

CASE 63. Etienne Kabila, a 6-year-old boy, presents with a history of fever for 3 days. There are no other symptoms. On examination he has a temperature of 39°C and appears moderately ill. There is no pallor, cyanosis, jaundice, lymphadenopathy, enlargement of liver or spleen, or rash. The rest of his examination is normal.

- *What is your differential diagnosis?*
- *How would you make a diagnosis?*
- *How would you treat the child?*

Differential diagnosis: The patient's name should suggest the possibility of travel to or of living in a country other than the United States, especially a former French or Belgian colony in Africa. This patient came to the United States 1 week earlier from Zaire (currently called the Democratic Republic of the Congo). This history suggests the possibility of exposure to several different infectious agents that are absent or less common in the United States, including the following:

Viruses: hepatitis A virus, Ebola virus, yellow fever virus, dengue virus

Bacteria: *Salmonella typhi* (typhoid fever), *Leptospira interrogans* (leptospirosis)

Protozoa: *Plasmodium* spp. (malaria), *Trypanosoma brucei* (African trypanosomiasis).

When evaluating a patient with a febrile illness who has traveled from an area endemic for infectious agents not endemic in your own area, you should consider possible (and multiple) diagnoses in terms of potential morbidity and mortality and public health implications. Of the above list, which is not exhaustive, that with the greatest public health implications is Ebola virus infection, which has the potential for significant nosocomial and community spread. Hepatitis A and *Salmonella typhi* infections are of importance but spread can be controlled with appropriate hygiene and enteric precautions. Ebola fever and yellow fever have extremely high case fatality rates. Malaria, caused by *Plasmodium falciparum*, can be fatal if the patient is untreated, as can typhoid fever and trypanosomiasis.

Management should consist of appropriate isolation while evaluation is taking place, and performance of a blood smear to diagnose malaria and trypanosomiasis, and a blood culture to diagnose typhoid fever. Serum chemistries, in particular serum transaminases, may provide a screen for the viral infections listed above. When viral hemorrhagic fevers are considered as possible diagnoses, the laboratory should be notified, and the appropriate

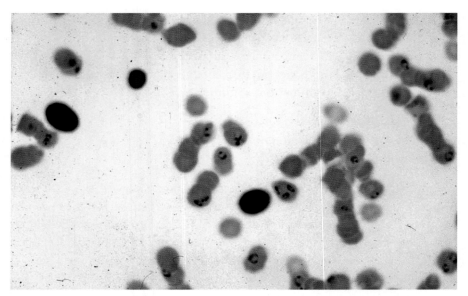

FIG. 63.1.   Thin blood smear showing numerous ring forms of Plasmodium falciparum.

public health authority should be consulted. In the United States, this is the Centers for Disease Control and Prevention in Atlanta.

Figure 63.1. shows the thin blood smear of another child with the same problem as this patient, and Figure 63.2 shows this child's thick blood smear.

The blood smear revealed a heavy parasitemia with *Plasmodium falciparum*.

He was treated with quinine for 5 days and a single dose of pyrimethamine and sulfadoxine, and he made an uneventful recovery.

Malaria is one of the most important diseases of humankind, considering the number of individuals at risk of infection, the number of individuals actually infected, and the number of deaths it causes (>1 million per year), especially among children. It occurs across the tropics and subtropics of the world, its distribution being shown in Figures 63.3 and 63.4.

There are four species of plasmodium that cause malaria in human beings: *P. falciparum, P. vivax, P. ovale,* and *P. malariae*. Their life cycle is shown in Figure 63.5.

The vector, a female mosquito of the *Anopheles* genus, injects a sporozoite into the bloodstream of the vertebrate host, while she is taking a blood meal. This rapidly enters a hepatocyte, where it multiplies by binary fission into many merozoites. These leave the hepatocyte and enter erythrocytes, where they progress from ring forms (trophozoites) to schizonts. By binary fission

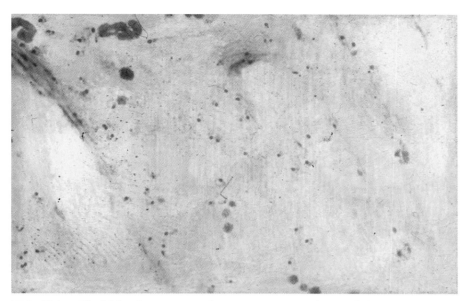

*FIG. 63.2.   **Thick blood smear revealing numerous ring forms of** Plasmodium falciparum.

these divide into 6–24 merozoites (depending on the species), which cause rupture of the erythrocytes. They then enter other erythrocytes. Thus there is an amplification process, which is asexual. During this process, some merozoites form male and female gametocytes, which are haploid cells. When a mosquito feeds and ingests this blood, the gametocytes unite forming a diploid oocyte, which forms an oocyst in the intestinal wall of the mosquito. Thus the mosquito, in which the sexual cycle is completed, is the definitive host, while the vertebrate is the intermediate host.

In the cases of *P. falciparum* and *P. malariae* all merozoites leave the liver at the same time. In the cases of *P. vivax* and *P. ovale* some of the liver stage parasites remain in the hepatocytes. These are called hypnozoites. They emerge from the liver at intervals over several months to a few years, accounting for clinical relapses.

The clinical manifestations of malaria can be explained by the following:

(a) destruction of erythrocytes (hemolysis), leading to hemolytic anemia, and hyperplasia of the reticuloendothelial system;

(b) elaboration of cytokines leading to chills and fever;

(c) in the case of *P. falciparum*, the species that causes the most severe disease and accounts for almost all malaria deaths, adhesion of infected erythrocytes to the endothelium. This results in vascular obstruction in

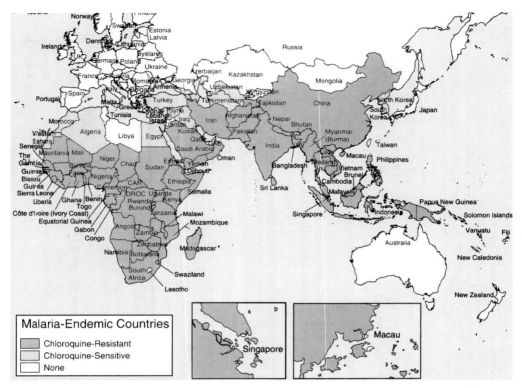

FIG. 63.3.   *Eastern hemisphere countries in which malaria is endemic in part or all of the country. (from Centers for Disease Control and Prevention. Health Information for International Travel 2005–2006. Atlanta: US Department of Health and Human Services. Public Health Service, 2005)*

all organs. The clinical manifestations include the following: (i) encephalopathy (cerebral malaria); (ii) acute renal failure; (iii) liver failure; (iv) diarrhea; (v) pulmonary edema; (vi) adrenal failure;

(d) immune stimulation, resulting in (i) splenomegaly – in areas where recurrent episodes occur, this can lead to chronic massive splenomegaly, a condition called tropical splenomegaly; (ii) autoantibody production, directed against erythrocytes, resulting in hemolysis of nonparasitized cells, and against platelets, resulting in thrombocytopenia; (iii) nephrotic syndrome complicating *P. malariae* infection.

As mentioned above, falciparum malaria is potentially a life-threatening disease. Therefore it constitutes a medical emergency. The causes of morbidity and mortality are organ failure, as described above, hypoglycemia, and severe anemia.

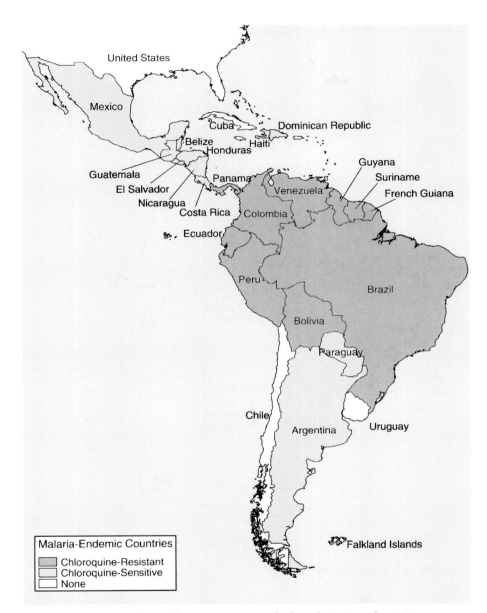

FIG. 63.4.   *Western hemisphere countries in which malaria is endemic in part or all of the country. (from Centers for Disease Control and Prevention. Health Information for International Travel 2005–2006. Atlanta: US Department of Health and Human Services. Public Health Service, 2005)*

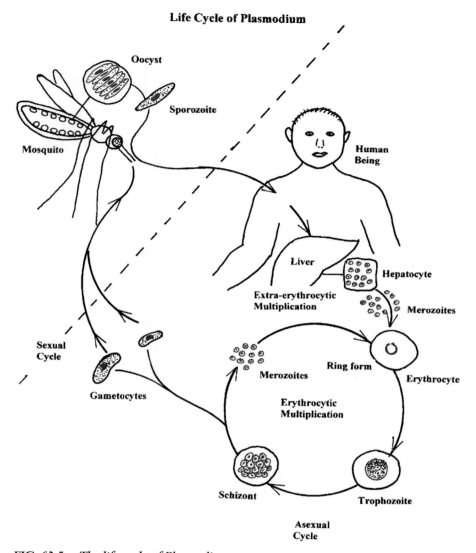

FIG. 63.5.   The life cycle of Plasmodium spp.

The diagnosis of malaria depends on demonstration of the organisms in a blood smear stained with a Romanowsky stain such as Giemsa stain. Two types of smear should be made:

(i)   A thin smear, which is fixed before staining, and in which the parasite morphology is well seen. This allows for speciation of the parasite. If parasites are seen on this smear, examination of a thick smear is unnecessary. Examination of this smear should enable one to estimate the degree of parasitemia (proportion of erythrocytes parasitized).

This is done by counting the numbers of parasitized and nonparasitized erythrocytes in a given number of fields. A more accurate method involves counting the numbers of parasites and of leukocytes seen in a given number of fields and using the results of a leukocyte count to calculate the proportion of erythrocytes parasitized.

(ii) A thick smear, which should be just thick enough for newsprint to be read through it. This is not fixed before staining. Because one looks through multiple layers of blood simultaneously, the sensitivity of the test is higher than that of a thin smear examination. However, the morphology of the parasites is not well seen. In *P. falciparum* infection the degree of parasitemia may reach greater than 5% of red cells (considered a heavy parasitemia), ring forms are usually the only forms seen in the peripheral blood, and more than one ring may be seen within one red cell (Figure 63.1). In infections caused by the other species of plasmodium, parasitemia rarely reaches 5% (unless the patient is asplenic), stages more advanced than ring forms can be seen in the peripheral blood (Figure 63.6), and more than one parasite per red cell is not seen. Other tests such as antigen detection have been used in the field but are not superior to blood smear examination. Genome detection can be done, but is not routinely available.

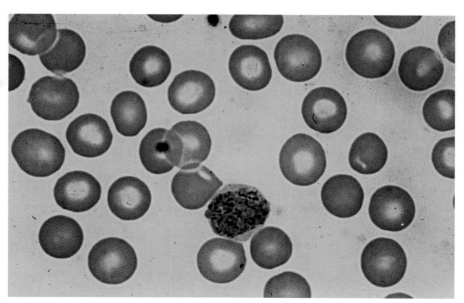

FIG. 63.6. *A thin blood smear showing a schizont of* Plasmodium vivax *from a patient with malaria acquired in India.*

Management:

(i)   *supportive care:* ensure adequate oxygenation, hydration, and hemo-globinization, and normoglycemia (both severe malaria itself, and therapy with quinine can cause hypoglycemia);

(ii) *antimicrobial therapy:* this consists of treatment of the acute attack, and, in the case of infection with *P. vivax* and *P. ovale*, "radical cure."

Treatment of the acute attack:

(a) *Falciparum malaria:* This formerly consisted of chloroquine. However, because chloroquine resistance in *P. falciparum* is so frequent in almost all malaria-endemic areas, one should assume chloroquine resistance. Currently recommended therapy in the United States is a fixed combination of atovoquone and proguanil. An alternative is quinine. When quinine is used, a second drug is also recommended. Doxycycline, sulfadoxine plus pyrimethamine or clindamycin can be used for this purpose. If the medication cannot be given by mouth or by nasogastric tube, for example if the patient is vomiting, then intravenous therapy should be given. Quinine for intravenous use is not available in the United States. Instead quinidine should be used. In such cases the patient should ideally be nursed in an intensive care unit, because the side effects of the drug include dysrhythmias. In other parts of the world single drugs and drug combinations that are used for treatment of malaria include mefloquine, artemether-lumefantrine, artesunate-mefloquine, artesunate-amodiaquine, and artesunate-sulfadoxine-pyrimethamine.

(b) *Other species:* Chloroquine can be used (although chloroquine-resistant *P. vivax* is reported in Asia and South America). However, if there is any concern about the possibility of falciparum malaria, quinine should be used. This is effective against non-falciparum species of plasmodium.

(c) *Radical cure for vivax and ovale malaria:* This is aimed at eliminating the hypnozoite stage in the liver and thus preventing relapses and consists of primaquine. This drug is contraindicated during pregnancy, and in individuals with glucose-6-phosphate dehydrogenase deficiency. In such individuals, relapses should be treated as described above.

(iii) *Contacts:* Malaria is not contagious from person-to-person, unless blood from a parasitemic individual is introduced into another individual, as can occur with shared needles or by blood transfusion. In such cases radical cure is not necessary because the liver stage of the life cycle has been omitted. However, when an individual is diagnosed with malaria outside of an endemic area, co-travelers should be observed for illness.

(iv) *Prevention:* Malaria can be largely prevented by the following methods: (a) Avoidance of mosquito bites by sleeping under insecticide-impregnated mosquito nets, keeping indoors from dusk to dawn, and use of mosquito repellents containing DEET on skin, and permethrins on clothing. (b) Chemoprophylaxis – several drugs are available for this purpose. Those recommended by the US Public Health Service for Americans traveling to endemic areas are mefloquine, atovoquone/proguanil, and doxycycline. (c) Reducing the ability of the mosquitoes to multiply, using insecticides, and draining of bodies of water.

Reading:

Greenwood BM, Bojang K, Whitty CJM, Targett GA: Malaria. Lancet 2005; 365: 1487–1498.

Baird JK: Effectiveness of antimalarial drugs. N Engl J Med 2005; 352: 1565–1577.

Stauffer W, Fischer PR: Diagnosis and treatment of malaria in children. Clin Infect Dis 2003; 37: 1340–1348.

Chen Q, Schlichtherle M, Wahlgren M: Molecular aspects of severe malaria. Clin Microbiol Rev 2000; 13: 439–450.

Hostetter MK: Epidemiology of travel-related morbidity and mortality in children. Pediatr Rev 1999; 20: 228–233.

Ryan ET, Wilson ME, Kain KC: Illness after international travel. N Engl J Med 2002; 347: 505–516.

McLellan SLF: Evaluation of fever in the returned traveler. Primary Care Clin Office Pract 2002; 29: 947–969.

CASE 64 (HYP). An 18-year-old boy presents with fever of 2 weeks' duration. One month ago he accompanied his father on a hunting trip to Botswana. During the trip he developed a sore on his arm, which he ascribed to an insect bite. On examination he is moderately ill-appearing with a temperature of 39°C. He has generalized lymphadenopathy, but no hepatomegaly or splenomegaly, and the rest of his examination is normal.

- *What is the differential diagnosis?*
- *What would you do?*

A sore suggests the possibility of a common skin infection following minor trauma, for example that due to *Staphylococcus aureus*. Such an infection would cause localized but not generalized lymphadenopathy. An arthropod bite might cause such trauma and might also provide a site of inoculation of an infectious agent. The travel and recreational history and such a sore should lead to consideration of anthrax, rickettsial infection (*Rickettsia africae* or *R. conori*), and African trypanosomiasis (sleeping sickness). In anthrax and rickettsial infection, the fever does not develop weeks after the appearance of the sore nor is generalized lymphadenopathy a feature of these infections. These features suggest trypanosomiasis. However, considering the patient's travel history, other ADDITIONAL infections should also be considered, in particular malaria.

The test for diagnosing trypanosomiasis is examination of a Giemsa-stained blood smear, and lymph node and skin lesion aspirate.

The smear of such a patient is shown in Figure 64.1.

This shows many flagellated protozoa, characteristic of *Trypanosoma brucei*, the cause of African trypanosomiasis or "sleeping sickness."

African sleeping sickness, which is present in many parts of tropical Africa, is one of the major global health problems. It is transmitted by the tsetse fly (*Glossina* spp.). The organism enters the lymphatics and then the circulation. It causes systemic disease characterized by fever, a rash, and

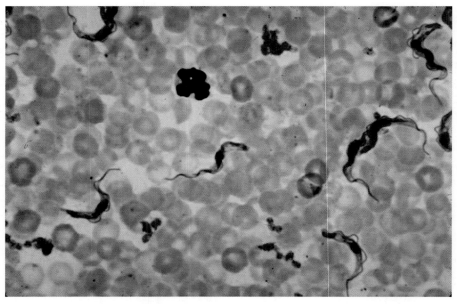

FIG. 64.1.   Blood smear showing Trypanosoma brucei. *(Courtesy of Dr Mae Melvin/Centers for Disease Control and Prevention)*

■TAB. 64.1: Treatments for African trypanosomiasis (*Trypanosoma brucei*) infection.

Subspecies	Hemolymphatic	Nervous system
T. b. gambiense	Pentamidine isethionate	Melarsoprol
	Suramin	Eflornithine
T. b. rhodesiense	Suramin	Melarsoprol

generalized lymphadenopathy. The organism eventually enters the central nervous system where it causes a progressive encephalitis, which is associated with disturbance of normal sleep patterns. This infection is fatal if untreated. Two subspecies of African trypanosomes infect human beings, namely *T. brucei rhodesiense* and *T. brucei gambiense*. The main reservoirs of *T. brucei rhodesiense* are cattle and antelope, while *T. brucei gambiense* is transmitted between human beings. *T. brucei rhodesiense* causes a more rapidly progressive infection than does *T. brucei gambiense*. The treatment according to the species and whether or not central nervous system disease has developed is shown in Table 64.1.

Reading:

Barrett MP, Burchmore RJS, Stich A et al: The trypanosomiases. Lancet 2003; 362: 1469–1480.

Uslan DZ, Jacobson KM, Kumar N et al: A woman with fever and rash after African safari. Clin Infect Dis 2006; 43: 609, 661–662.

Drugs for Parasitic Diseases. The Medical Letter. August 2004.

CASE 65 (HYP). A 4-month-old girl is noted to have developmental delay and strabismus. On examination she is microcephalic and her limbs are hypertonic. She does not interact with you and clearly has delayed motor and social milestones. The appearance of the optic fundus is similar to that shown in Figure 65.1.

Fundoscopy shows a scar from healed chorioretinitis over the posterior pole of the eye, involving the macula.

The differential diagnosis of microcephaly and psychomotor retardation in a 4-month-old infant can be considered in terms of intrauterine, intrapartum, and postnatal insults.

The major causes within each stage are shown in Table 65.1.

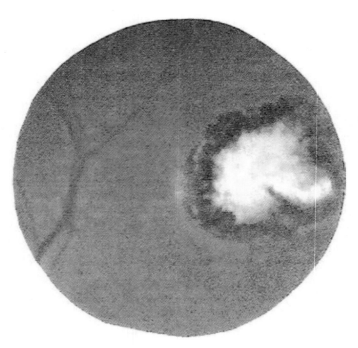

FIG. 65.1.   The posterior pole of the optic fundus. (Reprinted from: Scheie HG and Albert DM (editors): Adler's Textbook of Ophthalmology. 8th edition. WB Saunders, Philadelphia, 1969, p. 143, with permission from Elsevier.)

■**TAB. 65.1: Major intrauterine, intrapartum, and postnatal causes of psychomotor retardation.**

Intrauterine	Intrapartum	Postnatal
Infection		
Cytomegalovirus		
Rubella		
Herpes simplex (very unusual)	Herpes simplex	
Toxoplasmosis		
Lymphocytic choriomeningitis virus		
Varicella (uncommon)	Bacterial meningitis	Bacterial meningitis
Metabolic		
Hypoxia-ischemia	Hypoxia-ischemia	Hypoxia-ischemia
		Hypoglycemia
		Inborn error
Vascular		
Occlusion		Occlusion
		Hemorrhage
Trauma	Hemorrhage	Hemorrhage

Of the above causes, only cytomegalovirus and *Toxoplasma gondii* infections cause chorioretinitis. That caused by cytomegalovirus can affect any part of the retina, including the periphery, whereas that caused by toxoplasma typically occurs in the posterior pole, as shown in this case. The strabismus is probably due to very poor visual acuity, but could also be related to the psychomotor retardation.

Toxoplasmosis is caused by the sporozoan parasite *Toxoplasma gondii*. This organism has a life cycle similar to that of the other important sporozoans affecting human beings, namely *Cryptosporidium parvum* and *Plasmodium* spp. It is acquired by ingestion of infected meat (asexual cycle) or cat feces (sexual cycle). The organism is spread in the blood, in the form of tachyzoites (Figure 65.2), and can be deposited in any tissue, where it forms cysts containing many bradyzoites (Figure 65.3). These can remain dormant indefinitely, but can become active and cause disease in immunocompromised hosts such as individuals with AIDS.

The fetus can be infected transplacentally if the mother is infected. The main clinical features in the fetus are brain disease (brain atrophy, hydrocephalus), ocular disease, and disease of reticuloendothelial system (hepatosplenomegaly and anemia).

The diagnosis is confirmed serologically. This requires the demonstration of IgM or IgA antibodies in the infant's blood. Although imaging of the brain may show areas of calcification and volume loss, this is not likely to be of value in managing the infant. Treatment has been shown to ameliorate the

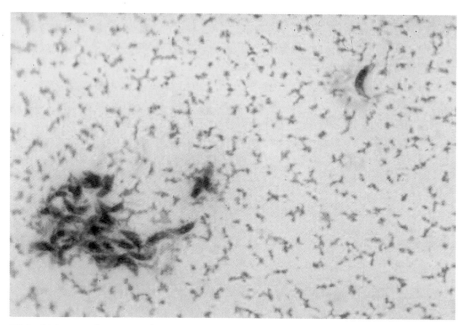

FIG. 65.2.   *Tachyzoites of* Toxoplasma gondii. *(Courtesy of Dr LL Moore, Jr, Centers for Disease Control and prevention)*

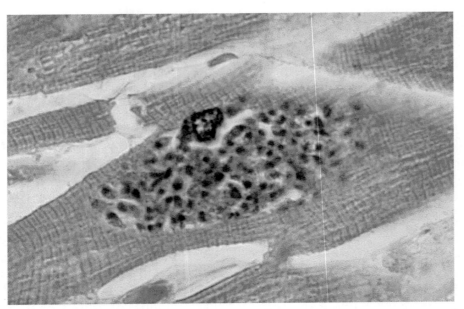

FIG. 65.3. *Bradyzoites of* Toxoplasma gondii *within a pseudocyst in cardiac muscle.*
(Courtesy of Dr Edwin P Ewing, Jr, Centers for Disease Control and Prevention)

disease or prevent progressive damage. This consists of a combination of pyrimethamine and sulfadiazine. Folinic acid supplements should be used concurrently to prevent folate deficiency.

Prevention depends on the mother avoiding eating undercooked meat and exposure to cat feces.

Reading:

Montoya JG, Liesenfeld O: Toxoplasmosis. Lancet 2004; 363: 1965–1976.

CASE 66. Maria Cortez, an 8-year-old girl, presents with a generalized seizure. She has a history of having had such seizures previously. Initially she is confused, but after a few hours she wakes up and then has a completely normal neurological and general examination.

- *What is your differential diagnosis?*
- *What risk factors for having seizures would you like to enquire about?*
- *What would you like to do?*

The differential diagnosis of seizures in a child can be considered in the following categories, shown in Table 66.1. Some of them can be eliminated from consideration on the basis of her rapid return to a normal state or her normal state prior to the event.

The patient's name suggests Hispanic ancestry and the possibility that she lived in Latin America.

Further history reveals that she grew up in Guatemala and has been in the United States for about 6 months.

In a patient presenting with a seizure, the most important aspects of management are to ensure that the patient has an adequate airway (A), is breathing adequately (B), has adequate circulation/perfusion (C), and an adequate blood glucose (dextrose) concentration (D).

In many parts of the world, including Latin America, one of the most common causes of seizures, where a cause is found, is neurocysticercosis, the larval stage of the pork tapeworm, *Taenia solium*. A computer tomography (CT) scan can demonstrate the cysts produced by these larvae. The CT scan of this patient's brain reveals multiple densities within the parenchyma, highly suggestive of this diagnosis (Figure 66.1).

■**TAB. 66.1: Differential diagnosis of seizures in a child.**

A. Structural abnormalities
      Cyst
      Lyssencephaly
B. Metabolic abnormality
      Hypoglycemia
      Hyponatremia
      Hypoxia
      Inborn metabolic error
C. Infection
      Meningitis
      Encephalitis
      Focal infection
         Brain abscess
         Neurocysticercosis
         Hydatid cyst
         Tuberculoma
D. Vascular lesion
      Arteriovenous malformation
      Vascular occlusion
      Hypoxic-ischemic insult (previous)
E. Neoplasm
F. Toxin/drug

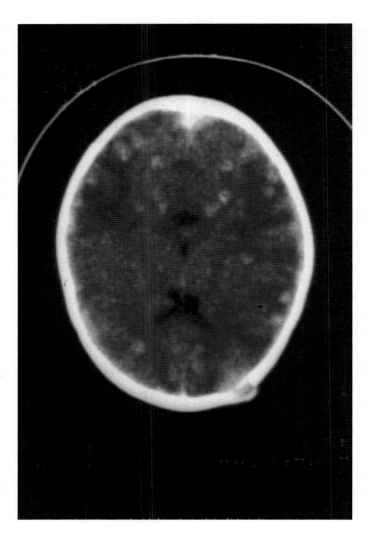

FIG. 66.1.   Computer tomography scan of the brain showing multiple cysts representing neurocysticercosis.

Cysticercosis is acquired in human beings when the human being acts as the intermediate host instead of the definitive host of *Taenia solium*. This means that the human is infected with the larva rather than the adult worm. The life cycle of the worm is as follows (Figure 66.2). The adult worm (in the human intestine) lays eggs, which are eaten by pigs, which are copraphagic. The eggs develop into larvae that penetrate the bowel mucosa, enter the portal blood, and become disseminated within the animal and form small cysts. When the uncooked pork is eaten by the human, the larvae grow into adult worms within the human intestine. If a human eats the feces (like the pig), it develops cysticercosis like the pig (Figure 66.2).

Life Cycle of *Taenia solium*

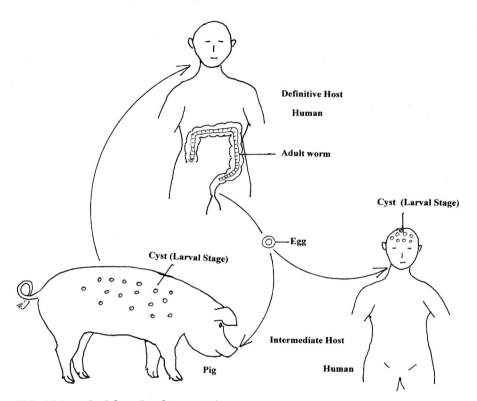

FIG. 66.2.   *The life cycle of* Taenia solium.

Therefore this disease is not due to eating uncooked pork but due to eating the feces (fecally contaminated food) of a person who has eaten un-cooked pork. Thus two conditions contribute toward the prevalence of this disease: (a) the eating of raw pork and (b) poor hygiene. The cysts often affect the brain. When the larvae die, the cyst contents leaks out, resulting in inflammation and focal edema, which results in many of the symptoms, including seizures.

Antimicrobial therapy with albendazole or praziquantel kills the larvae, which may lead to edema around the cyst. Therefore therapy has been controversial, the controversy revolving around whether treatment is bene-ficial or deleterious. Currently therapy is favored. If there are many cysts, corticosteroids (e.g. dexamethasone) should be given simultaneously with antimicrobial therapy to reduce cerebral edema.

Reading:

Garcia HH, Gonzalez AE, Evans CAW et al: *Taenia solium* cysticercosis. Lancet 2003; 361: 547–556.

CASE 67. Farouk Mahmoud, a 10-year-old boy, presents with a 1-month history of passing blood on urination. There is no history of fever. On examination he is completely normal. You collect urine from him in the examination room and notice something very interesting. At the beginning of urination the urine appears normal, but toward the end of urination it becomes red.

- *Where is the likely site of disease?*
- *What is its likely cause?*

This symptom is called terminal hematuria. It indicates pathology within the bladder. The differential diagnosis includes cystitis, a papilloma, and schistomiasis. The history alone might give a clue to the specific diagnosis. The patient's name suggests that he might be from North Africa or the Middle East.

He is, in fact, from Egypt, where schistosomiasis is very common. This is the cause of his illness. This fluke (trematode) infection is prevalent in most of Africa, parts of South America, and southeast Asia. It is one of the major global health problems. Several species of schistosome affect human beings. Their life cycle, which involves fresh water, is as follows.

Eggs are passed in urine or feces into fresh water, where the eggs hatch. The miracidia that are released enter a specific water snail where they multiply. The stage that emerges from the snail, the cercaria, requires a vertebrate host within 24 hours. The cercaria enter the vertebrate host through the skin, and travel through the lymphatics to the circulation whence they reach the respective venous plexuses (superior mesenteric in the case of *S. mansoni*, inferior mesenteric and superior hemorrhoidal in the case of *S. japonicum*, and vesical and periureteral in the case of *S. haematobium*), where they mature and mate. The female lays hundreds of eggs per day. While the female is attached to the wall of the venule, the eggs burrow through the wall of the respective organ (bowel in the case of *S. mansoni*, *S. japonicum*, and *S. mekongi*, or bladder in the in the case of *S. haematobium*). When she detaches herself from the endothelium, they are carried proximally to the liver.

The pathology is caused primarily by the eggs, which become trapped in tissue, and around which granulomas are formed (Figure 67.1). In the

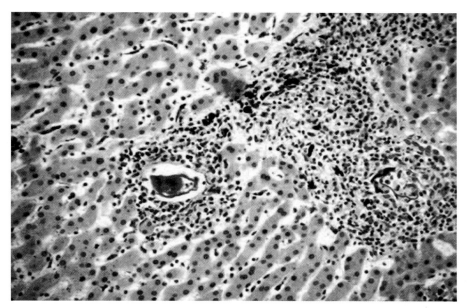

FIG. 67.1.   *The histology of schistosomiasis of the liver. Note the inflammation around the egg. (Courtesy of Dr Carlos Abramowsky, Emory University)*

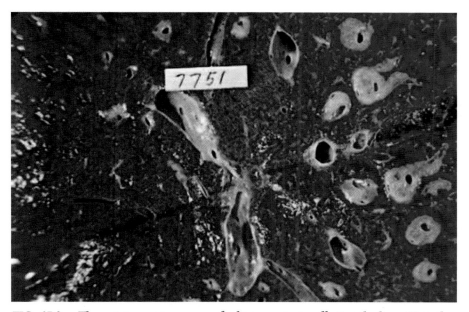

FIG. 67.2.   *The autopsy appearance of schistosomiasis affecting the liver. Note the "pipestem" fibrosis around the veins. (Courtesy of Dr Carlos Abramowsky, Emory University)*

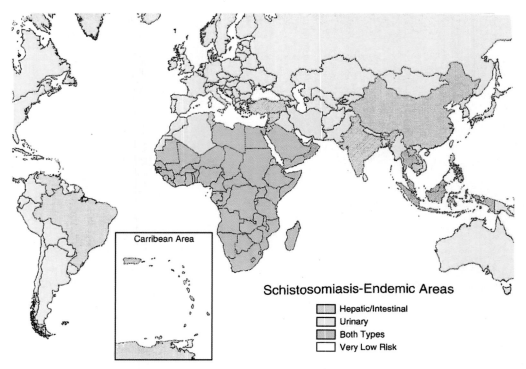

FIG. 67.3. Countries in which schistosomiasis occurs. (from Centers for Disease Control and Prevention. Health Information for International Travel 2005–2006. Atlanta: US Department of Health and Human Services. Public Health Service, 2005)

■TAB. 67.1: **Species, geographic distribution, venous plexus and organs affected, complications, and therapy of different schistosome infections.**

Species	Geography	Venous plexus	Organs	Complications	Therapy
S. mansoni	Africa	intestinal	liver, lung	portal hypertension	praziquantel
	S. America			pulmonary hypertension	oxamniquine
S. japonicum	East Asia	intestinal	"	"	praziquantel
S. mekongii	SE Asia	intestinal	"	"	praziquantel
S. haematobium	Africa		urinary bladder	urinary tract obstruction	praziquantel

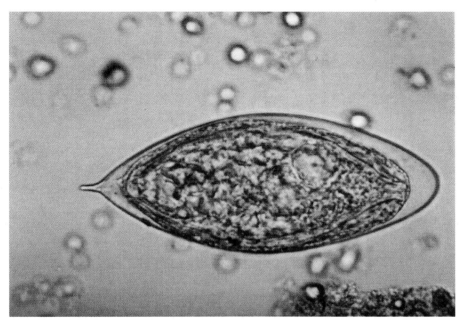

FIG. 67.4.   Microscopic appearance of Schistosoma haematobium *egg. Note the characteristic terminal spine. (Courtesy of the Centers for Disease Control and Prevention)*

liver this results in fibrosis (Figure 67.2) and the development of portal hypertension, while in the urinary tract this results in bladder scarring, urinary tract obstruction, and, ultimately, can lead to bladder cancer.

The world distribution of schistosomiasis is shown in the map (Figure 67.3), and the venous plexuses and organs that they affect, complications, and therapy are shown in Table 67.1.

The diagnosis of schistosomiasis is preferably made by the demonstration of ova in excreta, either urine, in the case of *S. haematobium* infection (Figure 67.4), or the stool in the cases of infection caused by the other species. Sometimes rectal biopsy is necessary to confirm the diagnosis of infection caused by non-haematobium species. Serology can demonstrate evidence of previous infection. The additional value of microscopy for ova is that the viability of the ova can be determined.

Antimicrobial treatment of the different species is shown in Table 67.1. In highly endemic areas, periodic mass population treatment is also used.

Reading:

Allen R, Bartley PB, Sleigh AC et al: Current concepts: schistosomiasis. N Engl J Med 2002; 346: 1212–1220.

Vennervald B, Dunne DW: Morbidity in Schisosomiasis: an update. Curr Opinion Infect Dis 2004; 17: 439–447.

CASE 68. A 3-year-old girl presents with difficulty breathing and fever. On examination she is found to be hypoxic and to have diffuse wheezing and crackles in her lungs. A blood count reveals a total leukocyte count of 20,000/mm^3 with 50% eosinophils, 25% neutrophils, and 25% lymphocytes.

- *What is your differential diagnosis?*
- *What would you do?*

This child has the clinical features of pneumonia together with airway obstruction. This might be caused by an infection or a hypersensitivity reaction. Her marked eosinophilia strongly suggests that she has a worm infection, although a hypersensitivity pneumonitis should still be considered. Further history should explore possible exposures to (i) worms: Does she eat or play in soil where animals or other human beings might have defecated? (ii) Is she exposed to moldy vegetation or dust from bird feathers?

Several intestinal roundworms affect the lung because, during their larval stage, they pass through this organ. Human beings become infected by eating soil contaminated with feces from infected animals or other human beings. The most important of these are the human, dog, and cat ascarids, namely *Ascaris lumbricoides*, *Toxocara canis*, and *Toxocara cati*, respectively. The dog and cat ascarids as well as the raccoon ascarid *Baylisascaris procyonis* cannot complete their life cycles in humans beings. The larval stages travel through the viscera but cannot reach the intestine. During this migration through the viscera, a condition called "visceral larva migrans," they can cause severe pneumonitis (as in this case) and affect the brain (particularly in the case of *B. procyonis*, which causes a severe encephalitis) and the eye, where they cause focal nodular lesions that can resemble retinoblastoma. The liver and spleen also may be enlarged. Children are the main victims because they play in contaminated dirt and lick their fingers. The diagnosis should be suspected in individuals with visceral disease and marked eosinophilia. Confirmation is not usually necessary but can be accomplished by serology.

Therapy should be supportive, for example with oxygen, and antimicrobial, namely with the antihelminthic agent albendazole.

Reading:

Despommier D: Toxocariasis: clinical aspects, epidemiology, medical ecology, and molecular aspects. Clin Microbiol Rev 2003; 16: 265–272.

Sorvillo F, Ash LR, Berlin OG et al: *Baylisascaris procyonis*: an emerging helminthic zoonosis. Emerging Infect Dis 2002; 8: 355–359.

CASE 69. A 16-year-old Mexican immigrant to the United States presents with a history of fatigue, headache, and weight loss for 2 weeks. On examination his height is 157 cm (<5th percentile), his weight is 51 kg (10th percentile), and he is afebrile. The rest of his examination is normal. A blood count reveals a hemoglobin concentration of 9.9 g/dl, an MCV of 61 fL, and a total leukocyte count of 10.9×10^6/l, with a differential count of 13% neutrophils, 30% lymphocytes, and 57% eosinophils.

* *What might explain these findings?*
* *What would you do?*

This patient has a microcytic anemia and marked eosinophilia (eosinophil count = 6200×10^6/l, normal <400). The most likely cause of marked eosinophilia is a worm infection. The anemia could be due to chronic infection, lead poisoning, nutritional iron deficiency, or blood loss. A unifying diagnosis is a worm infection that consumes blood. Hookworm infection could explain this. Therefore the stool should be examined for worm ova. This patient's stool contained many hookworm ova, with the appearance of that seen in Figure 69.1 (from a different patient).

He was treated with mebendazole, which was followed by a rapid drop in his eosinophil count.

Hookworms have a worldwide distribution. Two species infect human beings, *Ancylostoma duodenale* and *Necator americanum*. The adult worms attach themselves to the small bowel mucosa and suck blood, which results in blood loss and consequent protein and iron deficiency. The life cycle is as follows: the adult female worm lays eggs that pass out in the stool. In the soil the eggs hatch, giving rise to rhabditiform larvae. These undergo two molts, giving rise to filariform larvae, which enter the skin of a passing host. The larvae enter the circulation, pass through the lungs, where they break out of the circulation, ascend up the respiratory tract, and are swallowed. In the small intestine they undergo two further molts, becoming adults. Diagnosis, as in this case, depends on visualization of the eggs in a stool specimen. Treatment consists of albendazole, mebendazole, or pyrantel pamoate. Prevention requires use of latrines, so that individuals do not walk where others have defecated.

Hookworms of dogs and cats, for example, *Ancylostoma braziliense*, cannot complete their life cycle in human beings, and, after entry into the human skin, wander around the skin producing a serpiginous track of

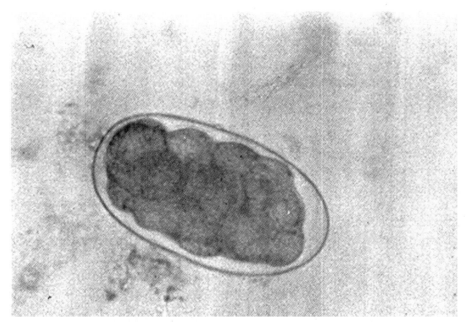

FIG. 69.1. A hookworm egg, containing an embryo. (From: Schneierson SS: Atlas of Diagnostic Microbiology. Publ: Abbott Laboratories, 1965, with permission.)

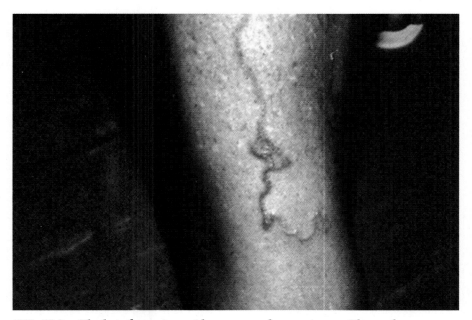

FIG. 69.2. The leg of a patient with cutaneous larva migrans. The erythematous line represents the inflammation along the track made by the migrating worm, not the worm itself.

inflammation that causes an intense itch. This condition is called cutaneous larva migrans or "creeping eruption" (Figure 69.2). The treatment consists of oral albendazole or ivermectin, or topically applied thiabendazole.

Reading:

Hotez PJ, Brooker S, Bethony JM et al: Hookworm infection. N Engl J Med 2004; 351: 799–807.

Bethony J, Brooker S, Albonico M et al: Soil-transmitted helminth infection: ascariasis, trichuriasis, and hookworm. Lancet 2006; 367: 1521–1532.

CASE 70. A 6-year-old Liberian girl presents with a swelling on her head. A dermoid cyst is diagnosed and removed. The histology is shown in Figure 70.1.

What is the diagnosis?

The histological section shows multiple cross sections of one or more worms. The multiplicity of cross sections suggests that the worms are curled up ("volved"). Considering that the patient came from Liberia, this suggests the presence of *Onchocerca volvulus*, the cause of onchocerciasis or river

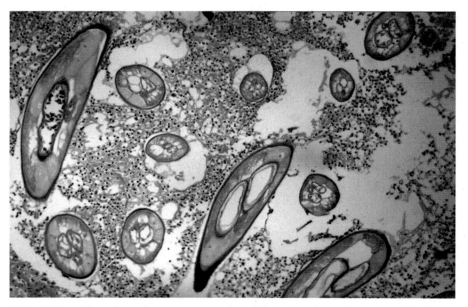

FIG. 70.1. *A histological section, stained with hematoxylin and eosin, of the "cyst."*

blindness. This filarial worm is endemic in parts of West Africa and Central America. The life cycle of the parasite is as follows: the vector is a black fly of the genus *Simulium*. It lives along the banks of rapidly flowing rivers and streams, hence "river blindness." When a fly bites a human being, larvae enter the subcutaneous tissue, where they mature into adults (both sexes) that become loculated within a nodule. The female produces microfilaria, which are infectious for the fly. The microfilariae are the cause of injury. They migrate through the skin, causing inflammation, and can reach the eye. They can migrate through any part of the eye, causing inflammation and blindness (Figure 70.2).

The increased chance of ocular damage with increasing age leads to the common sight in endemic areas of a child leading a blind adult (Figure 70.3).

The adult worms cannot readily be eliminated, but the microfilaria can be killed with ivermectin. This should be administered every 6–12 months for several years. Recent work has demonstrated that bacterial endosymbionts, *Wolbachia* spp., living within the parasites, are necessary for filarial fertility. They also play a role in the inflammation caused by the microfilaria. These

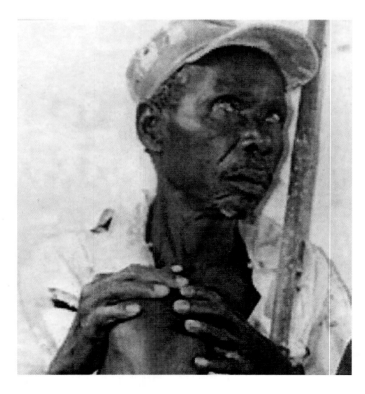

FIG. 70.2.   A 60-year-old man with blindness caused by onchocerciasis (with permission of The Carter Center/E Staub)

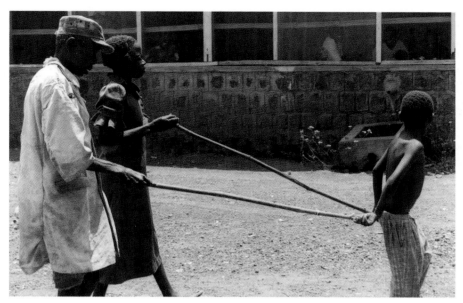

FIG. 70.3.   A child leading blind adults in Sudan. (with permission of The Carter Center/E Staub)

are targets for new modes of anti-onchocerca therapy, including doxycycline and azithromycin.

Reading:

Hoerauf A, Buttner DW, Adjei O, and Pearlman E: Onchocerciasis. Br Med J 2003; 326: 207–210.

Ryan ET, Felsenstein D, Aquino SL et al: Case 39-2005: A 63-year-old woman with a positive serologic test for syphilis and persistent eosinophilia. N Engl J Med 2005; 353: 2697–2705.

CASE 71. An 18-month-old child is found removing worms from his nose (Figure 71.1).

- *What are the worms?*
- *How did they get there?*
- *What complications could such worms cause?*

These worms are *Ascaris lumbricoides*, the human ascarid worm. Ascaris is one of the most common infections of humankind. Although visualizing such worms may be disturbing, they seldom cause problems. The life cycle

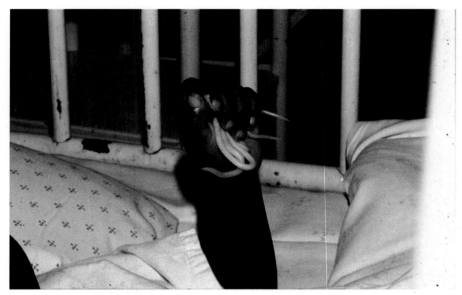

FIG. 71.1. The worms that the child had pulled out of his nose.

is as follows. The adult worm lives in the human intestine, where the female lays eggs, which are passed in the stool. These are very hardy and can remain viable in soil for prolonged periods. After the eggs are ingested, the larvae hatch in the small intestine. They pass through the intestinal mucosa and enter the circulation, which carries them to the lungs. There they break out of the circulation into the alveoli and ascend up the airway and are ultimately swallowed, finding their way back into the small intestine where they mature into adult worms, completing the cycle.

During the migrating stage they can cause severe pneumonitis (see Case 68). As with other worm infections, the development of symptoms depends on the number of worms in the host ("worm burden"), which, in turn, depends on the number of eggs (in this case) or larvae (e.g. schistosomiasis) entering the host. (This is different from protozoal infections in which case the parasite multiplies within the host.) Ascaris worms live in the small bowel. If there are many worms, they can cause intestinal obstruction. They can also migrate, for example up the bile duct, pancreatic duct, or esophagus (as in this case).

Diagnosis depends on direct visualization of the adult worm or microscopical visualization of the eggs in the stool (Figure 71.2).

Treatment of ascariasis consists of albendazole, mebendazole, or ivermectin.

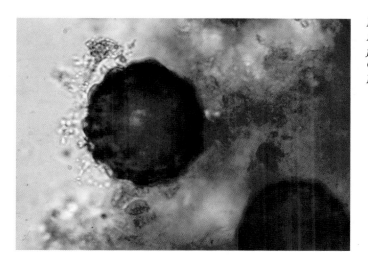

FIG. 71.2. An egg of Ascaris lumbricoides *in feces. (Courtesy of Dr Carlos Abramowsky, Emory University)*

Reading:

Bethony J, Brooker S, Albonico M et al: Soil-transmitted helminth infections: ascaris, trichuris, and hookworm. Lancet 2006; 367: 1521–1532.

CASE 72. A 2-year-old boy has been transferred to a tertiary care hospital with the following history: 2 weeks ago he became ill. He was diagnosed with otitis media and treated with amoxicillin. A week later he had not improved, but the treatment was continued. Another week later he became drowsy. He was transferred because of abnormal computer tomography (CT) scan and cerebrospinal fluid (CSF) findings. On examination he is very wasted and responds only to painful stimuli. He has no neck stiffness. The tone and deep tendon reflexes are increased and Babinski responses are present bilaterally. The pupils react to light only sluggishly, and a unilateral 6th nerve palsy is present. The lungs have crackles on the right side. The rest of the examination is normal.

- *Where is the disease?*
- *What is the differential diagnosis?*
- *What is the most likely diagnosis, and what is its pathogenesis?*
- *What would you do?*

The history suggests a subacute or chronic process. This patient has a disease affecting several parts of his brain: the sensorium, long tracts, and cranial nerves (II and/or III; VI). This must be due to either raised intracranial pressure, with falsely localizing signs affecting the III and VI nerves, or to a diffuse disease affecting multiple sites, including the cranial nerves. Only some form of meningitis can cause the latter. The absence of papilledema in a patient with a subacute or chronic illness argues against raised intracranial pressure as the cause of the clinical findings. Therefore the likely pathological diagnosis is *chronic meningitis*. The causes of chronic meningitis include tuberculosis (the most important), acute bacterial meningitis for which the patient has not received treatment, fungi, syphilis, systemic lupus erythematosus, and malignancies. Additional history may be helpful. The most important questions are related to possible tuberculosis exposures. These include the following: exposure to adults with tuberculosis, chronic cough, HIV infection, those who are immigrants, and those who have been incarcerated.

This child's uncle, who had suffered from AIDS, had died from tuberculosis 3 weeks earlier. This history makes the diagnosis of tuberculous meningitis (TBM) almost certain.

Management:

(a) supportive – this might entail artificial ventilation, as became necessary in this child.

(b) surgery – determine whether there is a neurosurgically correctible problem, for example, hydrocephalus, by performing a computer tomography (CT) scan. This showed marked hydrocephalus (Figure 72.1); the child therefore underwent ventricular drainage.

(c) Make a diagnosis:

(i) Chest X ray – to look for evidence of tuberculosis. Although the chest X ray might be normal in a case of tuberculous meningitis, it might show evidence of tuberculosis, including hilar lymphadenopathy, pulmonary infiltrates, diffuse mottling due to miliary tuberculosis, or pulmonary cavitation. This child's X ray is shown in Figure 72.2. It shows a right upper lobe cavity as well as a miliary pattern (which is not readily appreciated in the reproduction of the picture).

(ii) Obtain lumbar cerebrospinal fluid (CSF) for examination. In chronic meningitis the CSF pleocytosis usually shows a lymphocyte predominance, although early in the course of tuberculous meningitis it may show a neutrophil predominance. The protein concentration is elevated and the glucose concentration decreased. If there is significant arachnoiditis, there may be a block of CSF flow within the lumbar subarachnoid space (spinal block). If this occurs the protein concentration of lumbar CSF may be extremely high (1000–2000 mg/dl) and may produce a clot within the tube containing the CSF. If leukocytes are trapped within this clot, the cell

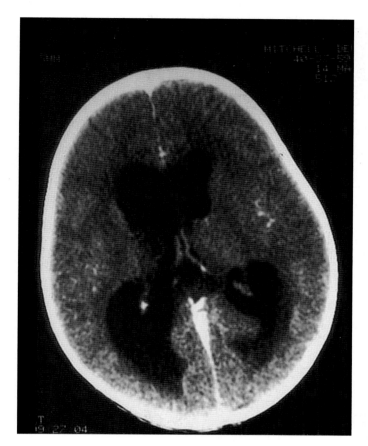

FIG. 72.1.   The head computer tomography scan of the patient, showing hydrocephalus and contrast enhancement of the basal meninges.

count will be falsely reduced. When TBM is suspected it is very important that a tube of CSF (5–10 ml) be sent to the laboratory specifically for culture for *Mycobacterium tuberculosis*.

In this patient the CSF revealed the following:

leukocyte count 126 cells/μl, with a differential count of 3 % neutrophils, 93 % lymphocytes, and 4% monocytes;

protein concentration 240 mg/dl and glucose concentration 16 mg/dl.

The culture was ultimately positive for *M. tuberculosis*.

(iii) Obtain sputum for microscopy and culture for *M. tuberculosis*. Because sputum cannot usually be obtained from children, early morning gastric washings should be used. If the child is ventilated, as was the case in this child, endotracheal aspirates should be used.

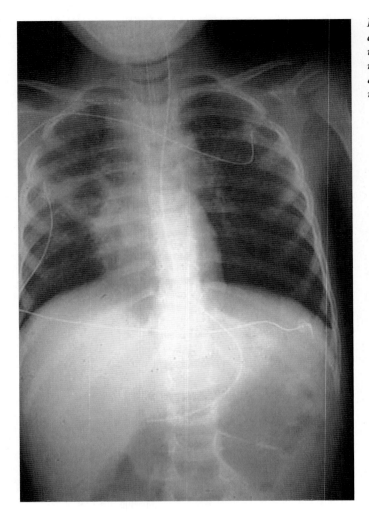

FIG. 72.2.   The child's chest X ray, showing a right upper lobe cavity. (The miliary pattern cannot be appreciated in the reproduction of the X ray.)

Tests for other causes of chronic meningitis:

Culture of the CSF for bacteria and fungi
Antigen test for *Cryptococcus neoformans*
Venereal Disease Research Laboratory test (VDRL) for syphilis
Cytopathology for malignant cells

(d) Antimicrobial therapy – Initially there may be some concern about the possibility of a chronic bacterial meningitis (acute bacterial meningitis for which the patient has not been treated). In this case antibacterial therapy should be instituted, such as with vancomycin and ceftriaxone. The treatment of tuberculous meningitis is the same as for other forms of tuberculosis, except that treatment should be extended for 9–12 months instead of

6 months. Treatment should be directly observed by a health-care worker (DOT). It should consist of the following drugs: isoniazid, rifampin, and pyrazinamide, daily for 2 months. After this period pyrazinamide should be discontinued and isoniazid and rifampin continued twice weekly. If there is a possibility of drug resistance, which is the case in most circumstances, a fourth drug (ethambutol or streptomycin) should also be used. Therefore it is very important to try to obtain cultures from the patient and the source patient in order to test for antimicrobial susceptibility.

(e) Antiinflammatory therapy – Corticosteroid therapy should be considered. Although this is somewhat controversial, I recommend its use, in the form of prednisone 2 mg/kg/day for about 6 weeks.

(f) Public health – The local health department should be contacted to trace the source and other contacts of the source. To prevent spread within the hospital, chest X rays must be performed on all family members who will be present in hospital. Anyone with an abnormal X ray must be excluded from the hospital.

Tuberculous meningitis (TBM) results from hematogenous spread of *Mycobacterium tuberculosis* organisms to the brain. There they cause subpial tubercles (Rich's foci). These can rupture into the subarachnoid space,

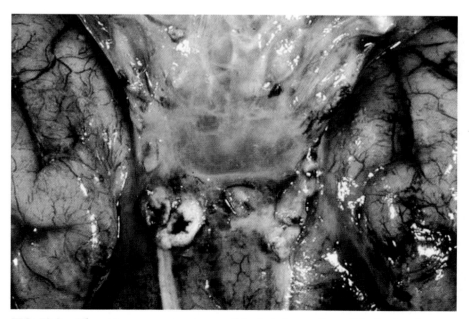

FIG. 72.3. *The appearance at autopsy of the inferior surface of the brain of a patient with tuberculous meningitis. (Courtesy of Dr Carlos Abramowsky, Emory University)*

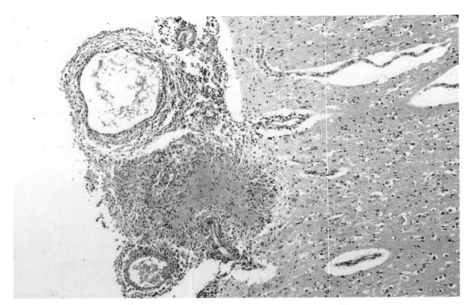

FIG. 72.4.   *The histology of tuberculous meningitis. Note the brain tissue on the right and the granulomatous inflammation on the left. (Courtesy of Dr Carlos Abramowsky, Emory University)*

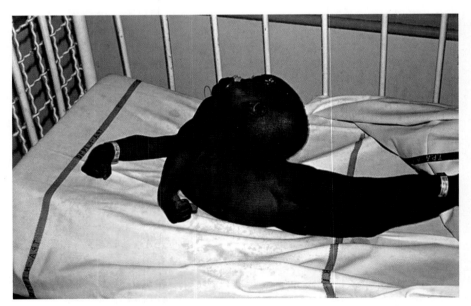

FIG. 72.5.   *A child with stage III tuberculous meningitis, showing opisthotonus.*

resulting in inflammation throughout the space, which is particularly severe in the basal meninges (Figures 72.3 and 72.4).

Because the main cerebral vessels and the cranial nerves traverse this area they are often injured by this process. In addition, the CSF pathways may be obstructed resulting in hydrocephalus, as seen this patient.

TBM can be categorized into three clinical stages, with progressively worse prognoses. Stage I: headache, malaise – no neurological signs; Stage II: neurological signs – hemiplegia, depressed level of consciousness, cranial nerve abnormalities such as poorly reactive pupils, paralysis of extraocular muscles; Stage III – coma (Figure 72.5, not this patient).

The patient presented above was in stage III.

Reading:

Smith KC: Tuberculosis in children. Curr Probl Pediatr. January 2001; 5–30.

Donald PR, Beyers N: Tuberculosis in Childhood. In: Davies PDO (editor). Clinical Tuberculosis. 2nd edition. Chapman and Hall Medical. London, 1998.

Small PM, Fujiwara PI: Management of tuberculosis in the United States. N Engl J Med 2001; 345: 189–200.

Thwaites GE: Tuberculous meningitis: many questions, too few answers. Lancet Neurology 2005; 4: 160–170.

CASE 73. An 18-month-old child, receiving treatment for miliary tuberculosis, presents with respiratory difficulty. On examination there is tachypnea, the lungs are resonant to percussion, and there are decreased breath sounds over the left lower lobe. The trachea is slightly deviated toward the right.

- *What are the causes of a localized area of decreased breath sounds?*
- *What is the pathogenesis of tuberculosis and how might it explain the clinical findings?*

The causes of decreased breath sounds and their associated clinical findings are shown in Table 73.1.

The pathogenesis of tuberculosis is as follows (see Figure 73.1 a–c):

1. The pathogen (*Mycobacterium tuberculosis*) is inhaled and enters the alveoli of the lung, where it is ingested by pulmonary macrophages but

■TAB. 73.1: Causes of localized decreased breath sounds and associated findings.

Abnormality	Percussion	Mediastinal shift
Lobar consolidation	dull	none
Collapse	dull	toward affected side
Obstruction (partial)	resonant	away from affected side
Obstruction (complete)	see collapse	
Pleural fluid	very dull	away from affected side
Pneumothorax	resonant	away from affected side

Pathogenesis of Pulmonary Tuberculosis in Children I

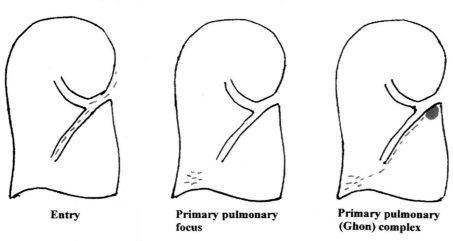

Entry   Primary pulmonary   Primary pulmonary
                     focus   (Ghon) complex

FIG. 73.1a.   The initial stages of the pathogenesis of tuberculosis.

not killed. An area of inflammation develops. This is called the primary focus.

2. The macrophages carry the organism to the hilar lymph nodes. The primary focus and the lymph node infection together constitute the primary (Ghon) complex.

3. Each of these foci may heal or may progress as follows:

   (a) the primary focus to pneumonia,

   (b) the lymph node enlarging to obstruct the bronchus or erode through the bronchus.

4. At any time organisms may enter the bloodstream and be deposited anywhere in the body.

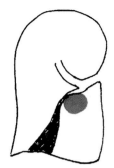
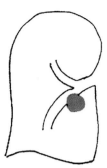
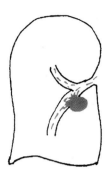

**Lymphadenopathy
With bronchial obstruction**

**Endobronchial
tuberculosis**

**Bronchogenic
spread**

FIG. 73.1b.   Subsequent stages of the pathogenesis of tuberculosis.

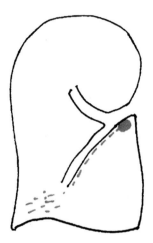
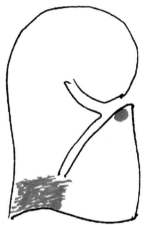
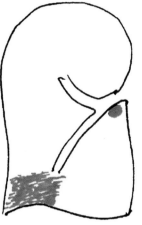

*FIG. 73.1c.   The
pathogenesis of progressive
primary tuberculosis.*

Primary complex

**Progressive primary
pulmonary tuberculosis**

*FIG. 73.2.   Chest X ray
showing increased lucency
and hyperinflation in the
left lower zone.*

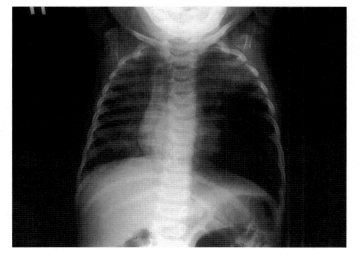

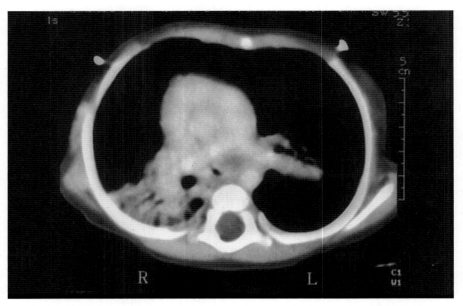

FIG. 73.3.   A computer tomography scan showing the left main bronchus markedly narrowed by lymphoid tissue.

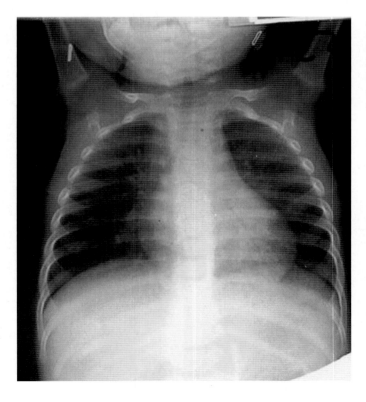

FIG. 73.4.   Chest X ray of a child with pulmonary tuberculosis, showing narrowing of the left main bronchus that could be easily missed on examination of the X ray.

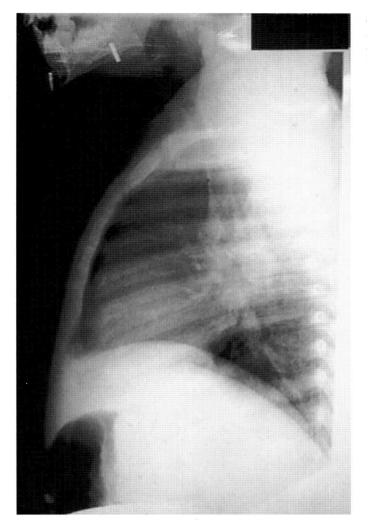

FIG. 73.5.   Lateral chest X ray of the same child showing hilar lymphadenopathy.

5. When large numbers of organisms enter the bloodstream, constituting tuberculous bacteremia, they may establish multiple foci of inflammation in many organs. These foci, called "tubercles," have the appearance of millet seeds, giving rise to the term miliary tuberculosis.

This child's trachea is shifted toward the right (away from the affected side) indicating a partial obstruction or a pneumothorax. The clinical background of tuberculosis suggests that there is probably an enlarged mediastinal lymph node partially obstructing the left lower lobe bronchus resulting in hyperinflation of that area of the lung. Such nodes may enlarge after the initiation of antituberculous therapy. This was confirmed by X ray and a computer tomography scan (see Figures 73.2 and 73.3).

She improved after corticosteroid therapy was instituted.

Many of the clinical features of tuberculosis in children are due to enlargement of hilar lymph nodes. This is not the case in adults. Because enlarged lymph nodes are *easier* (*not easy*) to visualize on a lateral chest X ray than on a posterior-anterior (PA) view, it is very important to obtain both PA and lateral films when evaluating a child for tuberculosis. This is illustrated by the following case. The chest X ray shown in Figure 73.4 might easily be thought to be normal, although narrowing of the left main bronchus can be seen behind the heart. However, on the lateral X ray (Figure 73.5) hilar lymph nodes can be readily seen.

Reading:

Frieden TR, Sterling TR, Munsiff SS et al: Tuberculosis. Lancet 2003; 362: 887–899.

CASE 74. An 11-year-old boy with advanced HIV disease is admitted to hospital with a 2-week history of weight loss and fever. He also has a cough. He has not been taking antiretroviral therapy. On examination he is very thin and has decreased breath sounds over the left lower lobe. Chest X rays taken 1 year before this admission and on this admission are shown in Figures 74.1 and 74.2, respectively.

- *What are the radiological findings?*
- *How would you evaluate him further?*

The initial X ray is normal. The current X ray shows pleural thickening on the left side, both laterally and medially (difficult to visualize medially). This pleural disease is most likely due to a chronic infection such as tuberculosis or other mycobacterial infection, or a fungal infection such as histoplasmosis. A computer tomography (CT) scan of the chest would be helpful to elucidate abnormalities within the mediastinum. This reveals massive lymph nodes in the mediastinum (Figure 74.3).

This finding suggests the possibility of lymphoma but is compatible with tuberculosis or other chronic infection. Making a definitive diagnosis in this case is essential for providing appropriate therapy and requires a biopsy. Although gastric washings showed acid-fast bacilli, given his immunocompromised state, this might not have explained his illness. A CT-guided percutaneous biopsy of the mediastinal nodes revealed granulomas containing acid-fast bacilli, which subsequently grew out *Mycobacterium tuberculosis*,

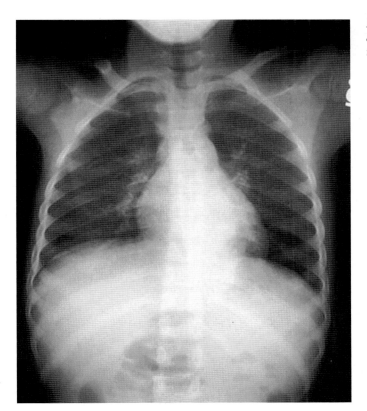

FIG. 74.1. The child's chest X ray 1 year before this presentation.

confirming the diagnosis of tuberculosis. The gastric washing isolate grew out *Mycobacterium avium* complex.

He was treated with isoniazid, rifabutin, pyrazinamide, and ethambutol, and antiretroviral therapy was initiated. A gastrostomy tube was also placed to facilitate continuous night-time feeds. His clinical condition improved markedly.

Tuberculosis in patients with HIV infection is associated with several specific problems:

(a) increased risk of tuberculous disease in individuals infected with *Mycobacterium tuberculosis*;

(b) atypical presentation of tuberculosis: this includes primary tuberculosis type of disease in adults, noncavitary pulmonary disease in adults (with lower contagiousness), a higher rate of extrapulmonary and disseminated disease, and more rapid progression of disease;

(c) a wide differential diagnosis of opportunistic lung infections;

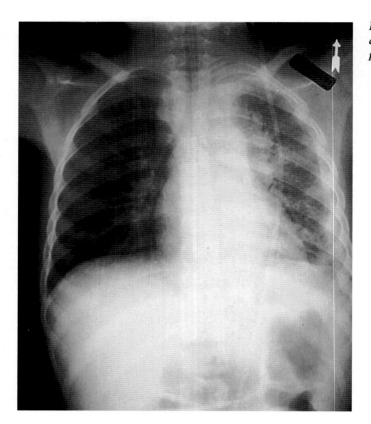

FIG. 74.2.   The child's chest X ray on this presentation.

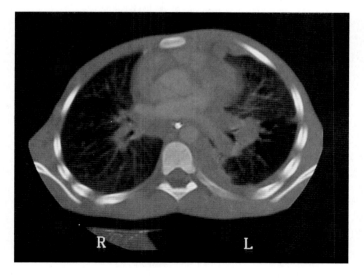

FIG. 74.3.   Chest computer tomography scan showing markedly enlarged anterior mediastinal lymph nodes.

(d) drug interactions between antituberculosis therapy, especially rifa-mycins, and antiretroviral therapy, especially protease inhibitors;

(e) a high rate of adverse drug reactions to antituberculosis medications;

(f) the immune reconstitution syndrome, manifesting with evidence of worsening tuberculous disease, in individuals receiving highly active antiretroviral therapy (HAART).

Reading:

Harries AD: The association between HIV and tuberculosis in the developing world with a specific focus on sub-Saharan Africa In: Davies PDO (editor): Clinical Tuberculosis. 3rd edition. Arnold, London, 1994, pp. 253–277.

Pzniak A: The association between HIV and tuberculosis in industrialized countries In: Davies PDO (editor): Clinical Tuberculosis. 3rd edition. Arnold, London, 1994, pp. 278–293.

CASE 75. A 2-year-old boy is diagnosed with probable tuberculous meningitis 1 day after admission to a pediatric intensive care unit.

- *What public health procedures should be performed regarding this patient?*

The goals:

(a) to identify who was the source of this patient's infection (most likely an adult such as a parent). This will allow for:

(b) tracing of other potential victims of spread from that source;

(c) treatment of the source case to prevent morbidity or mortality of the case; and

(d) prevention of further spread to other individuals.

Other contacts should undergo tuberculin skin testing. Those who are skin test positive (PPD ≥ 5 mm diameter) should have a chest X ray. Those with evidence of tuberculosis should be treated with a multidrug regimen. Children <5 years with skin test positivity only (normal chest X ray) should be treated with isoniazid only for 9 months (treatment of latent tuberculosis infection (LTBI)). Children <5 years with a negative skin test might still have become infected without having had enough time for development of a positive skin test. Therefore they should also receive isoniazid. If a repeat skin test performed 3 months later remains negative, isoniazid therapy may be discontinued. The

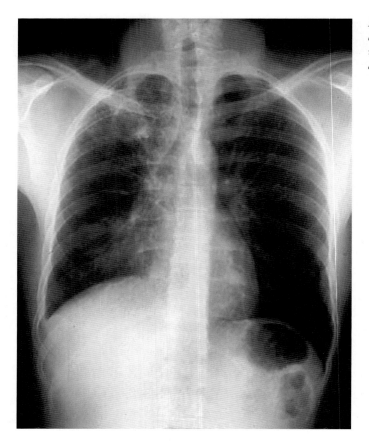

FIG. 75.1. The father's chest X ray, showing right upper lobe disease with a cavity.

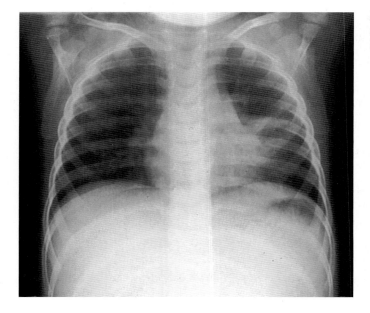

FIG. 75.2. The sibling's chest X ray, showing left lingular disease.

contact tracing and management should be done by the local health department. Therefore cases of tuberculosis must be notified to this department.

Within a hospital an infectious contact can continue to spread infection. Therefore all visitors who are potential sources of infection should have chest X rays performed, and only those with negative X rays should be allowed into the hospital. (The PPD status of visitors is of no importance regarding their contagiousness.) The most important individuals within this category are the parents. During this investigation, the patient should be nursed with airborne precautions (negative pressure room and 95 N masks).

The chest X rays of this patient's father and sibling are shown in Figures 75.1 and 75.2, respectively.

The father had a cavity in the right upper lobe, suggesting pulmonary tuberculosis with significant contagiousness. He was therefore the likely source of the index patient's infection. The sibling had an area of consolidation in the left lingula, probably representing pulmonary tuberculosis. Thus the diagnosis of tuberculosis in the index patient represented a sentinel event for the diagnosis of two other cases, namely the source case and another victim.

CASE 76. A 12-year-old boy presents with a history of neck pain for several months. On examination he is found to have an abnormal angulation at the lower end of his cervical spine (Figure 76.1). The rest of his examination is normal.

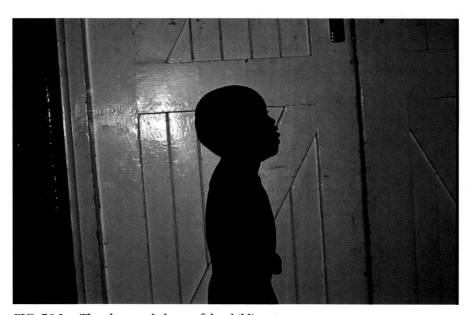

FIG. 76.1.   The abnormal shape of the child's spine.

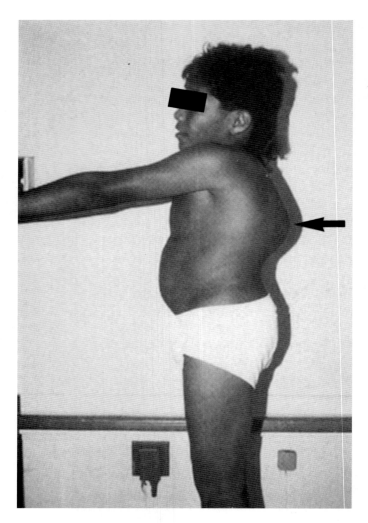

FIG. 76.2. A marked thoracic gibbus. (Reprinted, with permission, from: Shaw, B: Pott's disease with paraparesis. N Engl J Med 1996; 334: 958. Copyright © 1998 Massachusetts Medical Society. All rights reserved.)

- *What is the likely cause of this?*
- *What should be done?*

This child has collapse of one of the cervical vertebra. This is likely due to tuberculosis of the spine (tuberculous spondylitis, Pott's disease). The infecting organism reaches the spine hematogenously and results in destruction of the bone and intervertebral disc. The destruction of the vertebra and subsequent collapse, lead to the angulation of the spine called a gibbus (from the Latin for hump) (Figures 76.2 and 76.3).

The infection can extend into the tissues around the spine, resulting in, for example, a psoas abscess from lumbar disease and a retropharyngeal abscess

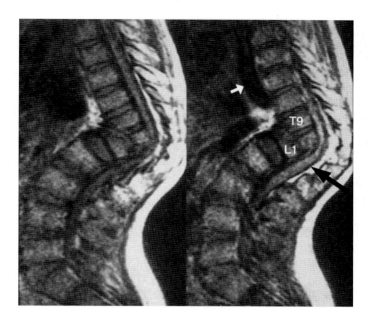

FIG. 76.3. Magnetic resonance imaging of the patient shown in Figure 76.2, showing vertebral destruction due to tuberculosis. (Reprinted with permission from: Shaw B: Pott's disease with paraparesis. N Engl J Med 1998; 334: 958. Copyright © 1998 Massachusetts Medical Society. All rights reserved.)

from cervical disease. Spinal cord damage causing paraplegia can complicate spinal tuberculosis. It usually results from extension of the infection into the spinal epidural space causing cord compression or from vascular injury and infarction, although vertebral collapse with dislocation can cause cord injury.

Management should entail attempts to confirm an etiological diagnosis by chest X ray and PPD, and antimicrobial therapy. Obtaining material for making a diagnosis from the site of disease can sometimes be accomplished using imaging guidance. This is particularly important when diseases other than tuberculosis are considered likely. Treatment consists primarily of antituberculosis therapy for 9–12 months. The role of surgery is controversial. The main indications for surgery are spinal instability and significant neurological deficit.

Reading:

Boachie-Adjei o, Squillante RG: Tuberculosis of the spine. Orthop Clin N Am 1996; 27: 95–103.

Jain AK: Treatment of tuberculosis of the spine with neurologic complications. Clin Orthop Relat Res 2002; 398: 75–84.

CASE 77. An 18-month-old boy presents with a history of fever starting 5 days ago. This was followed a day later by the development of red eyes and a rash. There is no history of cough or rhinorrhea. He has been immunized against diphtheria, pertussis, tetanus, smallpox, polio, and measles. On examination he is moderately ill-appearing and irritable. His temperature is 39°C, heart rate 130/minute, and his perfusion is good. His eyes, lips, skin, and hands are shown in Figures 77.1 through 77.5. In addition his buccal mucosa and pharynx are red, but there is no pharyngeal exudate.

- *What do these pictures demonstrate?*
- *What is the most likely diagnosis?*
- *What are the problems associated with this condition?*
- *How would you manage the patient?*

These pictures show the following:

(i)   marked conjunctival hyperemia, without apparent discharge, and with a clear zone around the limbus ("perilimbic sparing");

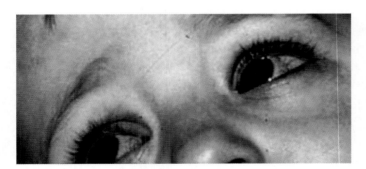

FIG. 77.1.   Note the appearance of the child's eyes.

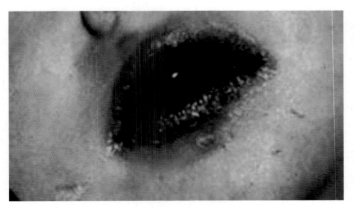

FIG. 77.2.   Note the appearance of the child's lips.

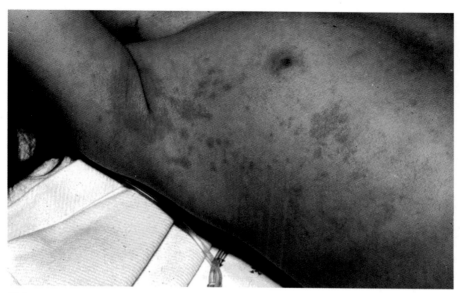

FIG. 77.3.   Note the rash.

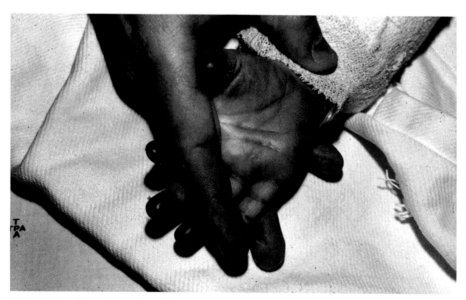

FIG. 77.4.   Note the color of the palms.

(ii)   red, cracked lips;

(iii)   a macular rash on the trunk, with severe dermatitis in the perineal
area;

(iv)   bright red palms.

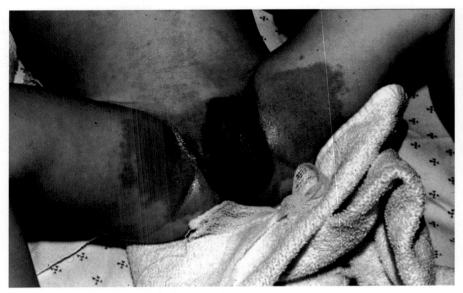

FIG. 77.5. Note the appearance of the perineal skin.

These findings, together with high fever, are highly suggestive of Kawasaki disease (formerly called mucocutaneous lymph node syndrome). This is an inflammatory disease of unknown etiology. Because there is no test for confirming the diagnosis, clinical criteria are used for making the diagnosis. These are as follows:

(I)   fever of at least 38.5°C for at least 5 days;
(II)   four of the following five clinical abnormalities:

      (i)   conjunctivitis (this is nonpurulent and is primarily bulbar);
      (ii)   mucosal inflammation (mouth, vagina, red and cracked lips)
      (iii)   cervical lymphadenitis, >1.5 cm diameter;
      (iv)   rash, which may be macular or polymorphic;
      (v)   swollen, red hands and feet;

(III) exclusion of other diagnoses. This constitutes the differential diagnosis; it is the criterion that is often difficult to meet, and includes the following:

measles (contact exposure, conjunctival discharge, and, most importantly, severe cough);
adenovirus infection;
streptococcal scarlet fever;
toxic shock syndrome;

Stevens–Johnson syndrome (pseudomembrane in mouth and eyes);
Rocky Mountain spotted fever;
leptospirosis.

The most important complication of Kawasaki disease, and the reason that it is important to diagnose and to provide treatment, is inflammation of the coronary arteries with subsequent aneurysm formation and thrombosis, leading to myocardial ischemia.

Other clinical features or complications include pericarditis, myocarditis, aseptic meningitis, arthritis, hydrops of the gallbladder, anterior uveitis, and rarely, peripheral gangrene.

The diagnosis is made clinically. The above criteria have been used for study purposes. However, not all patients meet all these criteria, thus constituting "incomplete cases." Considering the potential for a fatal complication (myocardial infarction) and the lack of a diagnostic test, patients presenting with some of the clinical features pose a very difficult clinical dilemma: to treat for Kawasaki disease or not. Diagnostic tests that can confirm or exclude alternative diagnoses are sometimes helpful. Tests of inflammation (e.g. total leukocyte count, C-reactive protein concentration, and erythrocyte sedimentation rate) may be helpful in that they are generally very abnormal in patients with Kawasaki disease. However, they are not specific. An echocardiogram should be performed to look for coronary aneurysms in suspected cases.

The treatment consists of an infusion (2 grams per kilogram) of intravenous immune globulin (IVIG) and high-dose aspirin (antiinflammatory dose). The dose of aspirin is reduced (anticoagulant dose) once the acute inflammation has abated or the platelet count has risen above normal, which usually occurs about 2 weeks after the onset of the illness.

Reading:

Newburger JW, Takahashi M, Gerber MA et al: Diagnosis, treatment, and long-term management of Kawasaki Disease: a statement for health professions from the Committee on Rheumatic Fever, Endocarditis, and Kawasaki Disease, Council on Cardiovascular Disease in the Young, American Heart Association. Pediatrics 2004; 114: 1708–1733.

CASE 78. A 5-year-old boy presents with shortness of breath of a few days duration. On examination he is tachypneic and has marked dullness to percussion and absent breath sounds on the right side of his chest. He is afebrile.

What are the possible causes of these physical findings?
How would you confirm your beliefs?
What are the possible specific etiologies of these abnormalities?

The physical findings indicate right lung consolidation and/or fluid in the right lung pleural space. Such fluid could be blood (hemothorax), a pleural effusion (exudate or transudate), or pus (empyema). A chest X ray should be performed. This is shown in Figure 78.1.

The X ray confirms the presence of a clinically suspected large pleural effusion.

The differential diagnosis includes:

(a) parapneumonic effusion or empyema due to an acute pneumonia caused by bacteria such as *Streptococcus pneumoniae* or *Staphylococcus aureus*; (these are unlikely in the absence of fever);

(b) tuberculosis;

(c) malignancy, especially lymphoma;

(d) transudate due to hypoproteinemia (unlikely considering that it is unilateral and there is no anasarca) or sympathetic to infradiaphragmatic disease such as a subphrenic abscess or pancreatitis;

(e) hemothorax secondary to trauma or malignancy.

Management of such a patient should entail a pleural tap to (a) relieve the symptoms, and (b) obtain fluid for diagnostic purposes. This should include microscopy for leukocytes and for malignant cells, measurement of protein concentration, and staining and culture for pyogenic bacteria and mycobacteria. In tuberculous pleural effusions, the fluid seldom reveals the causative

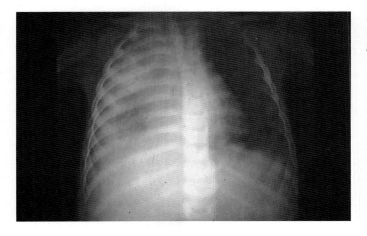

FIG. 78.1.   Chest X ray showing a large right pleural effusion.

organism. The yield is improved by pleural biopsy, which is seldom performed. A PPD should also be placed.

In this patient, in the face of a strongly positive PPD, a diagnosis of tuberculous pleural effusion was made, and multidrug therapy was instituted with isoniazid, rifampin, and pyrazinamide. The pleural effusion resolved and the patient's condition improved.

■CASE 79. An 8-year-old boy presented in 1975 to a hospital in Johannesburg, South Africa, with fever, weight loss, and weakness of 2 weeks' duration. There was no history of travel, animal or arthropod exposure, or blood transfusions. Examination revealed the following: temperature of 38.3°C, heart rate 120/minute, respiratory rate 50/minute, pallor, and extreme wasting. The heart was normal except for a 2/6 ejection systolic murmur, which sounded like a flow murmur, and the lungs were clear to auscultation. There was enlargement of his liver and spleen, but there was no jaundice or significant lymphadenopathy.

- *What is your differential diagnosis?*
- *What would you do?*

■TAB. 79.1: A list of conditions causing weight loss, anemia, fever, hepatosplenomegaly, and lung disease.

Infections
  Viral
    HIV infection
    HIV infection complicated by:
      Opportunistic infection
      Lymphocytic interstitial pneumonitis (LIP)
  Bacterial
    Tuberculosis (miliary)
    Brucellosis
    Typhoid fever
  Fungal (disseminated)
    Histoplasmosis
  Protozoal infection
    Visceral leishmaniasis (Kala-Azar) (not present in South Africa)
Malignancy
  Leukemia
  Lymphoma
  Langerhans histiocytosis
Inflammatory disease (noninfectious)
  Juvenile rheumatoid disease
  Systemic lupus erythematosus
  Sarcoidosis

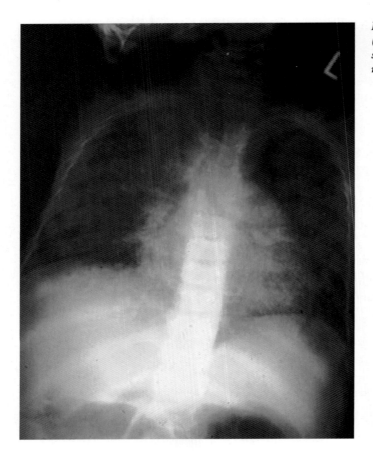

FIG. 79.1.   Chest X ray (posterior-anterior view) showing a diffuse reticulonodular pattern.

This child obviously is suffering from a systemic illness, affecting his hemopoietic system, his liver and spleen, and possibly his lungs. The fever suggests an infection, malignancy, or inflammatory disease, and the weight loss suggests a process that is subacute or chronic. An underlying immunodeficiency complicated by an opportunistic infection should also be considered. Nowadays HIV infection as an underlying disease would be a very important consideration, but this child presented before recognition of the pandemic of this infection. A differential diagnosis is listed in Table 79.1. Of note, infective endocarditis does not cause hepatomegaly unless the patient is in heart failure, and when malaria is associated with hepatomegaly, one would expect significant jaundice.

Management should be directed at diagnosing those conditions that are imminently fatal if untreated and have significant public health implications. In addition, the initial tests should be those that can provide answers quickly. Therefore a chest X ray and blood count should be performed first.

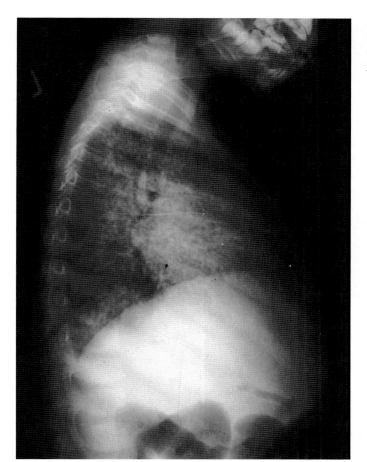

FIG. 79.2.   Chest X ray (lateral view) showing a diffuse reticulonodular pattern.

This child's PA and lateral chest X rays are shown in Figures 79.1 and 79.2, respectively.

The X ray shows a diffuse reticulonodular pattern. Although highly suggestive of miliary tuberculosis, this can be caused by other infections including disseminated fungal infections such as histoplasmosis and by neoplastic conditions such as Langerhans histiocytosis and lymphoma. Additional studies that should be employed to confirm the diagnosis of miliary tuberculosis are (a) sputum or gastric washings for stain and culture and (b) blood culture specifically for mycobacterial culture. (c) A PPD should be performed. However, this is negative in a significant proportion of patients with miliary tuberculosis. In patients suspected of having miliary tuberculosis, a lumbar puncture should be performed to look for evidence of meningitis, which may be subclinical initially.

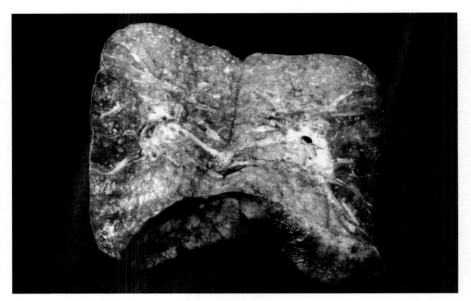

FIG. 79.3.   The lungs at autopsy revealing multiple tubercles.

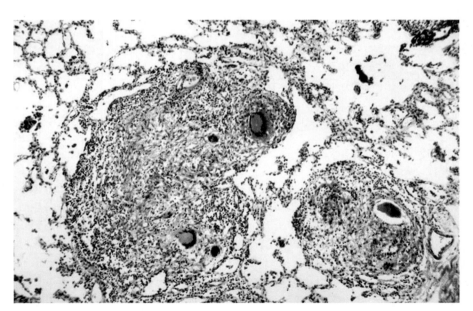

FIG. 79.4.   Histological section of lung of a patient with miliary tuberculosis showing granulomas representing tubercles. (Courtesy of Dr Carlos Abramowsky, Emory University)

In patients such as this in whom an accurate diagnosis is fairly urgent, examination of a tissue specimen can be very useful. The tissue that is easiest to sample and that would likely provide the answer in this case is the bone marrow. A bone marrow aspirate and biopsy should be performed, and specimens should be submitted for histology, cytopathology, as well as for culture and staining for mycobacteria and fungi. This is also applicable to any other tissue specimens that are obtained.

This patient was diagnosed with miliary tuberculosis, and he was treated with antituberculous therapy. However, he died. At autopsy the lungs showed widely distributed granulomas (tubercles) (Figure 79.3).

The histological appearance of the lung in miliary tuberculosis is shown in Figure 79.4 (not from this case).

Reading:

Shingadia D, Novelli V: Diagnosis and treatment of tuberculosis in children. Lancet Infect Dis 2003; 3: 624–632.

■**CASE 80.** A 9-year-old boy presents with swelling on the left side of his neck of several weeks' duration. He is born in the United States but has traveled to Mexico, his parents' native country, 2 years ago. There is no history of preceding trauma or upper respiratory tract symptoms. On examination he is well appearing and afebrile. The left side of his neck has a swelling of approximately 6 × 4 cm diameter just below the angle of the mandible. It is firm and mildly tender, but the overlying skin is not discolored. Movement of the neck is limited. The rest of the examination is normal.

- *What is the differential diagnosis?*
- *What would you do?*

This child has a subacute process in the submandibular area. The most likely focus of disease is in the upper cervical lymph node, but other possible foci include the submandibular salivary gland, a branchial cleft cyst, or extension of infection from the lateral pharyngeal space. If an infectious process is affecting a lymph node, the likely causative organisms are mycobacteria (*M. tuberculosis* or nontuberculous mycobacteria, such as *M. avium* complex) or cat-scratch disease. A malignancy, in particular a lymphoma should also be considered.

Therefore it is essential to make a specific diagnosis. Imaging might be helpful to determine the anatomical site of the disease. A computer tomography scan of his neck is shown in Figure 80.1.

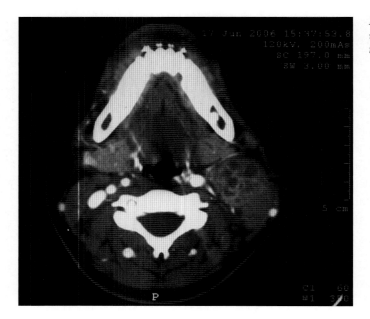

FIG. 80.1.   A large mass with hypodense areas on the left side of the neck.

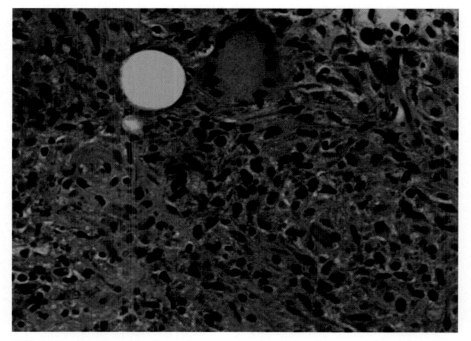

FIG. 80.2.   The hematoxylin and eosin stained section of a removed lymph node. Note the chronic inflammation and multinucleate giant cell. (Courtesy of Dr Marina Mosunjac, Emory University)

This shows a large mass with hypodense areas on the left side of the neck, probably representing lymphadenitis.

However, a biopsy will likely be necessary.

While these are being arranged, a PPD should be placed. If this is greater than 10 mm in diameter, a chest X ray should be performed, to look for other evidence of tuberculosis. When a biopsy is performed, it is essential that material be submitted to the laboratory both for histology as well as for culture of bacteria, anaerobic bacteria (in particular actinomyces), mycobacteria, and fungi.

This child's PPD was measured to be 20 mm. This size has a fairly high specificity for tuberculosis. His chest X ray was normal. He underwent biopsy of a lymph node, the appearance of which is shown in Figures 80.2 and 80.3.

The biopsy reveals chronic inflammation and granuloma formation with multinucleate giant cells. In addition, a few acid-fast bacteria are seen. This confirms a diagnosis of a mycobacterial lymphadenitis. The question remains: Is this infection tuberculosis or a nontuberculous mycobacterial infection?

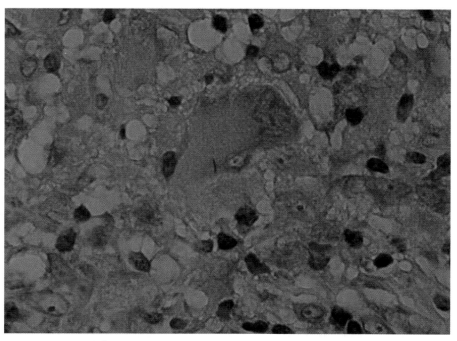

FIG. 80.3.   *Acid-fast–stained section showing an acid-fast bacillus in the center of the field. (Courtesy of Dr Marina Mosunjac, Emory University)*

If tuberculosis, he requires multidrug therapy, and the health department should be notified. If not tuberculosis, optimal therapy entails node removal (which was not accomplished in his case), although antimicrobial therapy might be effective. Such therapy depends on the species of mycobacterium isolated. For cases caused by *M. avium* complex, the commonest species causing this condition, a combination of clarithromycin and rifampin, with or without ethambutol should be used.

This child was treated as if he has tuberculosis with directly observed therapy with isoniazid, rifampin, pyrazinamide, and ethambutol. His mycobacterial culture was subsequently negative. A full course of anti-tuberculosis therapy was recommended.

CASE 81. A 10-month-old boy with kwashiorkor, who has received intravenous fluids containing electrolytes and glucose, and antimicrobial therapy, develops a high fever and swelling at the site of a peripheral intravenous catheter on the left arm (Figure 81.1). The intravenous catheter is removed and pus is expressed from the exit hole. The Gram stain is shown in Figure 81.2.

- *What is the diagnosis?*
- *What is the microbial cause?*
- *How should he be treated?*

Pus issuing from a vein confirms a diagnosis of suppurative (purulent) thrombophlebitis. This is a serious complication of intravenous catheters. The swelling in this child's upper limb indicates extension of the infection up the vein, causing a perivenous abscess. Therapy should entail immediate removal of the catheter, followed by drainage of the abscess, surgical removal of the affected segment of vein, and appropriate antimicrobial therapy.

The optimal antimicrobial therapy should be determined by the causative organism.

The main causative organisms are staphylococci, *Candida* spp. enterococci, and Gram-negative rods. Because the organism can be provisionally determined from the Gram stain, this procedure is essential and urgent.

In this case the Gram stain shows large oval-shaped Gram-positive organisms with elongated processes. These are characteristic of *Candida* spp. The oval bodies represent the yeasts, and the elongated processes are pseudohyphae.

Therapy can entail fluconazole or amphotericin B. This child was treated successfully with surgery and amphotericin B. (This case occurred before the advent of fluconazole.)

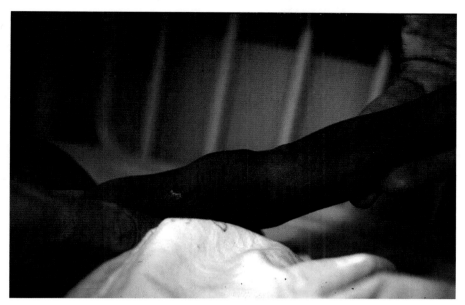

FIG. 81.1.   The swelling on the child's arm.

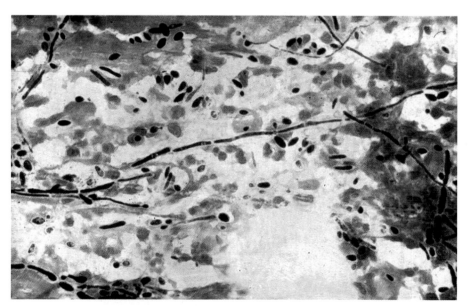

FIG. 81.2.   A Gram stain of the pus obtained from the vein.

Reading:

Khan EJ, Correa AG, Baker CJ: Suppurative thrombophlebitis in children: a ten-year experience. Pediatr Infect Dis J 1997; 16: 63–67.

CASE 82. A 2-year-old child with AIDS develops a sore over the elbow (Figure 82.1) where elastoplast has previously been attached to immobilize an intravenous catheter in the antecubital fossa.

- *What might have caused this?*
- *How would you proceed to evaluate the child's problem?*

This lesion is characterized by a blackish eschar, which suggests ischemic necrosis. In an immunocompromised individual such as this patient, such a lesion suggests an infection caused by an infectious agent that invades blood vessels. The agents that should be considered are fungi, notably Zygomycetes of the order Mucorales (which includes the genera *Rhizopus, Mucor, Rhizomucor, Absidia, Apophysomyces, Saksenaea, Syncephalastrum,* and *Cunninghamella*), *Aspergillus* species (including *A. fumigatus, A. flavus, A. niger,* and *A. terreus*), and the bacterial agent *Pseudomonas aeruginosa.*

It is very important that a biopsy be performed to obtain material for histology and culture for the above-mentioned pathogens.

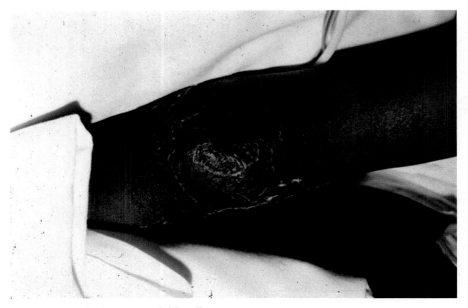

FIG. 82.1.   The lesion on child's elbow.

In this case histology of the biopsy revealed fungal hyphae with very few septa, (resembling those shown in Figure 82.2), and the culture grew out *Rhizopus* spp., confirming the diagnosis of mucormycosis. This child was treated with amphotericin B, and the lesion healed. In this case the infection was probably caused by contaminated elastoplast used in the dressing on the elbow.

Mucomycosis is an infection affecting primarily immunocompromised individuals, such as those with neutropenia, those posttransplant, and those with diabetic keto-acidosis. The Mucorales cause cutaneous infections, pneumonia, and infections of the paranasal sinuses. Infection of the paranasal sinuses can spread rapidly to involve the orbit and brain. A clue to the presence of this organism in the sinus is black discoloration around the nose. Mucormycosis is rapidly progressive and destructive. Therefore making a diagnosis in a suspected case and initiating appropriate therapy is an emergency. Making a diagnosis requires performing a biopsy of tissue, such as sinus mucosa, for histology and for culture for fungi and bacteria. Surface cultures are not appropriate. Histology is more sensitive than culture.

Therapy consists of the following three elements: (i) correcting the underlying defect to the extent possible, (ii) surgical debridement,

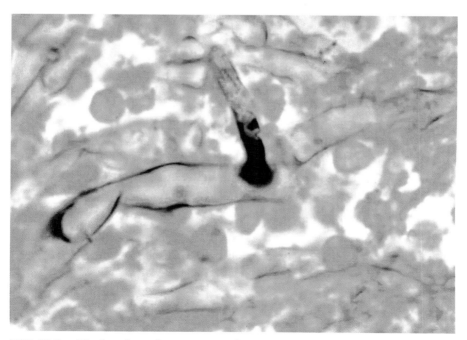

FIG. 82.2.   The histological appearance of a zygomycete in tissue. (Courtesy of the Centers for Disease Control and Prevention/Dr Libero Ajello)

(iii) antifungal therapy. Antifungal therapy should consist of amphotericin B or one of its lipid-based derivatives. Of the antifungal azoles, only posaconazole is active against the zygomycetes.

Reading:

Greenberg RN, Scott LJ, Vaughn HH et al: Zygomycosis (mucormycosis): emerging clinical importance and new treatments. Curr Opin Infect Dis 2004; 17: 517–525.

Gonzalez CE, Rinaldi MG, Sugar AM: Zygomycosis. Infect Dis Clin N Am 2002; 16: 895–914.

CASE 83. A 15-month-old girl presents with a 1-day history of fever and vomiting. There is no diarrhea or cough, and no other members of the family are ill. There is no history of foreign travel, day-care attendance, or exposure to animals. On examination she is moderately ill-appearing, but alert and perfusing well. Her temperature is 39.1°C, heart rate 140/minute, and respiratory rate 30/minute. The heart, lungs, ears, throat, and limbs are normal, and there is no lymphadenopathy or neck stiffness. There is mild abdominal tenderness, particularly in the left upper quadrant and flank. However, no masses or enlargement of the liver or spleen can be detected.

- *What is your differential diagnosis?*
- *What would you do?*

This child has a febrile illness with localizing signs in the abdomen. Disease of several different organs can give rise to abdominal pain or tenderness, but those that cause pain in the left upper quadrant are the left lung, colon, spleen, and kidney. The high fever suggests an infection. The absence of diarrhea after 24 hours of symptoms makes enteric infection unlikely; the absence of respiratory symptoms and findings makes pneumonia unlikely; infection of the spleen itself is very rare, and infection in the subphrenic space would imply previous bowel perforation. The most likely cause of this child's symptoms and signs is pyelonephritis. Therefore the tests that are most likely to confirm the diagnosis are chemical analysis, microscopy, and culture of the urine.

The results of these tests showed the following: 2+ protein, 3+ leukocyte esterase, 3+ hemoglobin, leukocytes too numerous to count, 50 red cells per high power field, and many bacteria.

This is sufficient information on which to base a provisional diagnosis of a urinary tract infection, although a culture is the definitive diagnostic test.

On the following day the urine culture grew out *Escherichia coli*, >100,000 organisms per milliliter.

This confirms the diagnosis of a urinary tract infection. Although the urine findings do not determine the site of infection within the urinary tract, the symptoms of high fever, and the signs referable to the left kidney, indicate a diagnosis of pyelonephritis.

Urinary tract infections are usually caused by *Escherichia coli*. In children who have not previously been treated for urinary tract infection, other causative organisms are other enteric rods, in particular *Klebsiella* spp., and *Enterococcus faecalis*.

Making the diagnosis of a urinary tract infection in an infant or young child is often difficult for the following reasons:

(i)   there may be no focal symptoms or signs. When present, focal clinical features include urinary frequency, crying on urination, and suprapubic or abdominal pain or tenderness.

(ii)   obtaining a specimen of urine that is not contaminated with feces, smegma, or vulval flora requires the performance of a suprapubic bladder puncture (in infants only) or bladder catheterization. These require that there is urine in the bladder at the time of the procedure.

Diagnosing a urinary tract infection and treating the patient is important for the following reasons:

(i)   it can be complicated by bacteremia;

(ii)   it indicates the possibility of an underlying urinary tract malformation that has predisposed the patient to the infection, in particular vesicoureteral reflux;

(iii) it can lead to renal scarring and, over a long period, to chronic renal damage.

Therefore in infants and young children with fever and no apparent site of infection, urinary tract infection should be considered. Because of the above implications of diagnosing this condition, an appropriate specimen of urine must be obtained. If such an infection is diagnosed, further investigation, looking for evidence of a urinary tract abnormality should be performed. This usually consists of a renal ultrasound and a voiding cystourethrogram.

Management consists of antimicrobial therapy directed at the most likely pathogen, namely *Escherichia coli*. In the past ampicillin was active against most strains of this organism. However, this is no longer the case. Therefore therapy should consist of trimethoprim/sulfamethoxazole (to which there is also a rising rate of resistance) or a cephalosporin. Although parenterally administered third-generation cephalosporins, such as ceftriaxone or cefotaxime are appropriate for ill children, they have not been shown to be superior to oral therapy with cefixime. If imaging reveals a urinary tract malformation that might predispose to urinary tract infection, such as vesicoureteral reflux, the child should receive long-term antimicrobial prophylaxis and be referred to a urologist. Prophylaxis should consist of a drug that does not have significant effects on the bowel flora, for example, trimethoprim/sulfamethoxazole, at about one-fourth the usual therapeutic dosage. Whether such prophylaxis is clearly of benefit is currently being questioned.

Reading:

American Academy of Pediatrics, Committee on quality improvement: practice parameter: the diagnosis, treatment, and evaluation of the initial urinary tract infection in febrile infants and young children. Pediatrics 1999; 103: 843–852.

Hoberman A, Wald ER, Hickey RW et al: Oral versus intravenous therapy for urinary tract infections in young febrile children. Pediatrics 1999; 104: 79–86.

Wald ER: Vesicoureteral reflux: The role of antibiotic prophylaxis. Pediatrics 2006; 117: 919–922.

CASE 84. A 2-year-old girl presents with a history of cough and fever for 2 days.

On examination she has a temperature of 39°C, a respiratory rate of 50/minute, dullness to percussion, and bronchial breathing (tubular breath sounds) over the right upper lobe anteriorly. The rest of her examination is normal.

- *What is the likely diagnosis?*
- *How would you manage her?*

In a child with fever, cough, and tachypnea the most likely diagnosis is pneumonia. The additional findings of dullness to percussion and bronchial breath sounds indicate pulmonary consolidation. Dullness with decreased breath sounds could indicate consolidation and/or the presence of pleural fluid. However, pleural fluid, being dependent, is usually detected over the lower lobes. Pneumonia associated with pulmonary consolidation indicates lobar pneumonia. In such a patient the most likely causative agent is

Streptococcus pneumoniae, although *Haemophilus influenzae* (type b or non-typeable), *Staphylococcus aureus*, *Mycoplasma pneumoniae*, or respiratory viruses are also possible causes. An attempt to make a microbiological diagnosis should be made by blood culture. Sputum cannot be obtained from young children, but in those older than about 6 years, an attempt should be made to obtain sputum for Gram stain and culture. Detecting respiratory viral antigens or culturing these viruses from nasopharyngeal secretions can be performed. However, they are useful only for isolation procedures for hospitalized patients and for witholding antibiotics in those patients with positive results.

A microbiological diagnosis is important in immunocompromised children in whom the diagnostic possibilities are broad. In such cases invasive procedures such as lung puncture, bronchoalveolar lavage, or lung biopsy may be indicated.

Although a chest X ray may not be essential for initial management, it is of use for the following reasons:

(a) as a baseline, in case the patient does not improve as expected;

(b) to evaluate for complications;

(c) to determine whether there is an underlying lung problem predisposing the child to pneumonia. Radiological evidence of consolidation should have cleared within 6–8 weeks. Failure of this to occur should alert one to the possibility of an underlying abnormality, such as bronchial obstruction.

The chest X ray of this child is shown in Figure 84.1.

Management consists of supportive care, ensuring that the child is adequately oxygenated and hydrated, and antimicrobial therapy. Initial antimicrobial therapy should consist of a penicillin, for example, amoxicillin or a third-generation cephalosporin.

Pneumonia means inflammation of the alveoli. This is usually caused by an infectious agent, but it may also be caused by other noxious agents, such as toxins, for example kerosene. Pathologically pneumonia may be patchy (bronchopneumonia) or be localized to a segment or lobe of the lung (lobar pneumonia). These may have different clinical features (see below). The differential diagnosis of pneumonia and associated physical findings are listed in the Table 84.1. The main microbial causes of pneumonia in children of different ages and in those with different risk factors are shown in Table 84.2.

Pathogenesis of pneumonia: Microorganisms can reach the alveoli by descending from the upper airway (aerogenous), the usual route, or hematogenously. In aerogenous pneumonia, there may be descent of organisms

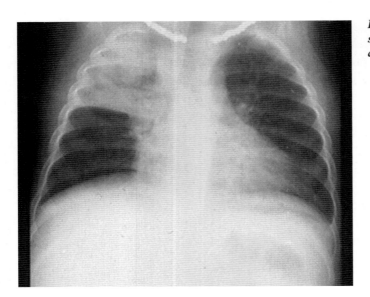

FIG. 84.1. Chest X ray showing right upper lobe consolidation.

into many parts of the lung or spread within a lobe through the pores of Kohn.

Clinical features: Fever and tachypnea are the hallmark features of pneumonia in infants and young children. Tachypnea is the most important physical finding in pulmonary disease because it is more sensitive than other findings, such as auscultatory findings. In addition, the respiratory rate is an objective physical finding. Crackles are often present in both patchy and lobar pneumonia, but signs of consolidation are present in only lobar pneumonia. There may be additional signs of respiratory distress or failure, or of the sepsis syndrome. These include intercostal and subcostal retractions, use of accessory muscles of respiration, cyanosis, depressed level of consciousness, agitation, poor perfusion, and hypotension. Lobar pneumonia may be associated with the symptom of localized chest pain and/or tenderness. In the case of pneumonia abutting on the diaphragm, there may be very severe abdominal pain, suggesting the possibility of an acute abdominal emergency. In children with upper lobe pneumonia neck stiffness may be present, suggesting the presence of meningitis. The signs of lobar consolidation include the following: dullness to percussion, decreased intensity but a higher pitch of the breath sounds ("bronchial" or "tubular" breath sounds), "E- to-A changes," crackles, and increased vocal resonance over the involved area.

Complications of pneumonia may be present at the time the patient presents or may develop during the course of treatment. These can be considered in terms of local spread and distant spread of the infection and of complications specific to the causative organism.

■TAB 84.1:   The differential diagnosis of pneumonia and associated findings.

Bronchiolitis	fever, tachypnea, crackles, wheeze, hyperinflation
Pulmonary infarction	fever, focal chest pain, tachypnea, consolidation[a]
Acute chest syndrome (sickle cell disease)	fever, focal chest pain, tachypnea, consolidation[a]
Pulmonary edema	tachypnea, crackles
Atelectasis	tachypnea, decreased breath sounds, consolidation[a]
Bronchial obstruction (total)	see atelectasis, mediastinal shift toward the side of obstruction
Bronchial obstruction (partial)	tachypnea, decreased breath sounds, hyperinflation of affected side, mediastinal shift away from the side of obstruction
Pleural fluid	dullness, decreased breath sounds, shift away from the side of the fluid
Pneumothorax	resonance, decreased breath sounds, shift away from the side of the pneumothorax
Tumor	decreased breath sounds, dullness

[a]Signs of consolidation: dullness to percussion, bronchial breathing ("tubular" breath sounds), and decreased breath sounds.

1. Local spread:

   (a) *Pleural effusion*: This may occur with bacterial or nonbacterial pneumonia, adjacent to the site of pneumonia. It is termed a "parapneumonic effusion." However, in the case of bacterial pneumonia, infection may spread to the pleural space, leading to a pleural empyema. This is associated with persistent fever in patients whom one would have expected to improve with therapy. Infection-related pleural effusions can develop in the absence of pneumonia as a result of infradiaphragmatic infection such as a subphrenic abscess, liver abscess, or perforated esophagus. A pericardial effusion can also complicate pneumonia.

   (b) *Lung abscess*: This results from necrosis of lung tissue caused by bacterial pneumonia, especially in cases caused by *Staphylococcus aureus* or anaerobic bacteria (Figure 84.2).

2. Hematogenous spread of infection can occur with any bacterial infection. This is a particular problem in cases of bacteremia caused by

■**TAB 84.2:   Causes of pneumonia in children, according to age and risk factors.**

Infectious causes
  Normal host, community-acquired
Newborns
  Streptococcus agalactiae (group B)
  Escherichia coli and other enteric Gram-negative bacilli
  Listeria monocytogenes
  Herpes simplex virus
  Chlamydia trachomatis
  The role of *Mycoplasma hominis* and *Ureaplasma urealyticum* in neonatal pneumonia is controversial
Infants and toddlers
  Respiratory syncytial virus
  Other respiratory viruses
    Adenovirus
    Parainfluenza virus
    Influenza virus
    Metapneumovirus
  Streptococcus pneumoniae
  Haemophilus influenzae
  Staphylococcus aureus
School aged children and teenagers
  Mycoplasma pneumoniae
  Chlamydia pneumoniae
  Streptococcus pneumoniae
Organisms requiring specific exposures that can often be determined by history
  Measles
  Coxiella burnetii (Q fever)
  Chlamydia psittaci
Hospital-acquired
  Respiratory syncytial virus
  Other respiratory viruses
  Enteric Gram-negative bacilli
  Pseudomonas aeruginosa
  Staphylococcus aureus
Immunocompromised patients:(neutropenia, cancer chemotherapy, transplantation, HIV infection)
  All of the above *PLUS*:
  Pneumocystis jiroveci (formerly *P. carinii*)
  Cytomelgalovirus
  Fungi, especially *Aspergillus*
  Nocardia species
  Rhodococcus equi
Cystic fibrosis
  Staphylococcus aureus
  Haemophilus influenzae
  Pseudomonas aeruginosa
  Burkholderia cepacia
  Stenotrophomonas maltophilia
  Nontuberculous mycobacteria

(Continued)

(Continued)

Subacute and chronic
  Mycobacterium tuberculosis
  Endemic mycoses
    Histoplasma capsulatum
    Blastomyces dermatitidis
    Coccidioides immitis
Pulmonary infiltrates + eosinophilia
  Visceral larva migrans – *Ascaris lumbricoides*, *Toxocara canis*, *T. cati*
Noninfectious causes of pulmonary infiltrates
  Food/milk aspiration
  Hypersensitivity pneumonia e.g. bird fancier disease
  Toxic e.g. kerosene ingestion, paraquat ingestion, chlorine inhalation, cancer chemotherapy
  Vasculitis e.g. Goodpasture's syndrome, Wegener's granulomatosis, systemic lupus
    erythematosus
  Pulmonary infarction (thrombus/embolus)
  Pulmonary contusion (trauma)
  Acute chest syndrome (sickle cell disease)
  Heart failure (pulmonary edema)
  Malignancy

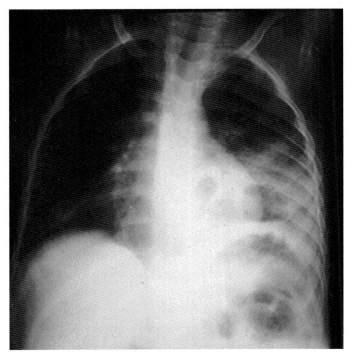

FIG. 84.2.   Chest X ray of a child showing left lower lobe consolidation with cavitation due to an abscess.

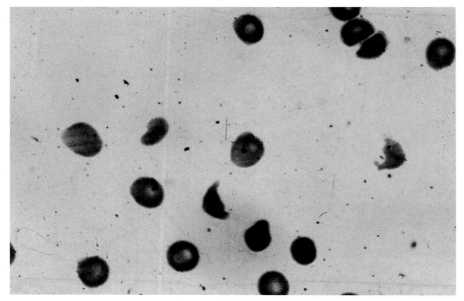

FIG. 84.3.   A blood smear from a child with hemolytic uremic syndrome complicating pneumococcal pneumonia. Note the wide spaces between the cells, indicating severe anemia (the hemoglobin concentration was 1.8 g/dl), and fragmented red cells.

Staphylococcus aureus and *Fusobacterium necrophorum* (Lemierre syndrome).

3.   Complications related to specific organisms:

(a) *Streptococcus pneumoniae*:   This organism may cause the hemolytic uremic syndrome. The mechanism, which is different from that in cases caused by Shiga-like toxin of enterohemorrhagic *E. coli*, is related to bacterial neuraminidase injuring cell membranes of host cells (Figure 84.3).

(b) *Mycoplasma pneumoniae* can cause a cold antibody autoimmune hemolytic anemia, as well as erythema multiforme and encephalitis.

Management of complications of pneumonia

Empyema: When this is suspected, a chest radiograph should be taken, preferably in the erect and lateral decubitus positions, in order to determine whether there is fluid in the pleural space and whether it flows or is loculated. If fluid is present, it should be aspirated for the purpose of confirming the diagnosis and with the hope of obtaining a culture of the causative organism. (This is seldom accomplished if the patient has already received antimicrobial therapy.) Ultrasound can also be helpful in localizing the pleural fluid. If empyema is present, the treatment is surgical, either by closed chest tube drainage or by thoracoscopy-directed debridement. This latter procedure is associated with a shorter hospital course.

Lung abscess: Treatment in this case entails antimicrobial therapy for several weeks. Surgical management is seldom necessary.

Reading:

Bradley JS: Old and new antibiotics for pediatric pneumonia. Semin Respir Infect 2002; 17: 57–64.

CASE 85. An 18-month-old girl presents with a history of fever for 4 days and bilious vomiting for 1 day. She has not defecated for 3 days. She was seen in an emergency room 1 day ago and was treated with ceftriaxone. On examination she is moderately ill-appearing, but alert and perfusing well. The examination is normal except for the abdominal examination which reveals mild distension and marked generalized tenderness, particularly marked on the right side, especially inferiorly.

- *What is the differential diagnosis?*
- *How would you manage the child?*

This child has three main clinical features: fever, vomiting, and marked abdominal tenderness. This suggests an infectious process within the abdominal cavity. Although acute lobar pneumonia can cause abdominal pain, tenderness, and fever, tenderness in that case is mainly upper abdominal. The absence of respiratory symptoms and signs are also against the diagnosis of pneumonia. Organs within the abdominal cavity that are potential foci of disease include the kidneys, the liver, the gallbladder, the intestine, and the pancreas. The absence of diarrhea is against the diagnosis of acute gastroenteritis, but the infections related to the intestine that can present in this fashion are those associated with inflammation of the subepithelial layers, such as typhoid fever or acute appendicitis, especially if perforation has occurred. The most likely diagnosis is a perforated appendix with abscess formation. The bile-stained vomitus suggests the possibility of a high bowel obstruction as might occur with a midgut volvulus, associated with intestinal malrotation. Although this is the most serious consideration, a patient with this condition is likely to be very ill-appearing due to bowel ischemia and systemic acidosis.

Management should entail the following:

(a) ensuring adequate perfusion and hydration;

(b) nasogastric drainage;

(c) laboratory tests: blood culture; electrolyte concentrations; serum amylase and lipase; urinalysis and urine culture;

(d) antimicrobial therapy directed against enteric rods and anaerobes should be initiated, such as a combination of a third-generation cephalosporin and metronidazole.

(e) imaging studies, which should be done in the following sequence:

(i)   plain abdominal X ray with the X ray beam horizontal, to look for free gas. If this is seen the child should undergo laparotomy immediately.

(ii)   contrast study of the upper gastrointestinal tract to look for malrotation, which is the predisposing factor to midgut volvulus. If this is abnormal, the child should undergo laparotomy immediately.

(iii)   computer tomography (CT) scan of the abdomen and pelvis with intravenous and intrabowel contrast to look for foci of intra-abdominal infection. This might need to be delayed if the contrast used in the earlier upper gastrointestinal study interferes with the imaging.

In this case the plain abdominal X ray and upper gastrointestinal contrast study were unrevealing. After 2 days, during which the child received antimicrobial therapy as described above, and during which her condition

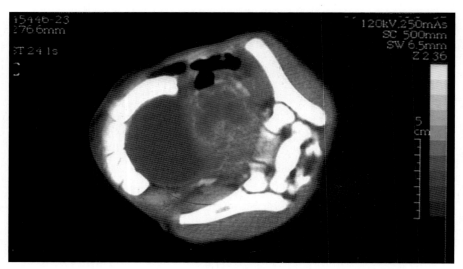

FIG. 85.1.   *CT scan showing a large pelvic abscess resulting from a perforated appendix.*

improved, a CT scan was performed, revealing a pelvic abscess probably arising from a perforated appendix (Figure 85.1).

She was treated with antimicrobial therapy for 10 days and made an uneventful recovery. The diseased appendix was removed laparoscopically 4 weeks later.

Reading:

Solemkin JS, Mazuski JF, Baron EJ et al: Guidelines for the selection of anti-infective agents for complicated intra-abdominal infections. Clin Infect Dis 2003; 37: 999–1005.

CASE 86 (COMP). An 11-year-old boy presents with fever and severe headache, followed by confusion. He had a "cold" about 2 weeks ago. On examination he is febrile, drowsy, and has mild swelling and erythema of the right upper eyelid. The eyes have normal movements, but there is papilledema on the right. There is some neck stiffness and slight weakness of the left upper and lower limbs. During the examination he suffers a seizure, which is controlled with intravenous clonazepam.

- *What is the differential diagnosis?*
- *What would you do?*

The clinical features of fever, headache, and changes in mental state strongly suggest an infection affecting the brain. The swelling and erythema around the right eye suggest bacterial sinusitis, and the papilledema indicates raised intracranial pressure. This whole clinical picture indicates that bacterial sinusitis has been complicated by intracranial suppuration such as a subdural or epidural empyema, a brain abscess, and/or meningitis. The intracranial empyemas in this circumstance can be present over the convexity of the brain or within the interhemispheric fissure, while abscesses affect the frontal lobes. Had external ophthalmoplegia been present, this would have suggested the additional possibly of orbital cellulitis, while the presence of internal and external ophthalmoplegia and chemosis would have suggested the complication of cavernous sinus thrombosis.

Management should consist of the following:

(a) *Supportive care*: Controlling the seizure, ensuring an adequate airway and breathing, and reducing the intracranial pressure;

(b) Initiating antimicrobial therapy directed at the most likely pathogens, which include *Streptococcus pneumoniae*, other streptococci, in particular those belonging to the *Streptococcus milleri* group,

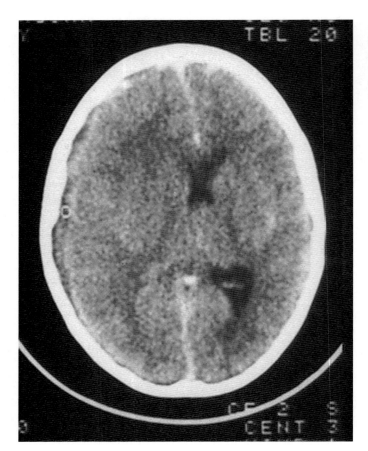

FIG. 86.1.   CT of the patient's head showing a right epidural empyema and right hemispheric brain swelling with midline shift, complicating sinusitis.

Haemophilus influenzae, Staphylococcus aureus, anaerobes, and Gram-negative bacilli, including enteric bacilli. A combination of vancomycin, a third-generation cephalosporin and metronidazole, or a combination of vancomycin and meropenem is suitable.

(c) *Confirming and clarifying the diagnosis*: This involves imaging the head by a computer tomography (CT) scan, with contrast, or by magnetic resonance imaging (MRI) (Figure 86.1); this shows a right hemisphere epidural empyema, with right hemisphere swelling and shift of the midline.

(d) *Surgery*: The need for drainage of an abscess will depend on the actual findings on imaging. Specimens should be sent to the laboratory for Gram stain, and aerobic and anaerobic bacterial culture.

Similar complications can occur with middle ear infection. In this case the brain abscess affects the temporal lobe or cerebellum, and thrombosis affects the lateral sinuses.

This patient illustrates several very important points:

(i)   Eyelid swelling is an important feature of paranasal sinusitis; this is not an ocular problem.

(ii) Severe headache or vomiting in individuals with sinusitis or otitis media suggests the possibility of intracranial complications of the infection. These include osteomyelitis of the skull, cerebral venous sinus thrombosis, epidural empyema, subdural, empyema, meningitis, and brain abscess.

Reading:

Piccirillo JF: Acute bacterial sinusitis. N Engl J Med 2004: 351: 902–910.

Bair-Merritt MH, Shah SS, Zaoutis TE et al: Suppurative intracranial complications of sinusitis in previously healthy children. Pediatr Infect Dis J 2005, 24: 384–386.

Subcommittee on Management of Sinusitis and Committee on Quality Improvement, American Academy of Pediatrics: Clinical practice guideline: management of sinusitis. Pediatrics. 2001: 108;798–808.

CASE 87 (COMP). A 6-year-old previously healthy boy presents to a hospital in South Africa with a history of fever and abdominal pain for 1 week, and extreme fatigue for 1 day. There is no diarrhea or hematochezia. On examination he is moderately ill-appearing, with a temperature of 39°C, heart rate of 120/minute, blood pressure of 100/50 mm Hg, good peripheral perfusion, mild jaundice, and marked mucosal pallor. The heart and lungs are normal. The abdominal examination reveals mild generalized tenderness, and the spleen is palpable 3 cm below the left costal margin. The rectal examination is normal, and the stool appears normal and tests negative for occult blood. There is no significant lymphadenopathy, and the neuromuscular examination is also normal. The urine is pink, and tests positive for hemoglobin.

- *What are the diagnostic possibilities?*
- *What should be done to differentiate between them?*

There are several abnormalities. Can they be linked in a single unifying diagnosis?

(a) *Fever*: This is most likely caused by an infectious process, whether viral, bacterial, fungal, or parasitic.

(b) *Abdominal tenderness*: This is not severe, tending to exclude generalized peritonitis, and diffuse, tending to exclude a focal process in a site such as the liver or appendix. In young children, however, the lack of focality of abdominal tenderness may be misleading, both because they cannot vocalize their symptoms, and, in young infants, because the omentum is not large enough to seal perforations of the bowel. The organ that is present in every area of the abdominal cavity is the bowel. These symptoms may be compatible with bowel inflammation or distension.

(c) *Jaundice*: This suggests either cholestasis, as might occur with hepatitis or biliary duct disease (unusual in previously healthy children), failure of conjugation, as occurs with hepatitis, or an excessive bilirubin load, as occurs with hemolysis.

(d) *Pallor*: In the absence of shock this indicates anemia. The history suggests an acute anemia. This can be due to acute blood loss (for which there is no evidence), acute hemolysis, or acute bone marrow failure. Because there are abdominal symptoms, bleeding into the intestine should be considered. Acute anemia due to bone marrow failure caused by parvovirus B 19 ("aplastic crisis") can occur in an individual with a shortened red cell lifespan due to a chronic hemolytic state such as sickle cell disease or hereditary spherocytosis, of which there is no history in this child.

(e) *Pink urine*: This can be caused by certain foods, such as beetroots, but in the context of an ill patient should be considered likely due to blood, free hemoglobin, or myoglobin. All of these give a positive test for hemoglobin. If the urine is pink and turbid, this suggests hematuria, as occurs with disease of the urinary tract; if it is pink and clear (like rosé wine), this indicates hemoglobinuria or myoglobinuria. Hemoglobinuria is due to intravascular hemolysis, while myoglobinuria is due to rhabdomyolysis, of which there is no clinical evidence.

The acute anemia, jaundice, and pink urine suggest the likelihood of intravascular hemolysis. The few disorders that cause this include some autoimmune hemolytic anemias, which may complicate several different infections; macroangiopathic hemolytic anemia due to heart valve abnormalities (for which there is no evidence); microangiopathic hemolytic anemia, as occurs with hemolytic uremic syndrome, a possibility; and glucose-6-phosphate dehydrogenase (G6PD) deficiency, also a possibility. Hemolytic crises in individuals with G6PD deficiency are usually precipitated by infections but may be precipitated by oxidant drugs.

What infection might the child have? Of systemic viral infections infectious mononucleosis due to Epstein–Barr virus (EBV) might explain the

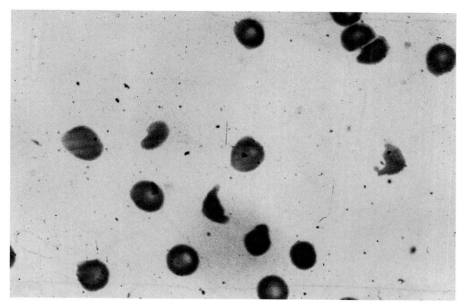

FIG. 87.1.   Schistocytes in the blood of a child with microangiopathic hemolytic anemia associated with hemolytic uremic syndrome. Note the large spaces between the red cells, indicating severe anemia. (The hemoglobin concentration was 1.8 g/dl.)

anemia, jaundice, and splenomegaly best but not the abdominal tenderness, unless there is splenic rupture. If anemia were due to splenic rupture, there would likely be features of shock. The systemic bacterial infections that would best explain the abdominal pain, tenderness, and splenomegaly is typhoid fever (*Salmonella typhi* infection). Although malaria causes fever, hemolytic anemia, and splenomegaly, the hemolysis in this infection is generally not intravascular. A few tests might provide all the necessary information for a complete diagnosis of this child's problems:

hemoglobin concentration – to determine the severity of the anemia;

blood smear for red cell morphology and parasites – for schistocytes of angiopathic hemolysis;

hemolysis (Figure 87.1), "bite" cells of G6PD deficiency (Figure 87.2), malaria parasites (see Case 63), and Downy cells of infectious mononucleosis (see Case 6);

Coomb's test – to diagnose autoimmune hemolysis;

urine dipstix and microscopy – to differentiate between causes of pink urine;

blood culture – to diagnose bacteremia, especially that caused by *Salmonella typhi*;

heterophile antibody test – to diagnose infectious mononucleosis.

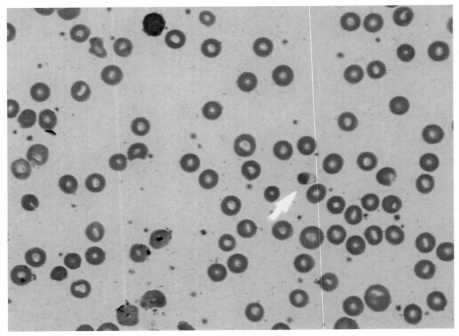

FIG. 87.2.   Blood smear of a child with hemolysis caused by glucose-6-phosphate dehydrogenase deficiency demonstrating a red cell with uneven distribution of hemoglobin within the cell ("bite cell"). (Courtesy of Dr Carlos Alvarado and Dr Carlos Abramowsky, Emory University)

Although management will depend on the likely diagnosis or diagnoses, supportive care should be instituted immediately. The most important element of this is to ensure adequate hemoglobinization with a blood transfusion.

The diagnosis in this child was typhoid fever with underlying glucose-6-phosphate dehydrogenase deficiency.

Reading:

Berkowitz FE: Hemolysis and infection: categories and mechanisms of their interrelationship. Rev Infect Dis 1991; 13: 1151–1162.

CASE 88. An 18-month-old girl presents with fever and swelling on the right side of her neck of 3 days' duration. There is no history of living in or visiting another country, trauma, or upper respiratory tract symptoms. On examination she is mildly ill-appearing, with a temperature of 38.5°C. The right side of her neck has a swelling of approximately 3 cm diameter just below the angle of the mandible. It is firm and tender, and the overlying skin is erythematous. Movement of the neck is limited. The rest of the examination is normal.

- *What is the differential diagnosis?*
- *What would you do?*

This child has an acute infection in the submandibular area. The most likely focus of infection is an upper cervical lymph node, but other possible foci include the submandibular salivary gland, a branchial cleft cyst, or extension of infection from the lateral pharyngeal space. The likely causative organisms are *Staphylococcus aureus*, *Streptococcus pyogenes*, and anaerobes. The possibility of a mycobacterial infection and cat-scratch disease affecting the cervical lymph node should also be considered.

There are several different strategies for managing such a patient. These are:

(i)   Administer antimicrobial therapy active against the above pathogens, especially against *Staphylococcus aureus*, and re-examine the child after 1 or 2 days. Such therapy would depend on the local prevalence of methicillin-resistant *Staphylococcus aureus*. This might be cephalexin, dicloxacillin, or clindamycin. Although trimethoprim/sulfamethoxazole is active against *Staphylococcus aureus*, it is not very active against *Streptococcus pyogenes*.

(ii) Aspirate the swelling and perform a Gram stain and culture of any aspirated material. If pus is aspirated this indicates the presence of an abscess, and adequate drainage should be performed. If no pus is aspirated, begin antimicrobial therapy as described above.

At the first visit a PPD should be placed.

If, at the follow-up visit, the abnormality has progressed, the following strategies, which are not mutually exclusive, should be considered:

(a) Aspiration of the swelling.

(b) Image the neck (by computer tomography) to determine more precisely the location of the disease. This should certainly be performed if conditions other than cervical lymphadenitis are considered likely. If an abscess is demonstrated this should be drained surgically.

(c) Admission of the patient to hospital for intravenous antimicrobial therapy and for observation of the course of illness. If there is no improvement or the disease progresses, surgical drainage or biopsy should be performed.

If the PPD is 5 mm or greater in diameter at 48 hours, a mycobacterial infection is likely. This should be addressed as follows, assuming that there is no specific tuberculosis exposure history: a specimen from the node for histology, acid-fast stain, and mycobacterial culture should be obtained, either by needle aspiration or biopsy, preferably excisional biopsy.

Also a chest X ray should be performed.

If the chest X ray suggests the possibility of pulmonary tuberculosis, three early morning gastric aspirate specimens for mycobacterial stain and culture should be obtained and antituberculosis therapy should be initiated. This strategy should also be used if there is a history of a tuberculosis contact.

If the chest X ray is normal:

(a) if the PPD is 5–9 mm in diameter, await the results of the culture. If a nontuberculous mycobacterium grows and the node has been removed, no further management is necessary; if the node could not be removed, antimicrobial therapy according to the organism's identity should be attempted.

(b) if the PPD is 10 mm or greater in diameter, initiate antituberculosis management while awaiting culture results. If the culture remains negative, a course of therapy for tuberculosis should be completed.

CASE 89. A 17-year-old boy presents with a 1-day history of back pain followed by loss of urinary and bowel control, ability to walk, and sensation in his legs. There is no history of preceding trauma, febrile illness, diarrhea, respiratory symptoms, foreign travel, or contact with other individuals with similar symptoms. He is, however, sexually active. He was fully immunized as a child. Examination reveals a generally healthy-appearing boy who is afebrile. The only abnormalities are referable to the nervous system. He cannot move his lower limbs or sit up unsupported, and the deep tendon reflexes in the lower limbs are absent. Sensory examination reveals a level in the mid-thoracic area below which he has decreased or absent sensation. The cremasteric and superficial abdominal reflexes are absent. The anal "wink" is absent, and he has lost bladder control. The upper limbs and cranial nerves are normal, as are his higher functions. There is no back tenderness.

- *What might this be due to?*
- *What should be done?*

This patient has acute paraplegia, indicating spinal cord disease. The differential diagnosis, in the absence of trauma, includes diseases within the cord itself (intramedullary) or outside the cord but within the spinal canal and compressing the cord (extramedullary). They include the following:

Abscess in the spinal epidural or subdural space. Such abscesses are hematogenous in origin and are usually caused by *Staphylococcus aureus*.

Hemorrhage (intra- or extramedullary) due to a tumor, cyst, or arteriovenous malformation.

Transverse myelitis: This may be due to an infection or due to an immune reaction to an infection. Several different infectious agents have been implicated, including Epstein–Barr virus, cytomegalovirus, human immunodeficiency virus (HIV), and *Schistosoma mansoni.*

Infarction of the cord, due to vasculitis, as can occur with spinal tuberculosis, or due to emboli.

Acute spinal cord disease constitutes a medical emergency. The most important elements of management are (a) to ensure adequate ventilation and perfusion, which was the case here, and (b) to diagnose or exclude immediately remediable causes of cord compression (compressive myelopathy), namely a tumor, an abscess, or a hemorrhage. This necessitates gadolinium-enhanced magnetic resonance imaging (MRI) of the spine and cord. If this cannot be performed, a computer tomography scan or a myelogram should be performed. Dexamethasone should be administered to reduce swelling of the cord. Compressive lesions should be treated surgically, with submission of any removed material for histology and for culture for bacteria, mycobacteria, and fungi. If a compressive myelopathy has been excluded, spinal fluid should be obtained to determine whether the disease is inflammatory or not. Further imaging may help to determine the extent of disease, and thus the particular nosologic entity, such as multiple sclerosis, neuromyelitis optica, acute disseminated encephalomyelopathy (ADEM), or only transverse myelitis.

In this patient the MRI showed an abnormal signal in the thoracic cord, with mild cord swelling, but no well-circumscribed lesion. This was most compatible with acute transverse myelitis. He was treated with dexamethasone, but showed very little improvement. He subsequently developed demyelination in his brain, leading to a diagnosis of ADEM. He has remained paraplegic and severely disabled.

Reference:

Kaplin AI, Krishnan C, Deshpande DM et al: Diagnosis and management of acute myelopathies. The Neurologist 2005; 11: 2–18.

CASE 90. An 18-month-old girl presents with a 1-day history of fever, unwillingness to eat, and inability to move her neck. Also her voice has developed a muffled quality. On examination she is mildly distressed from pain. Her temperature is 38.6°C, and her respiratory rate is 30/minute. She keeps her neck still, not flexing or moving it from side-to-side. There is mild cervical lymphadenopathy. Her throat is difficult to visualize due to the pooling of secretions there, and the cry is slightly muffled. However, she is not in any respiratory distress, and her lung examination is normal. Her neurological examination, including her mental status, is normal.

- *What is the differential diagnosis?*
- *What would you do?*

This child has an inflammatory disease, probably infectious, in the pharyngeal area. The differential diagnosis includes peritonsillar abscess, which is unusual in children as young as this child, retropharyngeal abscess, and lateral pharyngeal space abscess. These latter two conditions arise from infection spreading to the lymphoid tissue around the pharynx. A retropharyngeal abscess can also arise from infection in the cervical vertebra (e.g. due to tuberculosis) rupturing anteriorly. The presence of stridor and breathing difficulty, together with pooling of secretions would suggest the possibility of epiglottitis. Although meningitis can present with neck stiffness and fever, it is often associated with some change in mental status such as extreme irritability or depressed level of consciousness. In addition it is not associated with voice changes or with pooling of secretions in the pharynx (unless the patient is in coma).

Management of a patient such as this should entail ensuring an adequate airway (which is the case here) and establishing an anatomic diagnosis. The importance of making a diagnosis is for the consideration of surgical drainage of an abscess. A lateral X ray of the neck can demonstrate the airway and abnormal tissue impinging on it (Figure 90.1). Normally in this view, taken when the neck is in extension, the width of the retrophayngeal space is approximately equal to that of the anteroposterior width of the cervical vertebral body.

This figure shows the width of the retropharyngeal space far exceeding that of the vertebra and the airway being pushed forward. These are characteristic of a retropharyngeal abscess or retropharyngeal cellulitis (phlegmon). Better definition of the anatomy of the disease, which might be necessary for deciding about the need for surgical drainage, can be obtained with a computer tomography scan (CT) scan. This is shown in Figure 90.2.

This shows a large hypodense area behind the pharynx, suggestive of an abscess.

Therapy consists of two elements: antimicrobial and surgical drainage. In many cases the retropharyngeal infection consists of a phlegmon, without clear abscess formation. In such cases, antimicrobial therapy alone usually results in clinical improvement. This should be directed at *Staphylococcus aureus*, streptococci, anaerobes, and small Gram-negative rods, such as *Haemophilus influenzae* and *Eikenella corrodens*. A combination of clindamycin and a third-generation cephalosporin would be suitable. Surgical drainage

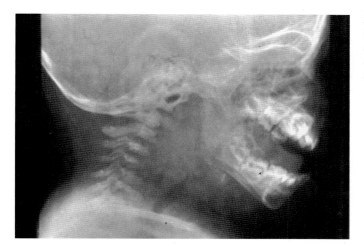

FIG. 90.1. Lateral neck X ray, showing abnormal swelling anterior to the cervical spine, pushing the airway anteriorly.

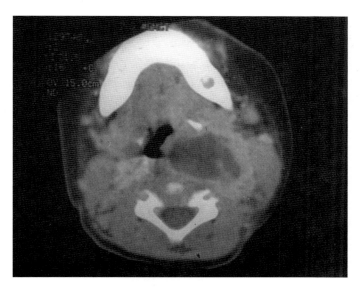

FIG. 90.2. A CT scan of the patient's neck, showing a large retropharyngeal abscess.

might become necessary in the case of a large abscess. This was performed in this child. The main complications of pharyngeal abscesses are impingement on the airway with airway obstruction, compression or erosion of the large vessels in the neck (jugular vein or carotid artery), and extension along the prevertebral fascia into the mediastinum.

Reading:

Craig FW, Schunk JE: Retropharyngeal abscess in children: clinical presentation, utility of imaging, and current management. Pediatrics 2003; 111: 1394–1398.

CASE 91. A 2-year-old boy presents with a history of limping and fever for 2 days. There is no history of trauma. On examination he is mildly ill-appearing with a temperature of 38.7°C. He has multiple mosquito bites on his legs. His gait suggests that he has pain when moving and bearing weight on his right lower limb. When he is examined lying supine, he does not allow the examiner to move his right thigh and hip. If the thigh is held still, movement of the ankle is normal. Movement of the knee cannot readily be tested without movement around the hip. Examination of the bones does not clearly reveal bony tenderness.

- *What is the differential diagnosis?*
- *What should be done?*

In making a diagnosis of the cause of a limp one should ask three questions: (a) Is the limp due to pain or weakness? (b) Where is the abnormality? (c) What is the pathology?

(a) In this case the limp seems to be due to pain, not to weakness.

(b) The areas that can give rise to pain on walking are, broadly, the back, pelvis, hip joint, thigh, knee joint, leg, ankle joint, foot, and shoe. In this case it seems to be the hip joint, the thigh, the knee joint, or proximal tibia.

(c) The presence of fever suggests that the cause is probably an infection, although a noninfectious, but inflammatory disease, for example, juvenile rheumatoid disease, or a malignancy, can also cause fever

The disease with the potential to cause the greatest damage is septic arthritis of the hip, which, if not appropriately treated, can result in avascular necrosis of the femoral head. The other important diagnostic considerations are septic arthritis of the knee and osteomyelitis of the femur or the tibia.

Therefore the child should be evaluated for these possibilities.

Septic arthritis of the hip joint: An ultrasound examination of the hip joint can be used to determine whether or not there is fluid in this joint. If this shows that fluid is present, the child should undergo aspiration of the hip joint, with cell count, Gram stain, and culture of the fluid obtained. If the fluid is purulent, the joint should be washed out. Antimicrobial therapy should be directed at *Staphylococcus aureus*, unless the Gram stain of the fluid suggests the presence of a different organism. In populations in which immunization against *Haemophilus influenzae* is not in widespread use, this organism is also a likely cause of septic arthritis in children. Other causes of septic arthritis in children are *Kingella kingae*, *Streptococcus pyogenes*, *Streptococcus pneumoniae*, and *Salmonella* spp.

If the hip ultrasound is normal further imaging studies should be performed. The optimal study is a magnetic resonance imaging (MRI) scan of the lower limb, which can demonstrate areas of osteomyelitis or arthritis. If this cannot be done a technetium bone scan should be performed. This can demonstrate increased blood flow around an inflamed joint or increased uptake in an area of osteomyelitis.

Although plain X rays can usually be performed rapidly, they are rarely helpful in the early stages of acute osteomyelitis because bony changes take 10–14 days to become manifest radiologically. Their value lies primarily in demonstrating fractures.

Management of skeletal infection consists of antimicrobial therapy, and, in the case of septic arthritis, washing out of the joint to reduce the damage caused by the inflammatory reaction to synovial cartilage. When to initiate antimicrobial therapy can be influenced greatly by the availability of the above imaging studies and the apparent severity of the child's clinical condition, which determines the urgency with which therapy should be initiated. Ideally, if a precise focus of bone or joint disease can be determined clinically, this should be aspirated, with specimens sent for Gram stain and culture, before antimicrobial therapy is started. The microbiological yield might be improved by injecting some of the specimen into a blood culture bottle. In patients such as the one presented, the site for aspiration should be guided by the results of imaging. Blood cultures should also be performed. However, they are positive in only about 50% of cases of osteomyelitis in children. If antimicrobial therapy is initiated before appropriate specimens are obtained, a microbiological diagnosis might never be made and the full course of therapy for skeletal infection will need to be empiric.

Antimicrobial therapy should be directed primarily at *Staphylococcus aureus*. In areas with low prevalence rates of methicillin-resistant *Staphylococcus aureus* (MRSA), an antistaphyloccal penicillin or first-generation cephalosporin should be used. In areas with high prevalence rates of MRSA, initial therapy should consist of vancomycin or clindamycin. Vancomycin should be chosen if the child is severely ill or if the prevalence rate of clindamycin-resistance is high. The duration of therapy should be at least 3 weeks for septic arthritis and 4 weeks for osteomyelitis. In cases in which an organism is identified and antibiotic susceptibilities can be determined, oral therapy can be used once the patient's condition has improved, provided that there is a suitable agent, for example, cephalexin or clindamycin.

Reading:

Hambleton S, Berendt AR: Bone and joint infections in children. In: Pollard AJ, McCracken GH, Jr Finn A (editors): Hot Topics in Infection and Immunity in Children. Kluwer Academic/Plenum Publishers, New York, 2004, pp. 47–62.

CASE 92. (HYP). A newborn boy is noted to have purple skin lesions at birth. He is born by normal vaginal delivery at term. The maternal history is normal, except that the mother had a mild febrile illness at about 24 weeks of pregnancy, lasting a few days. She also has a 3-year-old daughter who is well. On examination the baby is slightly lethargic. The weight is 2.6 kg, length 45 cm, and head circumference 32 cm. There is moderate pallor. The heart and lungs are normal, and the abdominal examination reveals marked enlargement of the liver and spleen. The skin shows diffuse petechiae. There is no lymphadenopathy.

- *What is the differential diagnosis?*
- *What would you do?*

There are three main immediate potential threats to this baby's life: bacteremia, complications from severe anemia, and hemorrhage. Therefore initial attention should be directed at detecting or quantifying these threats, by performing blood culture and urine cultures, blood count, blood smear, platelet count, Coombs test, prothrombin time (PT), and partial thromboplastin time (PTT). In view of the petechiae, a lumbar puncture should not be performed.

Bacteremia: Antibiotic therapy active against *Streptococcus agalactiae, Listeria monocytogenes*, and enteric bacilli should be administered intravenously.

Severe anemia: Considering the clinical findings, in particular hepatosplenomegaly, this might be caused by hemolytic disease of the newborn due to maternal–fetal blood group incompatibility. Arrange for Group O Rhesus negative blood, which might be necessary to transfuse into the infant before the cause of the anemia has been determined.

Hemorrhage: Management strategies to prevent or treat the infant for life-threatening hemorrhage will depend on the results of the above investigations.

Attention can now be paid to other diagnoses which are less threatening in the short term. These are:

(a) intrauterine infection of which the following are the most important:

    (i)   cytomegalovirus (CMV) infection. This is the most likely intrauterine infection because it is the most frequent;

(ii)   congenital rubella;

(iii)   congenital toxoplasmosis;

(iv)   congenital syphilis – this is often associated with maculopapular skin lesions, mucosal lesions, and lymphadenopathy. The manifestations might not be present at birth;

(v)   congenital human immunodeficiency virus (HIV) infection, which is also usually associated with lymphadenopathy.

Unusual congenital infections that can present in this fashion include malaria, tuberculosis, American trypanosomiasis, relapsing fever, and lymphocytic choriomeningitis virus infection.

(b)   congenital leukemia.

A good ophthalmological examination can be very helpful in distinguishing between several intrauterine infections. Congenital rubella causes diffuse speckled pigmentation of the retina ("salt-and-pepper" pigmentation), congenital CMV infection causes chorioretinitis in any area, while congenital toxoplasmosis causes chorioretinitis particularly at the posterior pole of the eye (see Case 65).

The use of serologic tests, utilizing IgM titers to differentiate maternal infection from fetal infection are of value in this clinical circumstance. These are used for diagnosing rubella, and toxoplasmosis, and may be helpful in diagnosing congenital syphilis. CMV infection should be diagnosed by culture of the infant's urine, and HIV infection is diagnosed by DNA PCR testing of the infant's blood.

Treatment is available for patients with the bacterial or protozoal infections, and HIV infection. Gancyclovir, which is active against CMV, has not been shown to be of significant benefit in cases of congenital CMV infection.

Reading:

Andrews JI: Diagnosis of fetal infections. Curr Opin Obstet Gynecol 2004; 16: 163–166.

CASE 93. An 18-month-old, previously healthy boy presents with fever and difficulty breathing. On examination he is ill-appearing, with grunting, a temperature of 39°C, heart rate of 180/minute, blood pressure of 80/40, and respiratory rate of 80/minute. The chest examination reveals intercostal, subcostal, and suprasternal retractions. The lungs are resonant to percussion and clear to auscultation. A diagnosis of pneumonia with possible bacteremia is made, and the child is hospitalized, given oxygen by nasal cannula, and treated with cefotaxime intravenously. A chest X ray is read as showing patchy right lower lobe pneumonia. Two days after admission he becomes obtunded. The peripheral pulse cannot be palpated, and the heart sounds are soft. He is intubated and ventilated, and given intravenous fluids and pressors. However, his pulse remains impalpable. Review of the initial chest X ray suggests cardiomegaly, and the admission blood culture is reported to be growing small Gram-negative rods. An electrocardiogram shows low amplitude complexes.

- *What might have happened?*
- *What would you do?*

The child is in shock, has cardiomegaly, soft heart sounds, low amplitude complexes on electrocardiogram, and has Gram-negative rod bacteremia.

Although Gram-negative sepsis might have explained shock on admission, it seems less likely to have developed after the child has received broad-spectrum antimicrobial therapy for 2 days. Refractory shock, soft heart sounds, and the radiologic appearance of cardiomegaly suggest myocarditis or pericarditis with cardiac tamponade.

Furthermore, the organism present in the blood could have localized within the pericardium causing a purulent (suppurative) pericarditis. Therefore an echocardiogram should be performed immediately to differentiate between myocarditis and pericarditis, and with a view to directing the immediate performance of pericardiocentesis.

In this case, due to the unavailability of echocardiography, a pericardiocentesis was performed at the bedside. After withdrawal of a few milliliters of purulent fluid, the blood pressure rose. A pericardiotomy was subsequently performed, and the child recovered. The blood culture isolate was *Haemophilus influenzae* type b.

Suppurative (purulent) pericarditis is a potentially lethal disease because it can cause cardiac tamponade. It is difficult to diagnose in children because its signs and symptoms are often ascribed to pneumonia, as initially occurred in this patient. Furthermore, it is relatively uncommon, and thus seldom considered as a diagnosis. The diagnosis is particularly difficult to make in young children. Older children can complain of chest pain that is worse on lying than sitting and that may radiate to the upper back or they may complain of abdominal pain. A pericardial rub may be heard. This is easier to detect when the patient is sitting up and leaning forward. Once a significant effusion has developed, the heart sounds are soft, and the signs of cardiac tamponade may be present, namely hypotension, elevated jugular venous pressure, and an increased pulsus paradoxus. Bacteria can reach the pericardium via several different routes, namely hematogenously, from infection in adjacent lung tissue, from the mediastinum, or from an infradiaphragmatic infection. The main causes are *Staphylococcus aureus*, *Haemophilus influenzae* type b, *Streptococcus pneumoniae*, and *Neisseria meningitidis*. In adults anaerobes are also important causes of purulent pericarditis.

Management consists of pericardiocentesis, both to establish the diagnosis and to relieve the tamponade, pericardial drainage, and antimicrobial therapy. This should be directed initially at the likely causative organisms and adjusted once an organism has been cultured. The optimal form of surgical drainage is controversial. Such procedures range from catheter drainage, the least invasive, through pericardiostomy tube drainage, to pericardiectomy, the most invasive. Constrictive pericarditis is a late sequela of this infection.

Reading:

Dupuis C, Gronnier P, Kachaner J et al: Bacterial pericarditis in infancy and childhood. Am J Cardiol 1994; 74: 807–809.

Park S, Bayer AS: Purulent pericarditis. Curr Top Infect Dis 1992; 12: 56–82.

CASE 94. A 5-year-old boy presents with a history of left-sided facial swelling and pain for 1 day. There is no history of rhinorrhea or of nasal congestion. On examination he has a temperature of 38°C but does not appear ill. He has fairly marked swelling and erythema of the left side of his face extending from the mouth to the lower eyelid, with some swelling of the lower eyelid. There is tenderness over the swollen area. There is no conjunctival injection, and the ocular movements are full. There is mild submandibular lymphadenopathy.

- *What is the differential diagnosis?*
- *What should be done at this time?*

The main differential diagnosis includes maxillary sinusitis and odontogenic infection. The above scenario does not include an oral examination, which is essential.

This shows severe and extensive dental caries, with swelling and marked tenderness of the gums in the left upper jaw. The diagnosis is an odontogenic abscess, and the treatment is antimicrobial therapy and surgical drainage of the abscess. A dental X ray can help in localizing the specific tooth affected (Figure 94.1), and a panoramic radiograph (orthopantomogram) is helpful in determining the extent of the dental and periodontal disease (Figure 94.2).

Such abscesses can spread through the bones of the jaw into several spaces around the mouth and the pharynx, including the lateral pharyngeal space, the sublingual space, the pterigomandibular space, the buccal space, the submandibular space, the submasseteric space, and the temporal space. A computer tomography scan can help to delineate such spread. In severe cases, as described here, the affected tooth or teeth must be removed. If there is evidence of abscess formation in one of the above-mentioned spaces, surgical drainage should be performed. Antimicrobial therapy should be directed mainly at streptococci and anaerobes. Although penicillin has been very effective in patients with such infections, there is a rising rate of resistance to this drug among anaerobes. Alternatives include amoxicillin/clavulanate (or ampicillin/sulbactam for parenteral therapy) or clindamycin.

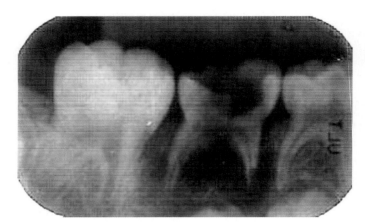

FIG. 94.1.   A dental abscess resulting from a carious tooth in a 6-year-old girl.

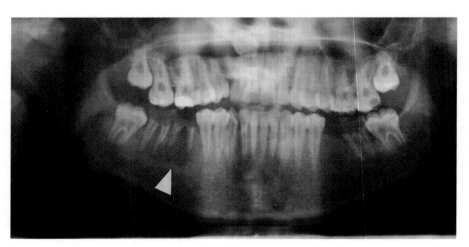

FIG. 94.2.   Orthopantomogram showing a lytic lesion of mandible due to an odontogenic abscess (arrow head).

Prevention depends on good dental hygiene and nutrition, including the drinking of fluoride-fortified water to prevent the development of dental caries.

Reading:

Flynn TR: The swollen face. Severe odontogenic infections. Emerg Med Clin N Am 2000; 18: 481–519.

Wayne DB, Trajtenberg CP, Hyman DH: Tooth and periodontal disease: a review for the primary-care physician. Southern Med J 2001; 94: 925–932.

CASE 95. A 2-year-old girl presents with a history of refusing to walk for 1 day and the suggestion of abdominal and back pain for a few days. There is no history of trauma or of preceding respiratory tract infection. On examination the child is afebrile and well appearing but in some discomfort. She is reluctant to bear weight on her legs and refuses to walk. The abdomen is soft and nontender; however, there is tenderness over the lumbar spine. Movement of the hips, knees, and ankles is normal, and a rectal examination is normal.

- *What is the differential diagnosis?*
- *What should be done?*

The clinical features suggest a problem in the lumbar spine. The possible disease entities include infections, injuries, and tumors. The most serious considerations are those diseases that can result in spinal cord compression, such as spinal epidural abscess or hematoma, which are rare in children, or a tumor such as neuroblastoma. The most likely infections of the spine are discitis and vertebral osteomyelitis. Several imaging studies may need to be employed to make a diagnosis:

(i) A plain X ray of the spine: this may show narrowing of the disc space in discitis, and bony erosion in osteomyelitis, but these changes are absent early on in these disease processes;

(ii) A technetium bone scan will often show increased uptake in the case of osteomyelitis, but may be normal in discitis;

(iii) A magnetic resonance imaging (MRI) scan of the spine has the advantage of assisting in the diagnosis of all the likely diagnoses, including osteomyeltis, discitis, as well as diseases of the soft tissue, epidural space, and spinal cord. If available, this is the study of choice.

In the case of discitis or osteomyelitis, it is optimal to obtain an aspirate of presumed infected material in order to make a microbiological diagnosis, and thus provide optimal antimicrobial therapy. This requires imaging guidance and is frequently not possible. A blood culture and a tuberculin skin test should be performed. Therapy should be directed at the most likely pathogen, namely *Staphylococcus aureus*. However, consideration should also be given to other pathogens such as *Kingella kingae* and *Salmonella enteritidis*.

Imaging studies in this child failed to show any abnormality. A provisional diagnosis of discitis was made. She was treated with analgesia and nafcillin and made a rapid recovery.

Discitis represents inflammation of the intervertebral disc. It affects mainly children younger than about 4 years of age and teenagers. There is controversy as to whether all cases are due to infection. In cases of infection, microorganisms are believed to reach the disc from the metaphyseal arteries supplying the vertebra. When a microorganism is isolated, the most common is *Staphylococcus aureus*. The main clinical findings are irritability, refusal to walk, abdominal pain, and back pain or tenderness. There may or may not be fever. These findings may have an insidious onset, over days or weeks.

Reading:

Early SD, Kay RM, Tolo VT: Childhood diskitis. J Am Acad Orthop Surg 2003; 11: 413–420.

CASE 96 (HYP). An 8-month-old girl presents to a South African hospital in 1976 with a history of fever and irritability. On examination she has a temperature of 39°C and is slightly obtunded. Her cerebrospinal fluid (CSF) reveals 2000 leukocytes per mm^3, of which 95% are neutrophils, and protein and glucose concentrations of 150 and 27 mg/dl, respectively. The Gram stain shows numerous Gram-positive diplococci. A provisional diagnosis of pneumococcal meningitis is made. She is treated with intravenous penicillin G, at a dosage of 300,000 units per kilogram per 24 hours divided into six doses. Her condition progressively deteriorates. Twenty-four hours after her admission the CSF cultures reveals *Streptococcus pneumoniae*. Her therapy is continued. However, her condition deteriorates progressively and she dies 36 hours after admission.

• *Why might her condition have deteriorated?*

Clinical deterioration in a patient thought to be treated appropriately may be due to:

(a) the natural progression of or a complication of the disease, irrespective of treatment;

(b) wrong diagnosis – in the case of an infection, this would include wrong microbial/etiological diagnosis ("wrong bug");

(c) in the case of an infection, the use of an antimicrobial agent to which the causative agent is resistant ("wrong drug").

In this case, the diagnosis was clearly pneumococcal meningitis. Deterioration might have been due to cerebral swelling or brain infarction, well-recognized complications of this disease. However, resistance of the organism to penicillin would be another possibility. In this case the minimal inhibitory concentration (MIC) of the isolate of *Streptococcus pneumoniae* to penicillin was >2 μg/ml. This indicates resistance to penicillin.

Historically and geographically, this child would have represented one of the early cases of the problem of penicillin-resistant *Streptococcus pneumoniae*, which became a major clinical, including nosocomial, problem in South Africa at that time, and which has since become a major problem worldwide.

Reference:

Jacobs MR, Koornhof HJ, Robins-Brown RM et al: Emergence of multiply resistant pneumococci. N Engl J Med 1978; 299: 735–740.

CASE 97 (HYP). A 10-year-old boy presents with fever and pain in his left leg, a few days after scraping the leg in a bicycle fall. On examination he has a temperature of 39°C, and swelling and erythema of the left leg, extending from the ankle to the mid-calf. He is treated with nafcillin 1 g every 6 hours intravenously and with elevation of the leg. After 48 hours he remains febrile and he complains of pain in his right knee. On examination there is marked tenderness just above the medial femoral condyle.

Why might he not be improving and why might he have developed new symptoms?

The initial presentation suggests a diagnosis of cellulitis, the most common causes of which are *Staphylococcus aureus* and *Streptococcus pyogenes*. Nafcillin would be expected to be active against both these organisms. Failure of the patient's condition to improve suggests:

(a) a complication, such as abscess formation, for which surgical drainage is necessary;

(b) a different causative organism, which is resistant to nafcillin, for example, a Gram-negative rod (very unlikely unless the injury had occurred in water or the wound had been contaminated with soil); or

(c) a resistant strain of staphylococcus or streptococcus. The new clinical manifestation, namely tenderness in the opposite femur, strongly suggests the development of osteomyelitis. Its manifestation during therapy provides further evidence that the initial causative organism is resistant to nafcillin. In 2005 methicillin-resistant *Staphylococcus aureus* strains (which are resistant to all penicillins and cephalosporins) are widespread in the United States. Penicillin-resistant strains of *Streptococcus pyogenes* have not yet been reported.

Discussion of cases 96 and 97

Antimicrobial resistance: There are two different definitions of this phenomenon:

(a) clinical resistance, in which the organism is resistant to the antimicrobial agent at a concentration attainable in infected tissue with the use of nontoxic dosages of the agent; and (b) microbiological resistance, in which the organism is more resistant than it was previously, even if it does not meet criteria for clinical resistance. Resistance affects antiviral, antibacterial, antifungal, and antiparasitic agents, but this discussion will be confined to antibacterial agents.

Bacteria develop resistance to antimicrobial agents by changing their genetic make-up. They accomplish this by acquiring genes from other sources, including from other bacteria, or by mutations. Mutations occur approximately every 10^8 to 10^9 divisions. For a single organism dividing every 30 minutes, it takes less than 1 day for a mutation to occur. Increase in the prevalence of resistant bacteria results from selective pressures placed on bacterial populations by their exposure to antimicrobial agents. The susceptible organisms are eliminated and the resistant ones survive, becoming the predominant population. This phenomenon (natural selection) was described by Charles Darwin in 1859, before bacteria had been identified.

How do resistant bacteria spread? The genetic material confirming resistance can spread among organisms, including across genera. More important, however, is spread of the resistant organisms themselves, in feces, secretions, and, of extreme significance within hospitals, on the hands of health-care workers.

Mechanisms of antimicrobial resistance in bacteria: There are four main mechanisms:

1. Barrier to entry of the organism into the bacterial cell. This operates mainly in Gram-negative bacteria, in which it is due to changes in porin proteins, which constitute the channels through which macromolecules enter the organism.

2. Efflux mechanisms: These are energy-dependent mechanisms whereby the organism pumps the antibiotic out of itself before the drug can exert its effect. This is important in resistance to tetracycline as well as to other agents.

3. Enzymatic alteration or destruction of the antibiotic: This mechanism is the most important mechanism of resistance to beta-lactams (the enzymes are beta-lactamases) and to aminoglycosides (the enzymes are acetylases, adenylylases, and phosphorylases). The following are examples: penicillin resistance in staphylococci (counteracted by antistaphylococcal penicillins such as oxacillin, cloxacillin, nafcillin, and methicillin); ampicillin resistance in *Haemophilus influenzae* and penicillin resistance in *Neisseria gonorrhoeae* (counteracted by third-generation cephalosporins); resistance to third-generation cephalosporins in enteric bacilli (conferred by "extended-spectrum beta-lactamases" and other types of beta-lactamases); resistance to aminoglycosides in enteric bacilli and *Pseudomonas aeruginosa*.

4. Alteration of the molecular targets of the antimicrobial agent, for example alteration of penicillin-binding proteins, resulting in penicillin resistance in pneumococci (Case 96), methicillin resistance in staphylococci (Case 97), and ampicillin resistance in enterococci.

More than one of the above mechanisms may operate in one organism synergistically.

Reading:

Berkowitz FE: Antibiotic resistance in bacteria. Southern Med J 1995; 88: 797–804.

Chambers HF: Community-associated MRSA – resistance and virulence converge. N Engl J Med 2005; 352: 1485–1487.

Kaplan SL: Treatment of community-associated methicillin-resistant *Staphylococcus aureus* infections. Pediatr Infect Dis J 2005; 24: 457–458.

CASE 98. A 17-year-old girl with short gut syndrome, a complication of systemic lupus erythematosus, is hospitalized with a tunnel infection of her Broviac catheter, used for hyperalimentation. Her weight is 56 kg. She is treated intravenously with vancomycin 1 g every 12 hours and amikacin 420 mg every 12 hours. Her catheter is removed. Her renal function deteriorates as shown by a serum creatinine rising from 0.8 to 3.2 mg/dl over a period of a few days.

- **What are the possible reasons for the deterioration in renal function?**

There are several possible reasons for her deterioration in renal function:

(a) underlying renal disease complicating systemic lupus. This is unlikely to have caused such a sudden change, however.

(b) infective endocarditis complicating the bacteremia and complicated by glomerulonephritis (infection of venous catheters has become an important cause of infective endocarditis).

(c) toxicity from the antibiotics. Both vancomycin and amikacin can cause nephrotoxicity. Because they have narrow therapeutic ranges, their blood concentrations should be checked, the peaks to ensure therapeutic concentrations and the troughs to ensure adequate clearance. This was the cause of the renal dysfunction in this patient.

CASE 99A (HYP). A 3-year-old boy had bacterial meningitis as an infant. This was complicated by hydrocephalus, for which he has a ventriculoperitoneal shunt, and epilepsy, which has been well controlled with phenytoin, 40 mg twice per day. He presents with fever, headache, and vomiting. Cerebrospinal fluid (CSF) from the shunt reveals 200 leukocytes per mm^3 with a Gram stain showing a few Gram-positive cocci in clusters. A shunt infection is diagnosed and the lower end of the shunt is externalized. Antimicrobial therapy with vancomycin intravenously and rifampin orally is initiated. The CSF culture grows out a coagulase-negative staphylococcus, and the antimicrobial therapy is continued. By the third day the child is afebrile and feeling much better, but on the fifth day he has a generalized seizure.

- **Why might he have had the seizure?**

Possible causes for seizures in a child whose seizures have previously been well controlled:

(a) brain injury resulting from the ventriculitis and meningitis. This is unlikely considering his improving condition.

(b) decreased serum concentration of phenytoin resulting from the drug interaction between the metabolisms of phenytoin and rifampin. Rifampin induces the enzyme responsible for phenytoin metabolism, resulting in an increased rate of phenytoin metabolism, and hence a decreased blood concentration of phenytoin, predisposing the child to a seizure.

CASE 99B (HYP). A 10-year-old boy with moderate persistent asthma, managed with albuterol inhalations and oral theophylline, presents with a cough and fever. He is diagnosed with pneumonia based on the finding of pulmonary infiltrates on chest X ray, and he is treated with erythromycin by mouth. After 4 days he develops vomiting and experiences a grand mal seizure.

What is the likely cause of these new clinical problems?

Vomiting and seizures are manifestations of theophylline toxicity. The likely cause of theophylline toxicity in this child is interference with theophylline metabolism by erythromycin, resulting in an increased blood concentration of theophylline.

CASE 99C (HYP). A 17-year-old girl weighing 65 kg is diagnosed with pulmonary tuberculosis and treated with isoniazid 300 mg, rifampin 600 mg, and pyrazinamide 1250 mg daily by directly observed therapy. She is sexually active and taking oral contraceptive pills. After 2 months on treatment she complains to her health-care worker of nausea and vomiting of 1 week's duration. On examination by a physician there are no abnormal findings, specifically no jaundice and no right upper quadrant tenderness nor hepatomegaly.

What are the possible causes of her symptoms?

The most important immediate consideration in an individual who is taking antituberculosis therapy and who develops nausea and vomiting is the possibility of drug-induced hepatotoxicity. If the therapy is not discontinued immediately, this can result in progression to hepatic failure that can prove fatal. Therefore when antituberculosis therapy is initiated, patients should be warned that if they suffer this symptom they should discontinue therapy and be seen by their physician immediately. Hepatotoxicity, which is rare in children, can be diagnosed by the demonstration of significantly elevated hepatic transaminase levels.

Another important cause of this symptom is pregnancy. According to the history she is sexually active and taking an oral contraceptive. This can be rendered less effective by rifampin due to the induction of enzymes by rifampin, leading to an increased rate of metabolism of the oral contraceptive.

Other considerations, unrelated to therapy, include gastritis and cholecystitis.

Therefore she should have tests of liver function and damage, and a pregnancy test.

Discussion of cases 98, 99A–C:

Drug interactions are important considerations in any individual receiving more than one drug, because they may result in significant toxicities or reduction in therapeutic effects. Most interactions are the result of pharmacokinetic effects, in which the presence of one drug affects the blood or tissue concentration of another drug, but a few can result from pharmacodynamic effects. There are a few broad mechanisms by which interactions affect drug pharmacokinetics:

(a) Drug A interferes with the intestinal absorption of drug B, thus reducing its activity, for example, aluminum hydroxide interferes with the absorption of several cephalosporins, isoniazid, ethambutol, itraconazole, ketoconazole, rifampin, and tetracyclines.

(b) Drug A stimulates enzymes (particularly cytochrome oxidase P450 enzymes) that metabolize drug B, resulting in the increased rate of metabolism of drug B, and hence a decreased therapeutic effect of drug B, for example, rifampin causes a decreased therapeutic effect of atovaquone, benzodiazepines, oral contraceptives (Case 99C), corticosteroids, cyclosporine, several antiretrovirals, phenytoin (Case 99A), valproic acid, and warfarin.

(c) Drug A inhibits enzymes that metabolize drug B, resulting in toxicity of drug B, for example, erythromycin increases the blood concentrations of amiodarone, benzodiazepines, carbamazepine, digoxin, phenytoin, theophylline (Case 99B), valproic acid, and warfarin. This phenomenon can be used therapeutically.

(d) Drug A inhibits the excretion of drug B, for example, probenecid inhibits the excretion of penicillin. This is also used therapeutically in order to increase the serum concentration of penicillin.

(e) Drug A and drug B have similar toxicities, resulting in additive toxicities, for example, both vancomycin and aminoglycosides are nephrotoxic, and their use in combination may increase the risk of nephrotoxicity (Case 98).

(f) Drug A causes a toxicity that can affect the excretion of drug B, for example, amphotericin B causes renal dysfunction, which can result in decreased excretion of several other drugs, such as 5-flucytosine, vanco-mycin, and aminoglycosides.

Antimicrobial agents may have theoretical adverse pharmacodynamic interactions, the evidence for which is largely controversial. For example, a drug inhibiting protein synthesis, for example, tetracycline, could reduce the rate of production of bacterial cell wall, the site of action of beta-lactams, thus reducing the effect of the beta-lactam.

Therefore it is important to consider drug interactions whenever prescribing. Specific antimicrobial agents that are at particularly high risk for causing interactions include rifampin, triazoles, and protease inhibitors.

Reading:

Rang HP, Dale MM, Ritter JM, Moore PK: Pharmacology. 5th edition. Churchill Livingstone, Edinburgh, 2003, pp. 718–723.

CASE 100. An 11-year-old girl who has recently immigrated to the United States from Honduras presents with a history of pain and swelling of her left knee for about 3 weeks, which was preceded by injury to the knee. She has lost about 2 kg in weight in the past few weeks. She developed fever the night before presentation. She has no known contact with an individual with tuberculosis. On examination she is well appearing and afebrile. The proximal part of her left tibia is mildly swollen, erythematous, and tender. The knee joint has full range of movement and no fluid can be detected within the joint. Of note is the absence of pallor, jaundice, lymph-adenopathy, hepatomegaly, and splenomegaly. X rays of the knee are shown in Figures 100.1 and 100.2.

- *What is your differential diagnosis?*
- *What would you do?*

This child has several lucencies within the proximal tibial metaphysis. The differential diagnosis includes bone cysts, tumors, and infections. The indolent nature of the illness suggests that, if this is an infection, it may be caused by an organism that is slow-growing such as *Mycobacterium tuberculosis*. Nevertheless, pyogenic infections, such as those caused by *Staphylococcus aureus*, can become chronic in the absence of therapy.

It is important to make a specific diagnosis, by performing a biopsy, with performance of histology, routine bacterial cultures, and cultures for mycobacteria and fungi. The pace of this illness is slow, so there is no urgency in instituting any form of management.

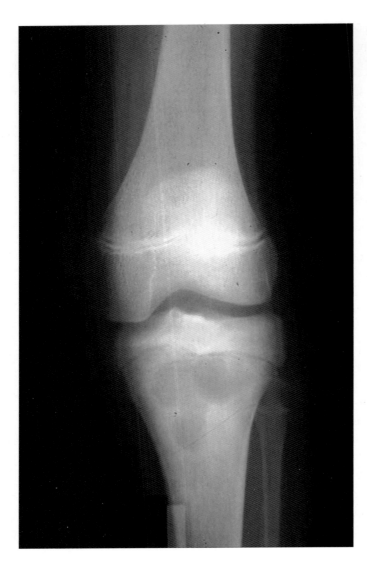

FIG. 100.1.   X ray
showing lucencies in the
proximal tibial metaphysis
(anterior-posterior view).

The child underwent a bone biopsy. The specimens revealed Gram-positive cocci, which were *Staphylococcus aureus*. This is a case of subacute or chronic staphylococcal osteomyelitis resulting in the formation of Brodie's abscesses. Chronic osteomyelitis is characterized by bone necrosis, due to ischemia. This area of bone, the sequestrum, becomes surrounded by new bone formation, the involucrum.

There are several different types of subacute osteomyelitis, whose differential diagnosis varies according to the radiological appearance. These are shown in Table 100.1.

This child's X rays indicate Brodie's abscesses of type IA.

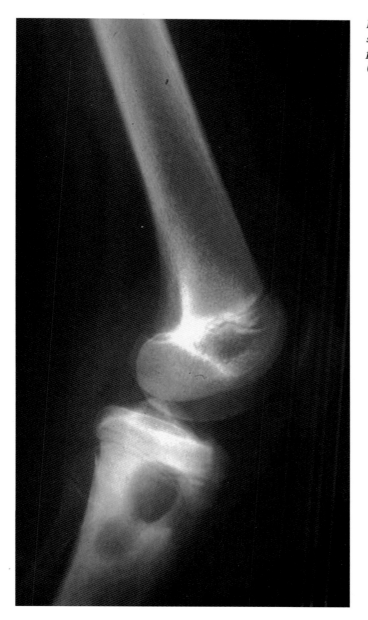

FIG. 100.2.   X ray showing lucencies in the proximal tibial metaphysis (lateral view).

As opposed to the treatment of patients with acute hematogenous osteomyelitis, which is medical (antimicrobial), the treatment of patients with chronic osteomyelitis entails surgical debridement of necrotic bone as well as antimicrobial therapy active against the causative organism. This should be prolonged and can usually be administered by the oral route (for about 3 months). However, there is a substantial chance of relapse.

■TAB. 100.1:   Different types of subacute osteomyelitis.

Type	Site	Radiologic appearance	Differential diagnosis
IA	metaphysis	lucency; no reactive bone	eosinophilic granuloma
IB	metaphysis	lucency; sclerotic margins	typical Brodie's abscess
II	metaphysis	cortical erosion	osteogenic sarcoma
III	diaphysis		osteoid osteoma
IV	diaphysis	"onion peel"	Ewing sarcoma

Reading:

Ramos OM: Chronic osteomyelitis in children. Pediatr Infect Dis J 2002; 21: 431–432.

Lopes TD, Reinus WR, Wilson AJ: Quantitative analysis of the plain radiographic appearance of Brodie's abscess. Invest Radiol 1997; 32: 51–58.

■**CASE 101** (COMP). Three days after undergoing an exchange transfusion for hyperbilirubinemia, a full-term, 3.1 kg boy develops temperature instability, vomiting, abdominal distension, and bloody stools. Examination reveals a very ill, gray-appearing, hyporesponsive infant, with poor perfusion, heart rate of 180/minute, blood pressure of 30/10 mm Hg, and respiratory rate of 80/minute. No abnormalities of the heart or lungs are detected. The abdomen is markedly distended, and bowel sounds are absent. The anterior abdominal wall is a deep red to purple color.

- *What do the history and physical examination indicate?*
- *What has caused this problem?*
- *How would you manage the child?*

The infant is in shock. He has peritonitis due to bowel perforation, which is the likely cause of the shock. The main causes of bowel perforation in a newborn infant are necrotizing enterocolitis or gastric perforation. In very low birthweight infants, isolated small bowel perforation may occur in the absence of necrotizing enterocolitis. The history in this patient is highly suggestive of the diagnosis of necrotizing enterocolitis. Although very rare, this is a recognized complication of exchange transfusion.

The immediate management should entail fluid resuscitation of the infant and artificial ventilation. During this time, antimicrobial therapy active against bowel organisms should be initiated, and abdominal X rays should be performed to attempt to clarify the cause of the problem. As soon as the infant is stable, an exploratory laparotomy should be performed.

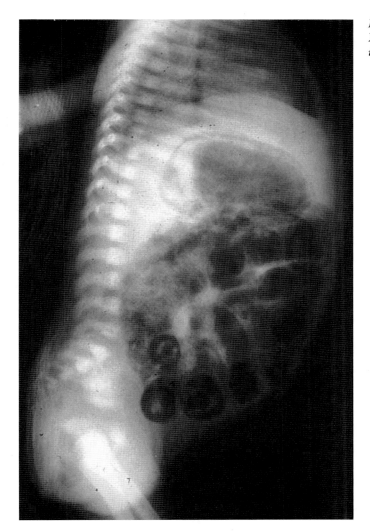

FIG. 101.1.   Abdominal X ray showing pneumatosis intestinalis.

Necrotizing enterocolitis is a disease of the bowel characterized by mucosal necrosis, with entry of bacteria and gas from the bowel lumen into the bowel wall. Although its pathogenesis is incompletely understood, it appears to be due to a combination of ischemia, infection, and the presence of protein within the bowel lumen. The vast majority of cases affect premature infants who have received some feeding, but conditions that affect intestinal blood flow, such as exchange transfusion and congenital heart disease, can also result in this disease.

The clinical features of necrotizing enterocolitis are vomiting (or increased gastric residuals in a tube-fed infant), abdominal distension, and hematochezia. There are often associated features suggesting a systemic infection such as hypothermia, apnea, and poor perfusion. The early radiological feature is dilated bowel loops, and the pathognomonic feature is pneumatosis intestinalis (gas within the bowel wall) (Figure 101.1).

If the disease progresses, intestinal perforation may occur, resulting in discoloration of the abdominal wall and scrotum, and free intraperitoneal gas (Figure 101.2).

Gas within the portal venous system and the liver may also be observed in severe cases (Figure 101.3).

Management consists of ensuring adequate perfusion, nasogastric tube suction, broad-spectrum antimicrobial therapy, directed at streptococci, enteric Gram-negative rods, and anaerobes, and frequent clinical and radiological monitoring for signs of progression, in which case surgery might be indicated. Such signs include free gas, intraperitoneal fluid, palpation of an abdominal mass, and persistence of dilated bowel loops.

Complications include the sepsis syndrome resulting from either the intestinal disease or vascular catheters required for management, enteric fistulae, short gut syndrome, and intestinal strictures.

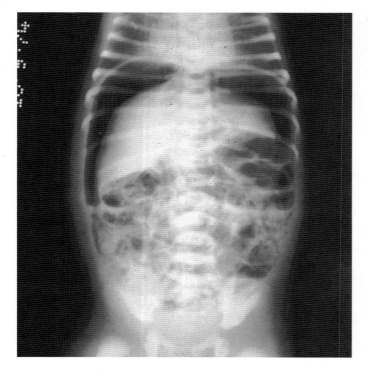

FIG. 101.2. Abdominal X ray showing free intraperitoneal gas.

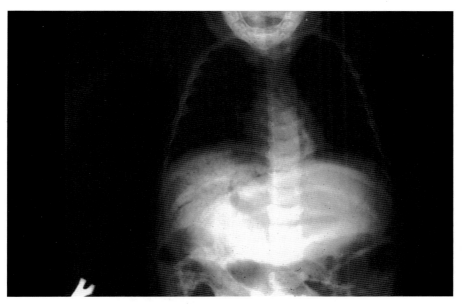

FIG. 101.3. *An abdominal X ray showing gas in the portal vein and the liver, resulting from necrotizing enterocolitis in a 9-month-old child who had suffered shock as a result of acute gastroenteritis.*

Reading:

Kafetsis DA, Skevaki C, Costalos C: Neonatal enterocolitis: an overview. Curr Opin Infect Dis 2003; 16: 349–355.

Caty MG, Azizkhan RG: Necrotizing enterocolitis. In: Ashcraft KW, Murphy JP, Sharp RJ, Sigalet DL, Snyder CL (editors): Pediatric Surgery. 3rd edition. WB Saunders, Philadelphia, 2000.

CASE 102. A 6-year-old shepherdess from rural South Africa presents with a 3-month history of abdominal discomfort. There are no other symptoms. On examination she is well appearing and afebrile. The only abnormality is a vague, nontender mass in the epigastrium, possibly within the liver (Figure 102.1).

- *What is your differential diagnosis?*
- *What would you do?*

A tender hepatic mass associated with fever would suggest the presence of a hepatic abscess, either bacterial or amebic in origin, while the findings in this child suggest a noninflammatory mass, such as a cyst or tumor in the liver or pancreas. The child's occupation exposes her to echinococcosis (infection with the dog tapeworm, *Echinococcus granulosus*).

A simple diagnostic test is an ultrasound of the abdomen (Figure 102.2).

This shows a large cyst within the liver, compatible with a hydatid cyst.

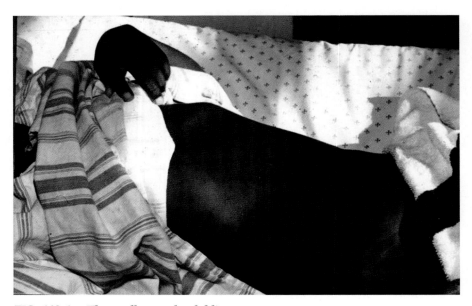

FIG. 102.1.   The swelling in the child's epigastrium.

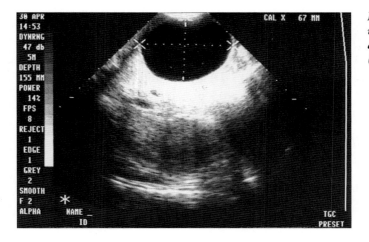

FIG. 102.2.   A large cyst within the liver, probably a hydatid cyst (Echinococcosis).

Life Cycle of *Echinococcus granulosus*

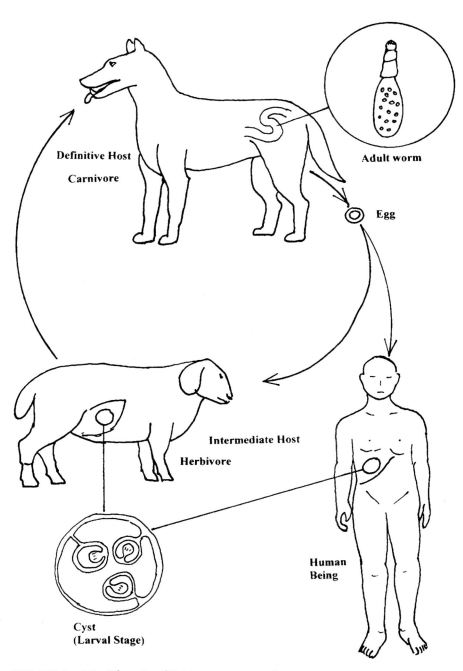

FIG. 102.3.   *The life cycle of* Echinococcus granulosus.

Hydatid disease is the larval stage of the small tapeworm *Echinococcus granulosus*. This worm has a carnivore (e.g. dog, wolf) as its definitive host and a herbivore (e.g. sheep, reindeer, camel) as the intermediate host. The larval stage forms the cyst. The life cycle is shown in the figure (Figure 102.3).

The adult worm lives in the intestine of the carnivore. Eggs are passed in its stool on to grass on which they are eaten by a herbivore and sometimes by a human being. The eggs hatch and the larvae enter the portal circulation and pass to the liver and sometimes on to the systemic circulation. The larvae form cysts that contain daughter larvae. These are infectious for the carnivore. The cysts may be multiple, and may become very large, causing disease by compression. Although usually located in the liver, they may also be present in lung, bone, or other viscera (Figure 102.4).

If a cyst ruptures, the contents form daughter cysts wherever the contents have spread to, such as throughout the peritoneal cavity. In addition, an anaphylactic reaction can occur.

Management consists of antimicrobial therapy with albendazole, followed, when necessary, by surgical removal. When surgery is performed, great care must be taken to prevent spilling of cyst contents and seeding of the field with larvae. Various techniques have been developed to minimize this risk. Prior antiparasitic treatment also reduces this risk.

This patient underwent surgical removal of the cyst. Microscopy of the cyst contents revealed hydatid "sand," with larvae showing hooklets (Figure 102.5).

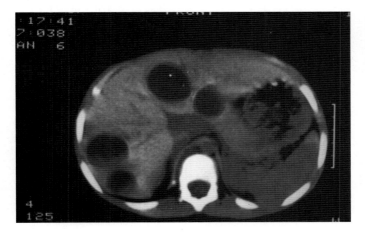

FIG. 102.4.   *Computer tomography scan showing multiple hepatic hydatid cysts.*

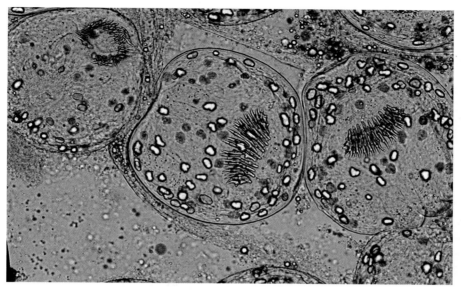

FIG. 102.5.   Contents of this patient's cyst, showing hydatid "sand." Note the row of hooklets on the larval segment.

Reading:

McManus DP, Zhang W, Li J et al: Echinococcosis. Lancet 2003; 362: 1295–1304.

CASE 103. A 9-year-old girl presents with a history of fever and joint pains for about 3 days and a rash for 1 day. On examination she is mildly ill-appearing, with a temperature of 38.7°C. She has pain on movement and swelling of her left ankle, and pain in her left knee. There is a macular rash on her limbs and trunk. The heart, lungs, abdomen, and nervous systems are normal, and there is no lymphadenopathy. The rash is shown in Figure 103.1.

· *What is your differential diagnosis?*
· *What would you like to know to help make a diagnosis?*

This patient has a clinical syndrome characterized by fever, arthritis, and a fairly diffuse macular rash. The differential diagnosis should include primarily infectious diseases but also rheumatologic diseases. In patients with diseases of unclear origin, knowledge about risk factors can be very helpful.

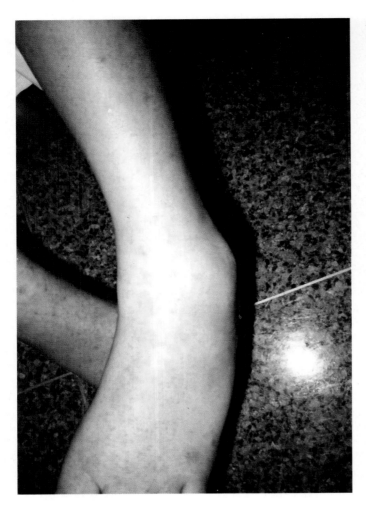

FIG. 103.1. *The child's rash.*

About 1 week before onset of her symptoms this patient had acquired a pet rat. She often kept it inside her shirt, where she had several scratch marks. This made the diagnosis of rat bite fever very likely.

There are two forms of rat bite fever. (a) That caused by *Streptobacillus moniliformis*, a Gram-negative bacillus that can be transmitted by ingestion as well as by skin inoculation. The incubation period is usually 3–10 days. (b) That caused by *Spirillum minus* (Soduku) occurs mainly in Asia. Both these infections are characterized by fever, a macular or petechial rash present mainly on the extremities, and polyarthralgia or arthritis. The main complications are severe visceral infections, especially infective endocarditis. A series of three fatal cases has recently been reported in the United States. Treatment consists of penicillin.

This patient responded rapidly to intravenous penicillin.

■TAB. 103.1: Diseases associated with fever, rash, and arthritis and their risk factors.

Infections characterized by diffuse rash and arthritis	Risk factor
Virus infections:	
arboviruses (including dengue, chikungunya, Onyong-nyong)	mosquitoes, travel
rubella	no immunization
parvovirus B19	contact with infected human
Bacterial infections:	
Septic arthritis associated with scarlet fever	*Streptococcus pyogenes, Staphylococcus aureus*
Meningococcal bacteremia	travel to area of high prevalence
Disseminated gonococcal infection	sexual activity
Infective endocarditis	heart disease
Leptospirosis	exposure to body of unclean water
Syphilis	sexual activity
Rat bite fever (*Streptobacillus moniliformis, Spirillum minus*)	rat exposure
Rocky Mountain spotted fever and other rickettsial diseases are associated with a rash similar to that observed in this patient, but are not associated with arthritis.	tick exposure
Rheumatological diseases to be considered are:	
systemic lupus erythematosus and rheumatoid arthritis	family history
juvenile rheumatoid disease	
acute rheumatic fever	prior pharyngitis

Reference:

CDC. Fatal rat-bite fever—Florida and Washington, 2003 MMWR 2005; 53: 1198–1202.

■CASE 104. A 21-year-old girl presents in shock and with renal failure to a community hospital. She is resuscitated, placed on a ventilator, and transferred to a tertiary care facility. Prior to transfer she had blood cultures drawn and antimicrobial therapy initiated with ceftazidime, vancomycin, and metronidazole.

Her history is as follows: at the age of 4 years she underwent repair of an atrial septal defect. As a result of a complete heart block, she had an intraventricular pacemaker placed. About 4 months before the current admission she had the power source of her pacemaker replaced. This was complicated, 1 month later, by a pocket space infection, which necessitated removal of the pacemaker and its replacement with an epicardial pacemaker. On examination she is very ill, sedated, and on a ventilator, requiring vasopressor therapy and continuous veno-venous hemofiltration. She has the following physical findings: subconjunctival hemorrhages, hemorrhagic skin lesions, hemorrhagic lesions on the tips of the fingers (Figure 104.1), splinter hemorrhages, purple discoloration of the distal third of the feet (Figure 104.2), and auscultation of her heart reveals a 3/6 holosytolic murmur at the apex.

- *What is the likely diagnosis?*
- *How might it have developed?*
- *How would you manage her?*

This patient has heart disease suggestive of mitral insufficiency and multiple conjunctival and cutaneous abnormalities indicative of emboli. These strongly suggest the diagnosis of infective endocarditis. The shock is probably due to a combination of cardiac failure and bacteremia (septic shock). The recent risk factor that might have caused the endocarditis is the pocket infection that could have led to infection of the intraventricular pacemaker. This is an entity called "pacemaker endocarditis."

Management should entail resuscitation and ventilation, as is described above, followed by attempts to make a microbiological diagnosis. This entails performance of blood cultures. Three cultures done a few minutes apart should be performed, and antimicrobial therapy, directed against the

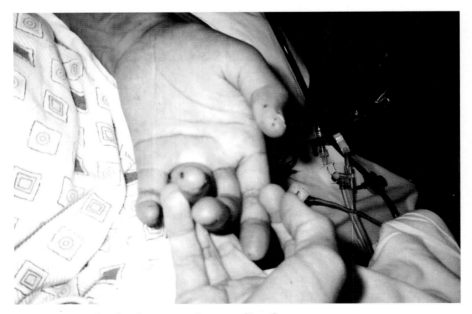

FIG. 104.1.   The skin lesions on the tips of her fingers.

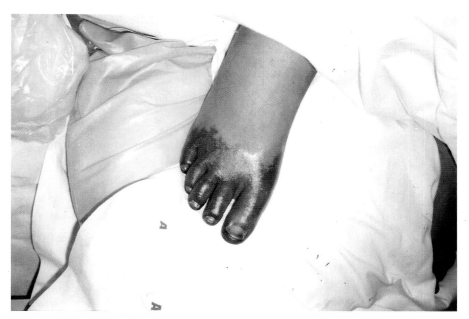

FIG. 104.2.   The appearance of her foot.

most likely pathogens, should be initiated. The most likely pathogens causing infective endocarditis are *Staphylococcus aureus* and viridans group streptococci. Empiric therapy should include vancomycin (for its activity against methicillin-resistant staphylococci), nafcillin (for its rapid activity against methicillin-susceptible staphylococci), gentamicin (for its synergistic activity against streptococci and enterococci), and a third-generation cephalosporin (for its activity against many Gram-negative rods) all dosed according to her renal function. Additional information can be provided by obtaining culture results from her prior hospitalization for the drainage of the pocket infection. In this case the pocket infection had been caused by *Pseudomonas aeruginosa*, which was subsequently cultured from the patient's blood on this admission. It is very important that any pacemaker leads from the original pacemaker be removed.

She was treated with ceftazidime and tobramycin, and after a difficult course, during which she suffered a cerebral embolus, she recovered from the infection.

A more complete discussion of endocarditis follows.

Infective endocarditis (IE) is an infection of the valvular or mural endocardium. It occurs mainly in individuals who have underlying structural heart disease but can affect previously normal hearts.

Pathogenesis: The first stage in the development of IE is the formation of a thrombus on the endocardium. Predisposing factors to this are turbulence, abnormal jets of blood, or trauma to the endocardium, for example, due to a catheter. If bacteremia is present at this time, the thrombus can become infected. This leads to accumulation of platelets and leukocytes at the site, within which are embedded the bacteria. This mass is called a vegetation (Figure 104.3).

The infection can result in local tissue injury, for example, valve destruction, and can spread to adjacent structures. Abnormal jets caused by the infection can result in infection in noncontiguous structures in the heart (e.g. spread from the aortic to the mitral valve). Pieces of vegetation can break off, resulting in emboli. In right-sided endocarditis, these usually impact in the lung, whereas in left-sided disease, they may impact anywhere in the systemic circulation.

Valvular endocarditis can result in valvular insufficiency or, if there is a large vegetation, in valvular obstruction.

Microbiology: The most common microorganisms causing IE are those that stick readily to the endocardium, namely staphylococci and viridans group streptococci. In native heart endocarditis (i.e. cases in which there is no underlying heart abnormality or prosthetic material) *Staphylococcus aureus* accounts for almost all cases of staphylococcal endocarditis. However,

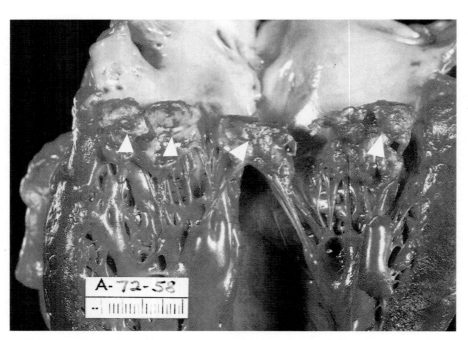

FIG. 104.3.   *Vegetations (arrows) on the mitral valve of a different patient with infective endocarditis. (Courtesy of the Centers for Disease Control and Prevention/Dr Edwin P Ewing, Jr)*

after heart surgery, coagulase-negative staphylococci are also important. Many cases of postsurgical endocarditis are nosocomial. In this circumstance *Candida* spp. and *Corynebacterium* spp., as well as staphylococci, are important. Gram-negative rods are important causes of nosocomial bacteremia in general, but less common causes of endocarditis. The "HACEK" group of organisms (**Haemophilus aphrophilus**, *Actinobacter actinomycetemcomitans*, **Cardiobacterium hominis**, *Eikenella corrodens*, and **Kingella kingae**) are rare causes of endocarditis, as are *Coxiella burnetii* and *Bartonella* spp.

Predisposing conditions: In infants and children the main underlying diseases predisposing to endocarditis are various congenital heart diseases. Because most predisposing conditions are either left-to-right shunts (ventricular septal defect, patent ductus arteriosus) or right-sided lesions (pulmonary stenosis, Fallot's tetralogy), most IE in children is right-sided. In countries where rheumatic heart disease is prevalent, this is also an important predisposing condition. Nosocomial bacteremia, particularly with *Staphylococcus aureus* and *Candida* spp., can lead to endocarditis, even in patients with normal hearts. An increasing number of cases of IE are associated with the presence of central venous catheters, which can remain in the superior vena cava or right atrium for prolonged periods.

Clinical manifestations: (a) General (systemic) symptoms and signs: fever is the most common and important feature of IE. Fatigue, malaise, digital clubbing, anemia, weight loss, and arthralgia may also occur. (b) Embolic and immune phenomena: splinter hemorrhages, Janeway lesions and Osler's nodes on the fingers, Roth spots in the retina (hemorrhages with a white center), petechiae, missing pulses, hematuria (due to immune-mediated glomerulonephritis), splenomegaly, and mental status changes. (c) Cardiac manifestations: the predisposing condition, changing or new heart murmur, chest pain due to coronary emboli, and heart failure.

Nowadays fewer cases are diagnosed after prolonged illness, when many of the classic signs of "subacute bacterial endocarditis (SBE)" would have developed, and more are diagnosed early. There are two main clinical syndromes: (1) acute infective endocarditis, usually caused by *Staphylococcus aureus*, in which the predominant manifestations are those of the sepsis syndrome, with hemodynamic instability, and (2) a less virulent form, in which prolonged fever occurs in an at-risk individual.

Differential diagnosis: As the manifestation of IE are protean, the differential diagnosis is broad. However, it generally includes conditions that are associated with fever and heart murmurs. They are shown in Table 104.1.

The diagnosis of IE is very important because, without treatment, the condition is almost universally fatal. On the other hand, treatment entails intravenous therapy for several weeks, which is undesirable in an individual

■**TAB. 104.1: Differential diagnosis of infective endocarditis.**

Fever and heart murmur
   Congenital heart disease + viral infection
   Flow murmur + infection
Heart murmur, arthralgia/arthritis
   Systemic lupus erythematosus
   Juvenile rheumatoid disease
   Acute rheumatic fever
Postcardiac surgery bacteremia
   Vascular catheter-associated
   Pneumonia-associated
   Wound-associated
   Urinary catheter associated
Other Postcardiac surgery fever
   Postpericardiotomy syndrome
   Post-by-pass infectious mononucleosis (postperfusion syndrome)
Heart murmur and emboli
   Atrial myxoma

without the condition. The main diagnostic test is blood culture. Three separate blood cultures should be taken, with a minimum of 5 ml of blood in each bottle. This is to demonstrate continuous bacteremia and to confirm or reject the hypothesis that a single positive culture is due to a contaminant (such as coagulase-negative staphylococcus). Echocardiography is useful to assist in the diagnosis, especially to demonstrate the location of the lesion and the extent of tissue damage that it has caused. A set of diagnostic criteria have been established in adults, which have been shown to be useful in children. These are known as the "Duke" criteria.

Management: The mainstay of management is antimicrobial. The role of surgery and prophylaxis is discussed later.

The main decision to make is to treat or not to treat, depending on how certain the diagnosis is. The disadvantage of treating a patient in whom the diagnosis is unclear is that once therapy has been instituted, if the blood cultures are subsequently negative, further blood culture information will not become available, and, in the absence of an alternative diagnosis, the course of therapy should be completed. Therefore, from a management viewpoint, I consider patients in three different categories. (a) Patients with suspected acute endocarditis. These patients should have three sets of blood cultures performed over a period of about 15 minutes, and therapy should then be started. (b) Patients with many features of endocarditis, whom one would treat irrespective of the blood culture results. These patients should have three sets of blood cultures performed over several hours, and then therapy should be started. (c) Patients who might have endocarditis (possible). These patients should have three sets of blood cultures over 24 hours but should NOT receive antimicrobial therapy. Their clinical course and blood culture results should be followed until a diagnosis of endocarditis or an alternative diagnosis can be made.

Choice of antimicrobial therpy: This should be bactericidal. Empiric therapy should be active against the likely pathogens (taking into account their likely resistance patterns). Once the pathogen and its resistance pattern becomes known, therapy can be adjusted. My initial empiric therapy is directed at *Staphylococcus aureus* that might be resistant to methicillin, streptococci (including enterococci), which might be relatively resistant to penicillin, and Gram-negative rods. Therefore I use a combination of vancomycin, nafcillin (optimal for methicillin-susceptible *Staphylococcus aureus* infection), ceftriaxone, and low-dose gentamicin.

Complication of IE: (a) Cardiac complications: The most important complication of IE is heart failure, which can lead to shock. Intractable heart failure is the main indication for surgery in patients with IE. It is usually due to valvular insufficiency but can be due to obstruction of a valve aperture caused by a massive vegetation. IE of the aortic valve can be associated with many different complications, mainly as a result of infection spreading through the valve ring. This can result in the following: spread to the conducting system, resulting in heart block; rupture into the pericardial space, resulting in tamponade; extension into the coronary sinus; extension to the mitral valve. (b) Emboli: These can occur anywhere. The most serious systemic emboli are those to the brain, resulting in a stroke; however, they can shoot to the heart itself, gut, kidney, or limbs, resulting in a threat to the function of those organs. Emboli from right-sided endocarditis usually lodge in the lungs.

Role of surgery in management: When a patient with IE has intractable heart failure, cardiogenic shock, or persistent bacteremia (at least 1 week's duration) despite optimal antimicrobial therapy, a cardiac surgeon should be consulted with a view to surgical removal of the infected tissue and replacement with prosthetic material.

Prevention of IE: Most patients with IE do not have a history of a preceding predisposing event (other than the cases following heart surgery). Nevertheless those at risk of IE should receive antibiotic prophylaxis when undergoing procedures that are associated with transient bacteremia. The benefit of this has not been shown in randomized controlled trials (it would require many thousands of cases to be studied to show a benefit). The recommendations of the American Heart Association regarding the types of underlying heart abnormalities, and types of procedures for which prophylaxis is recommended have been published. In patients with rheumatic heart disease, the prophylaxis against *Streptococcus pyogenes* should not be confused with prophylaxis against IE.

Reading:

Moreillon P: Infective endocarditis. Lancet 2004; 363: 139–149.

Durack DT, Lukes AS, Bright DK, Duke Endocarditis Service: New criteria for diagnosis of infective endocarditis: utilization of specific echocardiographic findings. Am J Med 1994; 96: 200–209.

Dajani AS, Taubert KA, Wilson W et al: Prevention of bacterial endocarditis. Recommendations by the American Heart Association. JAMA 1997; 277: 1794–1801.

CASE 105 (COMP). A 17-year-old boy develops fever, rash, and a severe headache 1 week after a safari in South Africa. On examination he is moderately ill-appearing with a temperature of 39.5°C; the other vital signs are normal. He has mild photophobia and mild conjunctival hyperemia but no neck stiffness. There is a macular rash on his trunk and limbs, and two eschars on his lower abdomen (Figures 105.1 and 105.2), and there is bilateral inguinal lymphadenopathy. The rest of his examination is normal.

- *What is the differential diagnosis?*
- *How would you manage him?*

The combination of a rash, fever, and headache suggest a systemic infection. The eschars suggest further that these sites might have been the inoculation site of an infectious agent, as a result of an injury or arthropod bite. An injury leading to focal and then systemic infection is likely due to *Staphylococcus aureus* or *Streptococcus pyogenes*. However, in that case the inoculation site would have more evidence of inflammation or suppuration than is present here. Furthermore the rash is not scarlatiniform as can occur with these infections and is too diffuse for embolic disease due to infective endocarditis. Therefore one should consider infection introduced by an arthropod. Many mosquito-borne virus infections (arbovirus infections) such as dengue and West Nile virus infection are associated with headache and rash, but they are not associated with eschars. *Trypanosoma brucei*, the cause of African sleeping sickness, which is transmitted by a Tsetse fly, is associated with an eschar at the bite site, fever, and rash, and generalized lymphadenopathy but is not transmitted in South Africa. This presentation is typical of

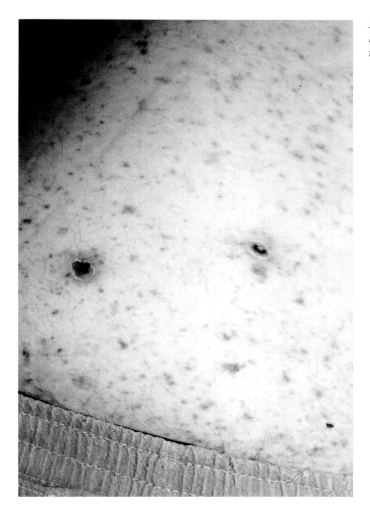

FIG. 105.1.   *The rash and lesions on the patient's trunk.*

certain tick-borne rickettsial infections, namely African tick bite fever, caused by *Rickettsia africae*, and Mediterranean spotted fever, caused by *Rickettsia conorii*.

As in the case of Rocky Mountain spotted fever, the decision to provide antimicrobial therapy (doxycycline) for patients suspected of having these infections should be based on clinical evaluation, not on any laboratory study.

The spotted fever rickettsiae have a worldwide distribution, with each geographic area having its particular species. They constitute an important and under-appreciated cause of febrile illness in travelers. They infect endothelial cells and consequently can affect any organ. Although African tick bite fever (African tick typhus) does not have the high case fatality rate associated with Rocky Mountain spotted fever, it can be fatal, the highest risk groups being infants and the elderly.

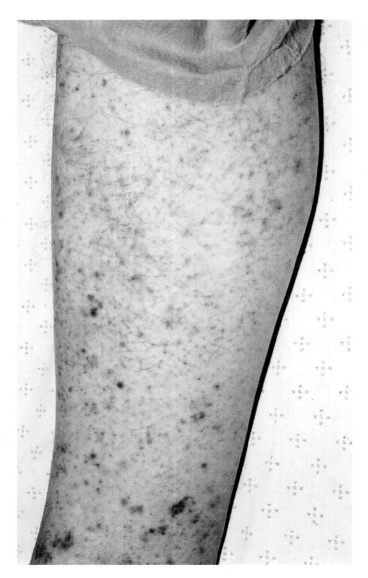

FIG. 105.2.   The rash on one of his limbs.

This patient was treated with doxycycline and he made a rapid recovery.

Reading:

Jensenius M, Fournier P-E, Kelly P et al: African tick bite fever. Lancet Infect Dis 2003; 3: 557–564.

Raoult D, Fournier PE, Fenollar F et al: *Rickettsia africae*, a tick-born pathogen in travelers to sub-Saharan Africa. N Engl J Med 2001; 344: 1504–1510.

CASE 106. A 10-year-old girl presents with a skin abnormality of several weeks' duration. It is not itchy and is only of esthetic concern to her. On examination it appears as seen in Figure 106.1. There are multiple areas of hypopigmentation with slight very superficial scaliness. The lesions have normal sensation.

- *What is the diagnosis?*
- *How can you confirm it?*
- *How would you treat the patient?*

This is the typical appearance of Pityriasis versicolor, which is a very superficial fungal infection caused by *Malassezia furfur*. This yeast can be part of the normal flora of the skin and causes lesions, as seen in the picture, mainly in adolescents, although it may affect younger children and adults. The infection usually affects the shoulders, neck, and upper trunk. The diagnosis can be confirmed by microscopic examination of a skin scraping stained with methylene blue stain or after clearing with potassium hydroxide. This shows round yeast cells and hyphae, the so called "spaghetti-and-meatballs" (Figure 106.2).

The treatment consists of selenium sulfide shampoo, applied for 10 minutes to the affected skin, daily for 1 week then weekly for 1 month.

This organism can cause invasive infection in individuals receiving total parenteral nutrition that includes a lipid preparation. The organism requires

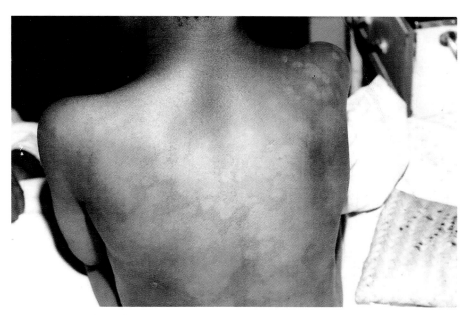

FIG. 106.1.   The child's rash.

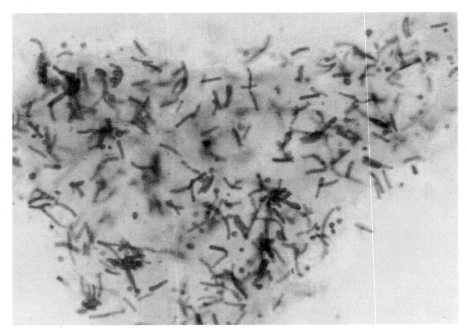

FIG. 106.2.   A photomicrograph of Malassezia furfur. (Courtesy of Dr Lucille K Georg/Centers for Disease Control and Prevention)

lipid for its growth. One of the methods used in the laboratory for identifying it is demonstration of growth in the presence of lipid, for example, olive oil, but no growth in its absence.

CASE 107. A 5-year-old girl presents with a history of having recurrent episodes of headache, abdominal pain, and stuffy nose, followed within a few hours by the onset of fever. This is associated with swelling of the lymph nodes in the neck and often with mouth ulcers. These episodes, which last about 4 days, occur every 4–6 weeks and have occurred her "whole life." She has been exposed to dogs, cats, hamsters, tropical fish, and ticks. No other family member has had similar symptoms. On examination she is well appearing and afebrile, and the only abnormal findings are enlarged, tender upper cervical lymph nodes, large tonsils, and a slightly enlarged spleen.

- *What is the differential diagnosis?*
- *How should she be managed?*

This child's current clinical findings suggest an infectious mononucleosis-like illness. This is caused by Epstein–Barr virus, cytomegalovirus, human immunodeficiency virus, and toxoplasmosis. These conditions do not, however, cause recurrent episodes of febrile illness over years. This child's symptoms suggest a "periodic fever" syndrome. This is a group of disorders characterized by recurrent episodes of fever without evidence of an infectious etiology. Some of them are inherited disorders of proteins involved in inflammation. The most important of these is Familial Mediterranean fever (FMF), which is characterized by recurrent episodes of fever, arthritis, and serositis. Affected individuals, who have ancestry from the eastern Mediterranean region, can develop amyloidosis. The cause is an abnormality of "pyrin," a protein involved in the inflammatory cascade. The treatment is colchicine. Other inherited disorders in this group are Muckle-Wells syndrome, also due to an abnormality of pyrin, Hibernian fever, due to an abnormality of the tumor necrosis factor receptor, and the Hyper IgD syndrome, due to a mutation of the enzyme mevalonate kinase.

This child's illness is highly suggested of a syndrome called the "Periodic Fever, Aphthous stomatitis, Pharyngitis, Cervical Adenitis" (PFAPA) syndrome. It does not appear to have serious sequelae, and there is no specific therapy.

Reading:

Feder, H: Periodic fever, aphthous stomatitis, pharyngitis, adenitis: a clinical review of a new syndrome. Curr Opin Pediatr 2000; 12: 252–256.

Scholl, P: Periodic fever syndromes. Curr Opin Pediatr. 2000; 12: 563–566.

Edwards MS, Millon JC, Perez MD: Recurrent fever in a healthy-appearing child. Semin Pediatr Infect Dis 2004; 15: 220, 229–234.

CASE 108. A 14-year-old previously healthy boy presents with a history of progressively worse pain in the left hip developing over the past 1 week, and fever for 3 days. He jumped off a porch 1 week ago but did not injure himself. On examination he is moderately ill-appearing with a temperature of 39.8°C, heart rate of 132 beats per minute, blood pressure of 111/64 mm Hg, and respiratory rate of 20 per minute. The most notable finding is warmth and tenderness over the left gluteal region and greater femoral trochanter area, and limitation and pain on rotation of the hip. Flexion and extension of the hip are fairly normal. There is a healed abrasion on the posterior aspect of the left thigh. There is mild conjunctival injection, and the heart examination is normal except for a 2/6 ejection systolic murmur. The rest of the examination is normal, in particular there are no enlargement of the liver or spleen, no lymphadenopathy, and no other skin lesions.

- *Where might the illness be located?*
- *What might its cause be?*
- *What would you do?*

In patients with pain around the hip, one should consider disease within the hip joint, the bones around the hip joint (pelvic bones, sacrum, and femora), the bones and soft tissue of the lower back, disease within the contents of the pelvic cavity (intestine, genital tract, urinary bladder, and muscles, including the obturator internus, pyriformis, gemelli, coccygeus, pubococcygeus, and levator ani), and disease affecting nerves around the hip.

Disease within the hip joint is very important to diagnose early because raised pressure within the joint from inflammation can lead to compromise of the vascular supply to the head of the femur and subsequent avascular necrosis. The ability of the patient to flex and extend the hip but not rotate it suggests that the disease is not within the hip joint itself, while tenderness over the gluteal region suggests the possibility of disease within the gluteal muscles.

Given the patient's fever, the most likely cause of the disease is an infection. The presence of a healed abrasion on the thigh suggests that the likely organism is *Staphylococcus aureus* or *Streptococcus pyogenes*. In addition to the local infection he could be bacteremic and at risk for the hemodynamic effects of bacteremia and for dissemination of the infection.

A specific clinical examination that should be performed in this situation is a rectal examination. This is the only clinical access available to examine the inside of the pelvis and the pelvic bones in males and prepubertal females. In this patient it revealed a boggy swelling anterior to the sacrum, suggesting that the problem is a pelvic abscess.

The clinical situation poses the following dilemma: should one immediately initiate antimicrobial therapy active against the most likely organisms in this moderately ill patient or should one first try to delineate the focus of disease by imaging, with the hope that this will enable a surgeon to aspirate or drain the infected material, after which antimicrobial therapy would be started?

In this child a blood culture was performed and antimicrobial therapy was initiated, directed against staphylococci, including methicillin-resistant *Staphylococcus aureus*, *Streptococcus pyogenes*, and enteric rods, with vancomycin, nafcillin, and cefotaxime. A magnetic resonance imaging (MRI) scan of the pelvis is shown in Figure 108.1.

This showed a large pelvic abscess compressing the rectum. There was also associated swelling around the posterior branch of the first sacral nerve root, which might have accounted for some of his pain. Although surgical

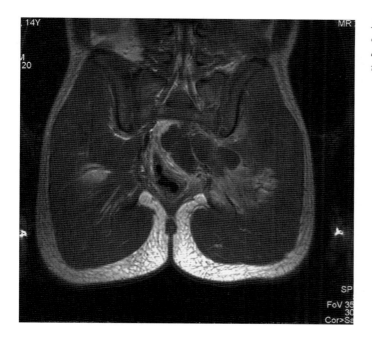

FIG. 108.1.   An MRI scan of the pelvis showing a large abscess compressing the rectum.

drainage was considered, the inaccessibility of the abscess led to a delay in performance of such a procedure.

The first blood culture grew out *Staphylococcus aureus*, susceptible to penicillin; the blood culture taken 2 days day after initiation of therapy, grew out the same organism but there were a few colonies that were methicillin resistant. He remained febrile, and a blood culture taken 3 days after initiation of therapy grew out a methicillin-resistant *Staphylococcus aureus*. He then underwent surgical drainage of the abscess through the rectum. The pus grew out methicillin-resistant *Staphylococcus aureus*. After the drainage he became afebrile and made a speedy recovery.

How did this abscess develop? Possibly he sustained an injury to one of the pelvic muscles when he jumped off the porch, causing a muscle hematoma. This might have become seeded during a transient staphylococcal bacteremia arising from the thigh abrasion.

This patient demonstrates the following:

(a) pain around the hip may be due to disease inside the pelvis;

(b) a rectal examination can help to locate disease around the hip;

(c) antimicrobial therapy may not be effective if pus is not drained;

(d) antibiotic resistance can emerge within a patient during antimicrobial therapy, due to natural selection of resistant organisms.

Staphylococcus aureus inhabits the skin and the anterior nares. It is an opportunist in that minor skin trauma may be followed by local infections. These include impetigo (pyoderma) and furuncles, which may progress to cellulitis and abscesses, and surgical wound infections. These foci can be associated with asymptomatic bacteremia. This bacteremia can, however, result in metastatic infections that can be severe, and, in turn, lead to severe symptomatic bacteremia. These foci include bone (osteomyeltitis), joint (septic arthritis), muscle (pyomyositis), lung (hematogenous pneumonia), and endocardium (infective endocarditis). Recently a syndrome of severe sepsis, associated with pneumonia and sometimes deep venous thrombosis, has been described, affecting particularly adolescent boys. This is caused by a community-acquired methicillin-resistant strain or strains of *Staphylococcus aureus* that produce a virulence factor called Pantin-Valentine leukocidin (pvl).

Although the above-described patient did not have manifestations of this syndrome, he was treated aggressively on presentation with the concern that this might develop.

Reading:

Crawford SE, Daum RS: Epidemic community-associated methicillin-resistant *Staphylococcus aureus*. Modern times for an ancient pathogen. Pediatr Infect Dis J 2005; 24: 459–460.

Gonzalez BE, Martinez-Aguilar G, Hulten KG et al: Severe staphylococcal sepsis in adolescents in the era of community-acquired methicillin-resistant *Staphylococcus aureus*. Pediatrics 2005; 115: 642–648.

Zetola N, Nuermberger EI, Bishai WR: Community-acquired methicillin-resistant *Staphylococcus aureus*: an emerging threat. Lancet Infect Dis 2005; 5: 275–286.

CASE 109. A 10-year-old boy, previously healthy, was diagnosed with pneumococcal meningitis caused by a fully susceptible strain of *Streptococcus pneumoniae*. He was treated with intravenous ceftriaxone and steadily improved. On the eighth day of therapy he complains of severe right upper quadrant pain and nausea. He lacks a cough or other respiratory tract symptoms. Examination is normal except for right upper quadrant tenderness. Of note is the fact that he is not jaundiced.

- *What might explain his problem?*
- *What additional information would you like?*
- *What would you do?*

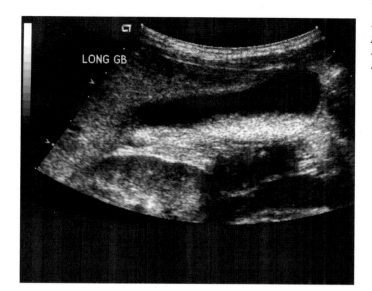

FIG. 109.1. An ultrasound picture of the gallbladder showing a large amount of sludge within the lumen.

The sites of disease most likely to cause the above symptoms are the liver, gallbladder, and lower lobe of the right lung. The lack of respiratory symptoms makes lung disease unlikely. A specific risk factor for disease of the gallbladder is cefriaxone, 50% of which is excreted in bile. It can cause the formation of "sludge" in the gallbladder where it is concentrated up to 120 times the serum concentration. The additional information of interest is the dosage of this drug that he received, which was 2 g every 12 hours. His weight was 45 kg. This dosage is the highest dose recommended for adults and was probably too high for him. An appropriate dose might have been 1.5 g every 12 hours. The presence of biliary sludge can be demonstrated by ultrasound. An ultrasound (Figure 109.1) revealed a large amount of sludge in the gallbladder.

Management should entail discontinuing the drug if appropriate or lowering its dosage. If symptoms persist or become worse, cholecystectomy might become necessary.

He improved initially after ceftriaxone therapy was discontinued. However, he presented a few weeks later with severe epigastric pain and was found the have acute pancreatitis. After this had resolved, he underwent cholecystectomy.

Reading:

Ko C, Sekijima JH, Sum P: Biliary sludge. Ann Intern Med 1999; 130: 301–311

CASE 110. A 4-year-old boy, previously diagnosed with autoimmune lymphoproliferative syndrome (ALPS) and being treated with systemic corticosteroids, presents with a history of fever and cough for a few days. There is no vomiting, diarrhea, dysuria, or bone pain, and he has not traveled outside his home town in Georgia, USA. On examination he is miserable and difficult to examine but not severely ill. His temperature is 39°C, and his vital signs are normal other than a heart rate of 120/minute. There is no pallor or jaundice. He has enlargement of cervical, axillary, and inguinal lymph nodes and a slightly enlarged spleen. After multiple attempts, his throat is visualized. This reveals inflamed tonsils covered with extensive exudates. The rest of his examination is normal.

- *What is your differential diagnosis?*
- *What would you do?*

This child is immunocompromised by virtue of receiving corticosteroids and possibly by his underlying disease itself. This places him at increased risk for severe viral infections. His only localizing finding is an exudative tonsillitis. This is the likely cause of his symptoms. This, together with the generalized lymphadenopathy and splenic enlargement suggests the diagnosis of infectious mononucleosis. However, the splenic enlargement could be due to his underlying disorder.

Other causes of tonsillitis are *Streptococcus pyogenes*, *Corynebacterium diphtheriae* (to which he has no known exposure risk), and several respiratory viruses, including adenovirus. *Arcanobacterium haemolyticum* infection of the pharynx is associated with a diffuse scarlatiniform rash, which this child lacks.

Therefore a test for streptococcal pharyngitis should be performed. If positive he should be treated with penicillin. If negative, specific tests for viruses, by antigen detection or by culture, should be considered. In most patients these are not of value because they do not influence therapy. However, in a child such as this, a positive test might restrain one from pursuing other diagnostic tests and from using antibiotics.

In this child, his fever persisted for several days. A culture from his throat grew out adenovirus.

There are more than 40 different serotypes of adenoviruses, which are large DNA viruses. Most of these cause mucosal disease, particularly of the respiratory tract and eye, but also of the urinary bladder. Specific serotypes, types 40 and 41, are well-recognized causes of acute gastroenteritis. Adenoviruses occasionally cause visceral disease such as hepatitis and severe pneumonia in normal hosts. However, they constitute a very important cause of severe and sometimes fatal pneumonia and hepatitis in immunocompromised hosts, in particular transplant patients.

Although antiviral therapy has not been clearly shown to be of benefit to affected patients, there are anecdotal reports of improvement in patients treated with cidofovir, which is a very toxic drug.

This child gradually improved without receiving any antiviral therapy.

Reading:

Leen AM, Looney CM: Adenovirus as an emerging pathogen in immunocompromised patients. Bri J Haematol 2004; 128: 135–144.

Ison MG: Adenovirus infection in transplant recipients. Clin Infect Dis 2006; 43: 331–339.

CASE 111. A 16-year-old boy presents with a 4-day history of fever, headache, generalized muscle aches, and weakness. He has also had odynophagia and upper abdominal pain. On examination he has a temperature of 38.4°C, heart rate of 93/minute, and blood pressure of 98/53. His conjunctivae are mildly inflamed, but the rest of his mucosae are normal. His abdomen is mildly tender with slight hepatomegaly but no splenomegaly. There are enlarged axillary, cervical, and inguinal lymph nodes. His strength is generally reduced and he has diffuse muscle tenderness. The rest of his examination is normal.

- *What is your differential diagnosis?*
- *What more would you like to know?*
- *What would you like to do?*

This patient clearly has a systemic disease associated with fever. An infectious etiology is most likely. The lymphadenopathy suggests an infectious mononucleosis-like illness. The differential diagnosis includes:

Viral infections
    Epstein–Barr virus (EBV)
    cytomegalovirus (CMV)
    human immunodeficiency virus (HIV)
    hepatitis A, B or C
Bacterial infections
    rickettsial or ehrlichial infection
    syphilis (secondary)
    leptospirosis

Parasitic infection
   toxoplasmosis
Noninfectious etiologies
   systemic lupus erythematosus
   leukemia

It is very important to enquire from him about possible exposures to these agents, in particular travel and recreational activities, including sexual activity. Laboratory studies should be used both to define the extent of organ system abnormalities and to determine possible etiologies, both for treatment and for public health reasons.

Such studies in his case revealed elevated hepatic transaminases (alanine aminotransferase 661 U and aspartate aminotransferase 935 U), indicating hepatitis, and elevated creatine phosphokinase (660 U), indicating myositis.

Serological studies revealed that he had evidence of a past infection with EBV and that he had a negative antibody test for HIV and *Toxoplasma gondii*.

Negative antibody studies do not exclude the diagnosis of acute (primary) HIV infection, because seroconversion can take 3–6 months from the time of infection. Therefore direct tests of viral presence should be performed. This generally means viral nucleic acid detection, by a polymerase chain reaction test, which was positive in his case. This is, in fact, a typical presentation of acute HIV infection. This occurs in about 70% of cases of horizontally acquired HIV infection. The symptoms and signs include fever and fatigue (almost all patients), night sweats, myalgia, arthralgia, nausea, vomiting, pharyngitis, lymphadenopathy, enlargement of liver or spleen, rash, oral or genital ulcers, oral thrush, headache, meningitis, myelitis, encephalopathy, peripheral neuropathy, and "cotton-wool" retinal spots.

The diagnosis should be considered in individuals who are at risk for HIV infection, and who have features of an infectious mononucleosis-like illness.

The importance of making a diagnosis is for long-term management and public health management, including counseling the patient about his risk of transmitting the infection to others and following-up .his sexual contacts. The overall benefit of antiretroviral therapy in such patients is controversial.

Reading:

Schacker T, Collier AC, Hughes J et al: Clinical and epidemiologic features of primary HIV infection. Ann Intern Med 1996; 125: 257–264.

Kahn JO, Walker BD: Acute human immunodeficiency virus type 1 infection. N Engl J Med 1998; 339: 33–39.

Perlmutter BL, Glaser JB, Oyugi SO: How to recognize and treat acute HIV syndrome. American Family Physician 1999; 60: 535–546.

CASE 112. A 4-year-old boy complains of sudden severe pain in his left eye while playing outside. At an initial evaluation, he is diagnosed with a corneal abrasion, but on the following day he has periorbital edema, proptosis, ophthalmoplegia, and markedly decreased visual acuity. There is a vitreous opacity, indicating a diagnosis of endophthalmitis. An ultrasound indicates the presence of a metallic foreign body in the eye. A surgical exploration of the eye is performed during which large necrotic areas of sclera and retina are noted. Therefore the eye is enucleated. Histology of the eye is shown in Figure 112.1, as is a Gram stain of the excised material (Figure 112.2).

- *What is the likely organism?*
- *Why did it cause such rapid destruction of the eye?*

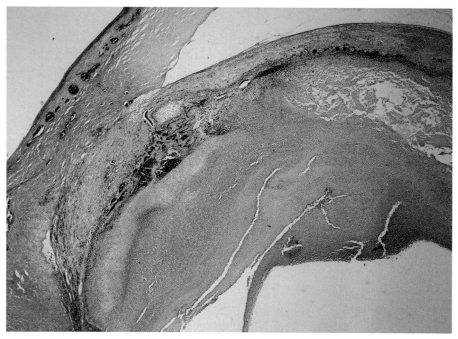

FIG. 112.1.   An abscess behind the iris (×100). (Courtesy of Dr Hans Grossniklaus, Department of Ophthalmology, Emory University)

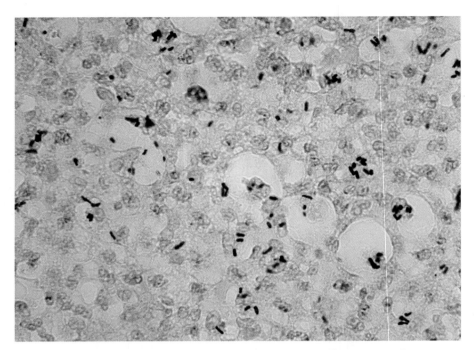

FIG. 112.2. A Gram-stained preparation of the contents of the intraocular abscess (×250). (Courtesy of Dr Hans Grossniklaus, Department of Ophthalmology, Emory University)

The organisms seen are large, fat, Gram-positive bacilli. This suggests a *Bacillus* spp. or a *Clostridium* spp. infection. (The culture subsequently grew out *Bacillus cereus*.) Both these organisms can cause infections complicating injuries, which must have occurred in this child, to explain the foreign body within his eye. This scenario is well described as being caused by *Bacillus cereus*, which is a very important cause of infection complicating penetrating eye injuries. This organism produces several exotoxins, including a lecithinase, which probably plays a role in the ocular damage. Endophthalmitis (inflammation of the intraocular structures) results from penetrating injury of the eye by trauma or surgery (such as cataract surgery) or from bloodstream infection with bacteria or fungi. Systemic antimicrobial therapy is not very effective for treatment of patients with this condition. Optimal therapy entails vitrectomy and instillation of antimicrobial agents, in particular vancomycin and amikacin, directly into the vitreous.

Bacillus cereus also causes other infections. In normal hosts it causes two acute food poisoning syndromes, namely an emetic syndrome and a diarrheal syndrome. The organism causes infections of vascular catheters and other indwelling devices, and, in severely compromised hosts, can cause bacteremia and other severe infections.

Reading:

David DB, Kirkby GR, Noble BA: *Bacillus cereus* endophthalmitis. Br J Ophthalmol 1994; 78: 577–580.

Gaur A, Shenep JL: The expanding spectrum of disease caused by *Bacillus cereus*. Pediatr Infect Dis J 2001; 20: 533–534.

CASE 113. A 12-year-old boy with nephrotic syndrome for several years presents with a 1-day history of fever and severe abdominal pain. He always has some edema and ascites. Treatment for his nephrotic syndrome consists of a low salt diet and prednisone. He requires infusions of albumin followed by furosemide when his ascites causes discomfort. There is no history of diarrhea or cough. On examination he is very ill-appearing and grunting. His heart rate is 120/minute, blood pressure 100/60 mm Hg, respiratory rate 40/minute, temperature 38.7°C, his peripheral perfusion is good, and he has marked anasarca. His lung examination reveals dullness to percussion and decreased breath sounds at both bases. His abdomen is distended and diffusely very tender. The rest of his examination is normal.

- *What is your differential diagnosis?*
- *How would you manage him?*

The child's nephrotic syndrome places him at risk for systemic infections, particularly those caused by *Streptococcus pneumoniae*, and for thromboses. In addition the corticosteroid therapy predisposes him to opportunistic infections, such as those caused by cytomegalovirus and *Pneumocystis jiroveci*. Individuals with ascites, whether due to nephrotic syndrome or liver disease, are at risk for the development of spontaneous bacterial peritonitis due to hematogenous spread of bacteria. In patients with nephrotic syndrome such infections are caused mainly by *Streptococcus pneumoniae*, other streptococci, and by enteric Gram-negative bacilli. Systemic infections are an important cause of morbidity and mortality in patients with nephritic syndrome, probably due to loss of immunoglobulin and complement through the urine.

His clinical picture strongly suggests an intraperitoneal infection and sepsis syndrome. Although peritonitis from a perforated bowel, such as the appendix, is possible, spontaneous bacterial peritonitis is much more likely in this case.

Management should consist of the following:

1. Ensuring adequate perfusion – Although he is edematous, his intravascular volume is likely depleted. An infusion of intravenous albumin would therefore be indicated.

2. Obtaining cultures of blood and the peritoneal fluid – Peritoneal fluid should be filtered and the filters cultured, because the concentration of organisms in the fluid is usually very low.

3. Antimicrobial therapy – This should include drugs that are active against pneumococci as well as enteric bacilli. A suitable drug is a third-generation cephalosporin, such as ceftriaxone or cefotaxime.

4. Prevention – Patients with the nephrotic syndrome should be immunized against pneumococcal infection with the heptavalent conjugate pneumococcal vaccine. Those older than 2 years should also receive the 23-valent polysaccharide vaccine.

This patient was treated as described here, and he recovered. The blood culture grew out *Streptococcus pneumoniae*.

Reading:

Gorensek MJ, Lebel MH, Nelson JD: Peritonitis in children with nephrotic syndrome. Pediatrics 1988; 81: 849–856.

Krensky AM, Ingelfinger JR, Grupe WE: Peritonitis in childhood nephrotic syndrome. Am J Dis Child 1982; 136: 732–736.

CASE 114. An 18-month-old girl presents at about 2 AM with a 1-day history of a noisy cough and fever. The illness started 2 days ago with a runny nose. There is no history of a choking episode. She is brought at this time because she has started having difficulty breathing and her breaths are noisy.

On examination she is in marked respiratory distress and has obvious inspiratory stridor. Her heart rate is 140/minute, respiratory rate 40/minute, and temperature 38.7°C. Although she is alert, she is very agitated and moving around a lot, while lying in her father's arms. She is mildly cyanosed and has a palpable pulsus paradoxus. Her respiratory tract examination reveals marked suprasternal and subcostal retractions on inspiration. The lungs are resonant to percussion, and, on auscultation, breath sounds are barely audible.

- *What is your initial assessment?*
- *What do you want to do?*
- *What is the differential diagnosis?*

This child is in respiratory failure, due to obstruction of the extrathoracic airway, and respiratory arrest is imminent. Therefore endotracheal intubation should be performed immediately. Once this has been accomplished and the child's condition has been stabilized, a differential diagnosis can be considered. The only condition which can present with stridor, and in which the management might be different, is a foreign body inhalation. In that case attempts should be made to dislodge it.

The mechanism of stridor and the differential diagnosis follows.

Stridor is an inspiratory noise that reflects obstruction of the larynx and extrathoracic trachea. Resistance to airflow is inversely proportional to the airway radius to the fourth power. Thus reduction of airway radius by one half causes a sixteenfold increase in airflow resistance. The noise and phase of respiration during which the noise occurs is very important in determining the site of respiratory obstruction. This is illustrated in Figure 114.1.

During inspiration, as the diaphragm descends and the thoracic wall moves outward, the lungs and intrathoracic airways expand; the airways outside the thorax (larynx and upper trachea) become narrower, due to the negative pressure within the lumen. Therefore any narrowing of the larynx or upper trachea, for example, that caused by mucosal swelling, is exacerbated during inspiration, resulting in stridor. During expiration the reverse occurs. Therefore narrowing in the intrathoracic airways, for example, asthma or bronchiolitis, is exacerbated during expiration. In such cases the noise produced is wheezing, which is more pronounced during expiration.

EXPIRATION   **INSPIRATION**

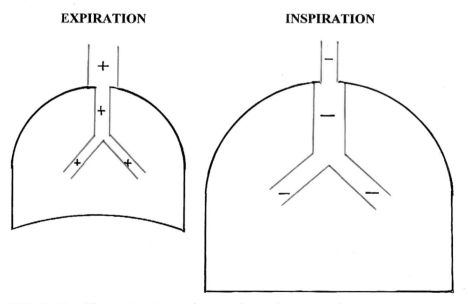

FIG. 114.1.   Changes in airway pressure during the stages of respiration (+, positive pressure; −, negative pressure).

■**TAB. 114.1: Differential diagnosis of acute stridor.**

1. Mechanical obstruction
    foreign body inhalation
2. Infections
    epiglottitis
    retropharyngeal abscess
    diphtheria
    viral croup (laryngotracheobronchitis)
    bacterial tracheitis
3. Chronic obstruction aggravated by a superimposed viral infection
    laryngotracheomalacia
    laryngeal web
    laryngeal cyst, tumor, hemangioma
    laryngeal papilloma
4. Bilateral recurrent laryngeal nerve palsy
5. Hypocalcemia
6. External pressure
    rapidly enlarging lymph node due to malignancy or tuberculosis

Clinical features indicating severe obstruction are:

mental status changes, including agitation
marked sternal , suprasternal, or subcostal retractions
palpable pulsus paradoxus
marked tachycardia
poor or absent breath sounds

The commonest cause of stridor is laryngotracheobronchitis, which was the diagnosis in this child.

A discussion of epiglottitis, viral croup, and bacterial tracheitis follows.

Epiglottitis: This is a bacterial infection of the epiglottis *and* the periepiglottic tissue. It was formerly caused mainly by *Haemophilus influenzae* type b, but as a result of widespread use of a vaccine against this organism, it is now caused mainly by *Streptococcus pneumoniae* and *Streptococcus pyogenes*. The disease is characterized by marked swelling of the epiglottis and aryepiglottic folds, resulting in a circle of swelling around the airway, which may totally occlude it. The clinical features are fever, cough, stridor, drooling, and respiratory distress. The child prefers to sit, with the neck forward. Because the airway in this condition can be severely compromised, this must be treated as an extreme emergency. When this condition is suspected, under ideal circumstances, the patient should be taken to an area, for example, operating room, where he/she can be have the airway examined by somebody skilled in endotracheal intubation. The airway obstruction can be so severe that the only clue to the presence of an airway is a bubble. The management is endotracheal intubation to secure the airway. Once this is accomplished, antimicrobial therapy can be addressed. This should be directed at *Haemophilus influenzae*, *Streptococcus pneumoniae*, and *Streptococcus pyogenes*. Ceftriaxone and cefotaxime are suitable choices.

Viral croup (Laryngotracheobronchitis): This is caused by several respiratory viruses, the most common of which is parainfluenza virus. Infants and young children present with a history of fever, a barking cough, and stridor, often preceded by rhinorrhea. The stridor often develops during the middle of the night. This diagnosis, which is usually made clinically, is the most common of those affecting the middle respiratory tract (larynx and extrathoracic trachea).

Management: Most patients require no specific treatment. Humidification of the atmosphere has been used traditionally and may be helpful, but its value has not been demonstrated in a clinical trial. Dexamethasone, administered orally or parentrally has been shown to bring about clinical improvement. Inhalation of epinephrine may also be of value in more severe cases. Inhalation of a 70% helium/30% oxygen mixture may help severe cases by lowering the resistance to airflow. Patients with the physical findings of severe disease, as described in the case scenario above, should undergo endotracheal intubation immediately.

Bacterial tracheitis: This is a severe infection in which the patient is toxic-appearing and has the features of middle respiratory tract obstruction. He/she coughs up (or is found at endotracheal intubation to have) large amounts of purulent secretions arising from the trachea. It usually complicates a previous epithelial injury such as that caused by a viral infection, in particular that caused by measles or influenza. The most common bacterial cause is *Staphylococcus aureus*. The diagnosis is based on clinical features and sometimes on findings at endoscopy. Treatment consists of establishing an adequate airway and of antibiotics directed at the likely agent. Examination of secretions by Gram stain is very important for choosing empiric antibiotic therapy.

Reading:

Brown JC: The management of croup. British Medical Bull 2002 ; 61: 189–202.

CASE 115. A 15-year-old previously healthy girl presents with a history of abdominal pain for 2 days. It started in the lower abdomen and has remained there. It is constant, aggravated by movement, but not crampy in nature. Her last menstrual period began 2 weeks ago and lasted 1 week.

There is nausea but no vomiting or diarrhea. There are no respiratory or urinary symptoms. On examination she is moderately ill-appearing. Her temperature is 37.9°C, and the rest of her vital signs are normal. The main finding is marked abdominal tenderness across the whole of the lower abdomen, on the right side more than the left side. She also has tenderness in the right upper quadrant, but neither the liver nor gallbladder can be palpated.

- *What is your differential diagnosis?*
- *What would you do?*

Pain in the lower abdomen is derived primarily from one of three organs, namely the intestine, urinary tract, or genital tract. In addition the organs that can give rise to right upper quadrant tenderness are the liver, gallbladder, pancreas, intestine, and kidney. Therefore the differential diagnosis is broad. Diseases of the liver, gallbladder, and pancreas do not, as a rule, cause lower abdominal pain, which is her main symptom. However, inflammatory disease of the Fallopian tubes can result in spread of inflammation up the right paracolic gutter to the perihepatic region, to cause perihepatitis (Fitz-Hugh-Curtis syndrome).

The differential diagnosis includes the following:

Intestinal disease
   acute appendicitis – her symptoms and signs are too diffuse, and she does not appear to have generalized peritonitis
Genital tract – salpingitis (pelvic inflammatory disease)
   ruptured ovarian cyst
   ovarian torsion
   ectopic pregnancy
   labor – this is crampy in nature
   endometriosis
Urinary tract
   infection – the symptoms seem too extensive for this condition

It is very important to enquire about a history of sexual intercourse (although denial by the patient does not necessarily exclude this possibility, and does not necessarily exclude the possibility of a sexually transmitted infection or pregnancy) and to perform a genital examination.

This patient was, indeed, sexually active. Pelvic examination revealed a purulent discharge issuing from the cervical os. In addition there was tenderness of the adnexa, and movement of the cervix elicited pain. These features strongly suggest the diagnosis of pelvic inflammatory disease.

The following tests should be performed:

(a) Microscopic examination of the discharge (wet preparation) to look for leukocytes, "clue cells," which are characteristic of bacterial vaginosis, and for *Trichomonas vaginalis*.

(b) A culture from the cervix for *Neisseria gonorrhoeae* and a test for *Chlamydia trachomatis* (antigen, nucleic acid). Although *Chlamydia trachomatis* can be cultured in tissue culture, this is expensive and should be reserved for use in prepubertal children (Figure 115.1).

(c) Screening tests for evidence of other sexually transmitted infections, including hepatitis B, syphilis, and human immunodeficiency virus (HIV) infection.

(d) A pregnancy test. A positive pregnancy test has the following implications:

   (i)   the diagnosis might be an ectopic pregnancy;

   (ii) if treatment for pelvic inflammatory disease is to be administered, a tetracycline should NOT be given;

   (iii) radiological (excluding ultrasound) procedures of the abdomen are contraindicated.

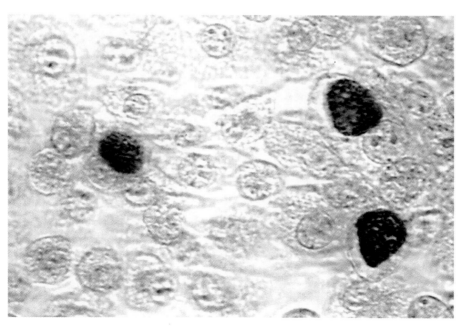

FIG. 115.1.   Tissue culture (McCoy cells) showing intracellular inclusions representing Chlamydia trachomatis. (Courtesy of the Centers for Disease Control and Prevention/Dr E Arum, Dr N Jacobs).

(e) Urinalysis, microscopy, and culture. However, if there is pus in the vagina, which can readily interfere with obtaining a clean urine specimen, these tests may show numerous leukocytes and the culture may be falsely positive.

If the pregnancy test is negative and there is no vaginal or cervical pus, the other diagnostic possibilities become more likely. Therefore, depending on the progression of her course, other diagnostic tests should be considered, including an abdominal and pelvic ultrasound or computer tomography scan.

This patient's pregnancy test was negative.

She was diagnosed with pelvic inflammatory disease, complicated by the Fitz-Hugh-Curtis syndrome.

She received antimicrobial therapy with cefoxitin and doxycycline, and she had largely recovered within 2 days. Her test for *Chlamydia trachomatis* was positive. She was counseled to use condoms during sexual intercourse and to advise her sexual partner(s) to seek medical treatment. Contraception was also discussed with her.

Pelvic Inflammatory Disease(PID) is the term used to refer to infection of the Fallopian tubes (salpingitis) and endometrium. It is an important cause of morbidity in adolescent girls and an important cause of infertility.

Pathogenesis: Infectious agents, primarily *Chlamydia trachomatis*, and, to a lesser extent, *Neisseria gonorrhoeae*, ascend from the cervix, into the uterus, and thence into the tubes, where they cause tubal epithelial damage. There is secondary invasion by normal vaginal flora, such as enteric rods, and anaerobes. The purulent discharge within the tubes can spread into the peritoneal cavity, resulting in localized peritonitis. A tubo-ovarian abscess may also develop. The discharge may extend to the capsule of the liver, resulting in perihepatitis. The main long-term complications resulting from the tubular damage are infertility and ectopic pregnancy. Adhesions resulting from the peritonitis can result in intestinal obstruction.

Diagnosis: The diagnosis is made clinically. Confirming the diagnosis is seldom accomplished because the "gold standard" for the diagnosis, namely visualizing the tubes at laparoscopy, is seldom done. Although the diagnostic features (adnexal tenderness, cervical motion tenderness, and lower abdominal pain) are suggestive, they are nonspecific. The differential diagnosis is discussed above.

Management: Whether patients should be hospitalized or not should be determined by their severity of illness and the degree of certainty of the diagnosis. I prefer to hospitalize patients with severe abdominal pain, until their symptoms have significantly improved. Firstly this allows for observation of the patient for improvement, particularly since deterioration would suggest an alternative diagnosis, for which they might require different management, and, secondly, it ensures that the patient complies with therapy initially.

The mainstay of therapy is antimicrobial. Several options are available. The chosen agents should provide antimicrobial activity against *Chlamydia trachomatis*, *Neisseria gonorrhoeae*, enteric rods, and anaerobic bacteria. I follow the recommendations of the US Public Health Service (see Reading). My preferred regimen is:

Doxycycline 100 mg every 12 hours, orally or intravenously,
    PLUS
Cefoxitin 2 g intravenously every 6 hours OR cefotetan 2 g every 12 hours intravenously

Once improvement has occurred, therapy can be completed on an out-patient basis with a course of doxycycline to complete 14 days of therapy.

Outcome: If the patient has not improved within 48 hours, one should consider the possibility that the diagnosis is mistaken or that a complication has developed, the most likely of which is a tubo-ovarian abscess. Imaging studies, in particular ultrasonography, may be helpful at this point.

Reading:

McCormack WM: Pelvic inflammatory disease. N Engl J Med 1994; 330: 115–119.

US Public Health Service. Guidelines for the treatment of sexually transmitted diseases. 2002. MMWR 2002; 51; RR-6: 48–52.

CASE 116 (HYP). A 12-year-old previously healthy boy presents with a history of fever and cough for about 5 days. In the past day he has become short of breath and weak. On examination he is ill-appearing, with a respiratory rate of 50 per minute, heart rate of 130 per minute, and blood pressure of 100/40, and he is perfusing well. His mucosae are pale, and he has mild jaundice. The heart is normal except for a 2/6 ejection systolic murmur, and the lungs are remarkable for retractions and diffuse crackles throughout the lower zones. The abdominal and neuromuscular examinations are normal.

- *What might be the problem?*
- *What would you do?*

The physiological problems are respiratory difficulty and pallor, but not shock. Therefore the first item of management is to provide additional oxygen. Pallor in the absence of shock indicates anemia. The findings of fever and pulmonary crackles suggest the presence of pneumonia. Although the crackles could be due to pulmonary edema, there are no signs of heart disease to suggest a cardiac cause for this problem. What might be causing pneumonia in a previously healthy boy? The preceding symptoms suggest a respiratory virus infection, such as influenza. What about the pallor and jaundice? These suggest a hemolytic anemia. The association of pulmonary disease and anemia should also suggest the possibility of pulmonary hemorrhage, as can occur with Goodpasture's syndrome and Wegener's granulomatosis. There is no preceding history of a genetic cause of hemolytic anemia, such as sickle cell disease. However, a sickle cell crisis affecting the lung (acute chest syndrome) could explain the child's condition very well. Infections can cause hemolysis by stimulating the production of autoantibodies, as in the case of *Mycoplasma pneumoniae* infection, or by precipitating a hemolytic crisis in the case of underlying glucose-6-phosphate-dehydrogenase (G6PD) deficiency. Making a hematologic diagnosis in this case is important for the following reasons: if there is an autoimmune hemolytic anemia, corticosteroid therapy might be beneficial; if this is a sickle cell acute chest crisis, there may be a very rapid deterioration, and a regular blood transfusion or an exchange transfusion

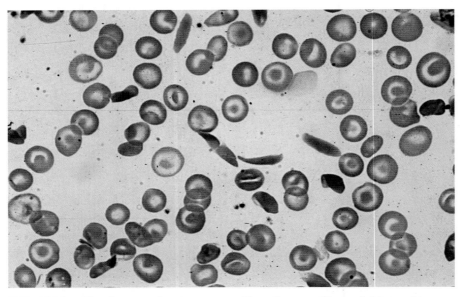

FIG. 116.1.   *Blood smear showing target cells, a feature of hemoglobinopathies, and sickle cells.*

might become necessary; if the diagnosis is G6PD deficiency, education about risk situations and drugs that can cause a hemolytic crisis is important.

Therefore tests that might help in making a diagnosis are a blood smear to examine the red cell morphology, a Coomb's test, hemoglobin electrophoresis and G6PD activity. The blood smear may show: diffuse basophilia (indicative of young red cells), agglutination of red cells in cold-agglutinin autoimmune hemolytic anemia, "bite cells," characteristic of G6PD deficiency, or sickle cells (Figure 116.1).

The patient nevertheless requires treatment for the pneumonia, with agents active against *Streptococcus pneumoniae* and *Mycoplasma pneumoniae*, such as a combination of a penicillin or third-generation cephalosporin together with a macrolide.

Reading:

Berkowitz FE: Hemolysis and infection: categories and mechanisms of their interrelationship. Rev Infect Dis 1991; 13: 1151–1162.

CASE 117. A 6-year-old girl presents with acute onset of fever and headache and is diagnosed with pneumococcal meningitis. Her left pupil does not respond to light, and the optic nerve is white and has a paucity of blood vessels. She has a history of a severe head injury as a result of a motor vehicle accident about 1 year ago. When examined a few days after institution of appropriate antimicrobial therapy, she is afebrile, alert, and has no nuchal rigidity.

- *Why might she have pneumococcal meningitis?*
- *How would you further evaluate her?*

The ocular findings are those of optic atrophy. This suggests that she indeed suffered a significant head injury, with damage to the optic nerve. Bacterial meningitis, in particular pneumococcal meningitis, after a significant head injury, strongly suggests a communication between the external environment and the subarachnoid space. When there is no obvious skull fracture, the likely site is a fracture through the base of the skull, either through the middle cranial fossa into the middle ear cavity or through the anterior cranial fossa through the cribriform plate. The latter can sometimes be demonstrated by having the patient lie prone with the head hanging over the edge of the bed. Cerebrospinal fluid (CSF) may begin to drip (CSF rhinorrhea). When performed on this patient, this maneuver elicited CSF rhinorrhea (Figure 117.1).

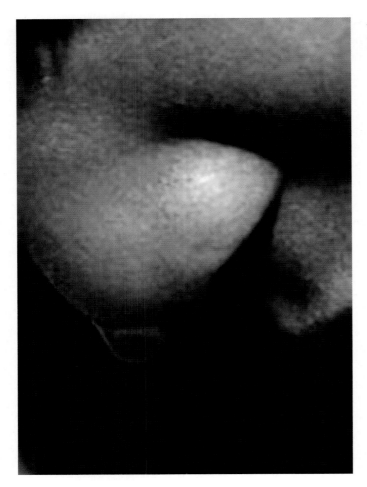

FIG. 117.1. The patient lying prone demonstrating CSF rhinorrhea.

A computer tomography scan with narrow cuts can demonstrate a bony defect in the cribriform plate, as was accomplished in this case. This was repaired surgically.

CASE 118. A 13-year-old girl presents with severe headache and fever. She has had a left earache and ear discharge for about 1 week. On examination she is ill-appearing and has a temperature of 39°C. She has mild neck stiffness. The left external auditory canal is occluded with a purulent discharge, but there is no pain on movement of the pinna. There is no swelling over the mastoid bone. The rest of the examination is normal.

- *What is the differential diagnosis?*
- *What should be done?*

This patient has several clinical features that should be cause for concern:

(a) A purulent auditory discharge suggests the possibilities of otitis externa or otitis media associated with a tympanic membrane perforation. The former is a very painful condition and is characterized by extreme pain elicited on movement of the pinna. Its absence indicates otitis media with perforation of the tympanic membrane.

(b) Severe headache in the presence of infection of the middle ear or paranasal sinus should suggest the possibility of intracranial extension of the infection.

(c) Neck stiffness supports the possibility of intracranial extension of infection, including meningitis, or a cerebellar abscess, or another site of intracranial suppuration with impending herniation. Intracranial suppuration from the middle ear or paranasal sinus can occur at any level: the epidural space, subdural space, subarachnoid space (meningitis), or brain parenchyma (cerebritis or brain abscess). Another intracranial complication of middle ear or paranasal sinus infection is dural sinus thrombosis.

Management:

Although it might be tempting to perform a lumbar puncture in such a case, the possibility of focal suppuration contraindicates this. Therefore management should consist of the following, in the following order:

(i) obtain blood cultures and culture and Gram stain of the auditory discharge;

(ii) initiate antimicrobial therapy (the drugs are discussed below);

(iii) brain imaging;

(iv) if no focal lesion or no significant cerebral edema are seen, lumbar puncture should be performed.

The computer tomography scan of this patient is shown in Figure 118.1.

This shows a large brain abscess in the temporal lobe. Brain abscesses arising from the middle ear occur in the temporal lobe or cerebellum. A wide variety of infectious agents can cause such abscesses, including *Streptococcus pneumoniae*, other streptococci, *Staphylococcus aureus*, anaerobes, such as *Bacteroides* spp. and *Fusobacterium* spp., and Gram-negative bacilli. The most common are streptococci and anaerobes.

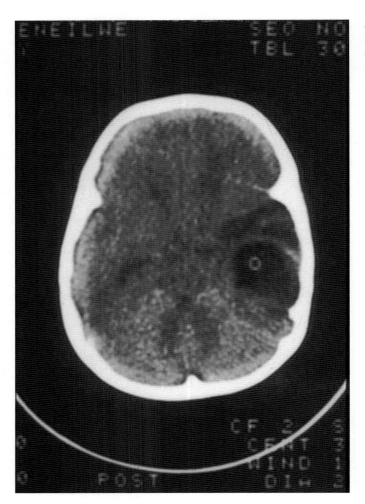

FIG. 118.1. The computer tomography scan showing a large brain abscess in the temporal lobe.

Treatment should consist of antimicrobial therapy directed at the likely pathogens and surgical drainage. Suitable antimicrobial therapy would include the following:

    ceftriaxone (or cefotaxime) + vancomycin + metronidazole

      or

    meropenem + vancomycin.

Reading:

Yogev R, Bar-Meir M: Management of brain abscess. Pediatr Infect Dis J 2004; 23: 157–159.

CASE 119. A 12-year-old previously well girl presents with a history of fever and cough for a few days, and difficulty breathing for 1 day. She lives in a rural area and has exposure to goats, cows, and many birds. (Her grandmother has an aviary.) She has no recent contact with sick individuals, and no knowledge of a tuberculosis contact. She has not been involved in any activities unusual for her. On examination she is very ill-appearing, with marked respiratory distress. There is mild cyanosis, but no pallor or jaundice. Her temperature is 38°C, heart rate 140/minute, and blood pressure 110/60, and her respiratory rate is 60/minute. The jugulo-venous pressure is not elevated and there is no peripheral edema. Examination of the chest shows marked intercostal retractions, and auscultation of the lungs reveals many crackles in both lower lobes. There are no signs of focal lung consolidation. The heart is not enlarged, the first and second heart sounds are normal, and there is no gallop. The rest of the examination is normal.

- *What is the differential diagnosis?*
- *What would you do?*

This patient has respiratory failure caused by a diffuse pulmonary disease, probably pneumonia. Although these pulmonary findings can also occur in left-sided heart failure, there are no other findings to indicate heart disease or a cause for heart disease. The most important action to take is to provide supplemental oxygen.

If this is indeed pneumonia, it is diffuse, a form that is sometimes referred as "atypical" pneumonia, which implies that it is not lobar. Although the patterns of pneumonia are not very specific for determining an etiological agent, this pattern does broaden the spectrum of agents that might be involved. The differential diagnosis includes the common causes of pneumonia in a 12-year-old girl, in particular *Mycoplasma pneumoniae, Chlamydia pneumoniae*, and *Streptococcus pneumoniae*, in addition to respiratory viruses such as influenza virus. Her exposures place her at particular risk for pneumonia caused by *Chlamydia psittaci* (from birds), *Coxiella burnetii* (from ungulates), and *Histoplasma capsulatum*. In addition she might have a hypersensitivity pneumonia caused by bird proteins ("bird fancier's disease"). If she were an immunocompromised host, then additional agents such as cytomegalovirus, *Legionella pneumophila*, and *Pneumocystis jiroveci* infection would be important additional considerations.

The most useful diagnostic test to determine the extent of the disease and to demonstrate any complications of the disease, such as pleural effusions or cavitation, is a chest X ray. Her chest X ray is shown in Figure 119.1.

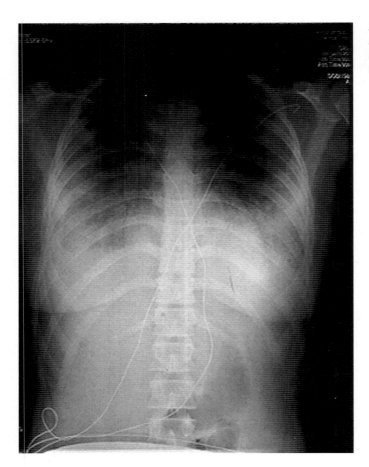

FIG. 119.1.   Chest X ray showing extensive, diffuse, bilateral pulmonary infiltrates.

In cases of pneumonia, the most useful test for reaching an etiologic diagnosis is examination of the sputum, by Gram stain and culture. The presence of numerous inflammatory cells and the absence of bacteria suggest an infection caused by an agent that is not stained by the Gram stain, such as *Mycoplasma pneumoniae*. Diagnosis of infections caused by *M. pneumoniae*, *C. pneumoniae*, *C. psittaci*, and *C. burnetii* depend largely on serology. Meanwhile she should be treated with a tetracycline (e.g. doxycycline) plus a third-generation cephalosporin or a penicillin; in addition a systemic corticosteroid should be administered in case this child has a hypersensitivity pneumonia.

This child was hospitalized in an intensive care unit. She required high concentrations of oxygen but did not require ventilation. She was treated with doxycyline and cefotaxime and improved over a few days. An etiology for her illness was not determined, despite extensive testing.

Reading:

Hindiyeh M, Carroll KC: Laboratory diagnosis of atypical pneumonia. Semin Resp Infect 2000; 15: 101–113.

CASE 120. A 12-year-old previously well boy presents with a history of fever, chills, sore throat, and neck pain for 5 days. He also has shortness of breath, nausea, and vomiting. He has had no exposures to animals and has not traveled outside his hometown in Georgia, USA. On examination he is moderately ill-appearing. His temperature is 39.1°C, heart rate 116/minute, respiratory rate 44/minute, and blood pressure 100/60 mm Hg, and his perfusion is good. He is not pale, but his sclerae are jaundiced. He has white patches on his tonsils, and examination of his lungs reveals crackles bilaterally. There is no lymphadenopathy and his cardiac examination and the rest of his examination are normal. He has a total leukocyte count of $12.5 \times 10^3/\mu l$, with 62% segmented neutrophils and 30% band forms, his total bilirubin is 4.1 mg/dl with a direct component of 3.6 mg/dl, and the aspartate aminotransaminase and alanine aminotransaminase are 58 and 35 units, respectively. His C-reactive protein concentration is 28 mg/dl.

He is admitted to hospital, and soon after admission he becomes hypotensive, necessitating his transfer to the intensive care unit.

- *What is your differential diagnosis?*
- *What would you do?*

This patient has evidence of septic shock, pharyngotonsillitis, pneumonia, and hepatitis. Which infections or infectious agents can cause this?

Viral agents:
  Epstein–Barr virus
  cytomegalovirus
  adenovirus

Although these viruses can cause pharyngotonsillitis, hepatitis, and pneumonia, they do not cause shock, except in the case of splenic rupture in cases of Epstein–Barr virus infection.

The laboratory findings in this child are very suggestive of a severe bacterial infection (marked left shift of leukocytes and markedly elevated C-reactive protein concentration).

Bacterial agents:

  Streptococcus pyogenes is the most important bacterial cause of pharyngotonsillitis. It can cause severe rapidly progressive pneumonia, but does not cause hepatitis, unless bacteremia or toxic shock-like syndrome is present. The latter condition, which carries a very high case fatality rate, is characterized by hypotension, diffuse erythroderma, and multiorgan dysfunction. Most cases have positive blood cultures for the organism.

Staphylococcus aureus does not cause tonsillitis but can be associated with abscesses in the peripharyngeal spaces. It is a very important cause of disseminated infection, with metastatic infection in many organs including the liver, lungs, and skeleton. It addition it can cause toxic shock syndrome.

Corynebacterium diphtheriae causes pharyngotonsillitis but does not cause pneumonia or hepatitis. Shock is due to diphtheria toxin causing a toxic cardiomyopathy, which develops 2–3 weeks after the onset of illness.

Fusobacterium necrophorum (Figure 120.1), which is a normal component of the oral flora, can cause invasion of the venous drainage of the throat, resulting in a septic thrombophlebitis of the jugular vein or its tributaries and sepsis syndrome. This is called Lemierre syndrome. The initial focus of infection is in the throat, which may have been initiated by another agent, such as Epstein–Barr virus. A peritonsillar abscess may be present.

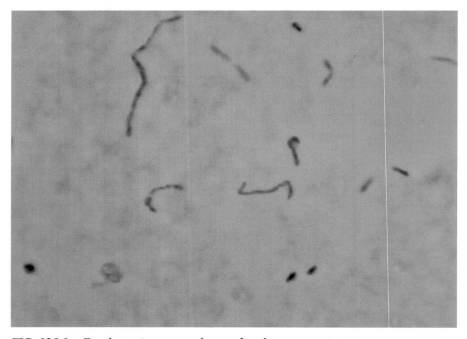

FIG. 120.1.   Fusobacterium necrophorum *by phase contrast microscopy.*
(Courtesy of the Centers for Disease Control and Prevention/Dr Lillian V Holderman)

Because the septic thrombophlebitis is an endovascular infection, it is frequently complicated by metastatic infection, particularly in the lung, but also in the liver, bone or joint, and skin. It may be associated with jaundice. The diagnosis is made clinically and can be confirmed by the demonstration of the organism on blood culture (Figure 120.1), and, sometimes, by demonstration of jugular vein occlusion by imaging. Therapy is primarily antimicrobial. Several antimicrobial agents are active against the organism, including clindamycin, metronidazole, a combination of a penicillin and a β-lactamase inhibitor, such as ampicillin/ sulbactam, or a carbapenem. Any abscess should be drained surgically. Anticoagulation should also be considered, although this is controversial.

Management of this patient should entail the following:

(a) ensuring adequate perfusion with aggressive intravenous fluid therapy and vasopressor therapy;

(b) ensuring adequate oxygenation; he required supplemental oxygen.

(c) antimicrobial therapy active against *Streptococcus pyogenes*, *Staphylococcus aureus*, and *Fusobacterium necrophorum*. He was treated initially with vancomycin, and meropenem was subsequently added to his regimen.

(d) attempting to make a diagnosis:

blood culture: this eventually grew out *Fusobacterium necrophorum*. chest X ray: this showed multiple foci of consolidation suggestive of embolic infection in the lungs (hematogenous pneumonia).

imaging of the neck, to look for evidence of venous occlusion: a Doppler ultrasound demonstrated a thrombus in the left internal jugular vein. As a result of this finding he was anticoagulated with low molecular weight heparin. Computer tomography imaging should be considered to look for evidence of a parapharyngeal abscess. This was not done.

He recovered and, after hospital discharge, was treated with oral clindamycin for 4 weeks.

Reading:

Ramirez S, Hild TG, Rudolph CN et al: Increased diagnosis of Lemierre's syndrome and other *Fusobacterium necrophorum* infections at a children's hospital. Pediatrics. 2003; 112: e380–385.

Venglarcik J: Lemierre's syndrome. Pediatr Infect Dis J 2003 2003; 22: 921–923.

Goldenberg NA, Knapp-Clevenger R, Hays T, Manco-Johnson MJ: Lemierre's and Lemierre's-like syndromes in children: survival and thromboembolic outcomes. Pediatrics 2005; 116: e543–548.

CASE 121. A 6-year-old girl underwent a major neurosurgical procedure 1 week ago to drain a large interhemispheric epidural abscess complicating sinusitis. A specimen of pus taken at surgery showed Gram-positive cocci in pairs, but the culture was negative. Because the parents had initially refused to grant permission for surgery, surgical drainage had been delayed for about 1 week. During this time the child was treated with vancomycin, ceftriaxone, and metronidazole, all intravenously, through a percutaneously inserted central venous catheter (PICC). After surgery her clinical condition improved markedly. However, despite broad-spectrum antimicrobial therapy for 2 weeks and surgical drainage, she has had a high fever. She feels well and has no other symptoms. On examination she is well appearing and very cooperative. Except for the large surgical scar along the length of her head, which is clean and without swelling, erythema, or drainage, examination of her head is normal. She has full range of ocular movements (initially she had a right third nerve palsy) and a normal neurological examination. The rest of her examination is normal.

- *What are the possible causes of fever in this child?*
- *What would you do?*

This child has several possible reasons for having fever:

(i)   intracranial infection which has not been adequately drained;

(ii)   infection introduced during the surgical procedure;

(iii)   nosocomial infection, particularly related to the intravascular catheter;

(iv)   drug fever.

The child's clinical improvement and lack of symptoms suggest that a continuing intracranial infection is unlikely. Nevertheless imaging to determine whether there is progression of the abscess should be performed. This showed the identical appearance to that seen a few days after surgery, which was a marked improvement over the preoperative appearance.

Possible sites of nosocomial should be sought clinically. Specifically the site of the intravascular catheter should be carefully examined for any signs of inflammation. In addition a blood culture drawn through the catheter should be performed. This clinical evaluation was normal, and the blood culture was negative.

The possibility of drug-induced fever should be considered. There are several different mechanisms by which drugs can cause fever:

(i)   altered thermoregulation, as can occur with anticholinergics;

(ii)   pyrogenic properties of the drug preparation such as amphotericin B deoxycholate, or contaminants within the drug preparation;

(iii)   pharmacologic effects of the drug, such as the Jarisch-Herxheimer reaction that occurs during therapy for certain infections and that is thought to be due to the release of endotoxin by dying bacteria;

(iv)   idiosyncratic reactions of certain individuals to anesthetic agents resulting in malignant hyperthermia;

(v)   presumed hypersensitivity or immune-mediated reactions: the mechanism is unknown. This is the type usually implied by the term "drug fever." Patients may have been taking the incriminated drug for a prolonged period before the problem occurs. Although the fever may be very high, the patient is not usually ill-appearing. In adults a relative bradycardia is common. The erythrocyte sedimentation is usually markedly elevated. Although many drugs can cause this, among antimicrobial agents, β-lactams are particularly important. The only way of diagnosing this problem is to discontinue the drug and to observe whether the fever abates, which occurs within 72 hours. This patient had been receiving ceftriaxone (in addition to other agents) for about 2 weeks. Since this was considered the most likely cause of drug fever in her, this drug and metronidazole were replaced by meropenem. Her fever abated within 48 hours. No further febrile episodes occurred.

Reading:

Johnson DH, Cunha BA: Drug Fever. Infect Dis Clin N Am 1996; 10: 85–91.

Part Three

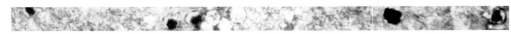

APPENDIX

■Table A1: Infectious diseases reportable in the United States.

Acquired immunodeficiency syndrome (AIDS)
Anthrax
Botulism
Brucellosis
Chancroid
Chlamydia trachomatis genital infection
Cholera
Coccidioidomycosis
Cryptosporidiosis
Cyclosporiasis
Diphtheria
Domestic arboviral disease – California, eastern equine, Powassan, St Louis, western equine
Ehrlichiosis
Enterohemorrhagic *Escherichia coli* O157:H7 and Shiga toxin-producing non-O157
Giardiasis
Gonorrhea
Haemophilus influenzae, invasive disease
Hansen's disease (leprosy)
Hantavirus pulmonary syndrome
Hemolytic uremic syndrome, postdiarrheal
Hepatitis A
Hepatitis B
Hepatitis C/non-A, non-B hepatitis
Human immunodeficiency virus infection (HIV)
Legionellosis
Listeriosis
Lyme disease
Malaria
Measles
Meningococcal disease

(continued)

(continued)

Mumps
Pertussis
Plague
Poliomyelitis, paralytic
Psittacosis
Q fever
Rabies, animal and human
Rocky Mountain spotted fever
Rubella (postnatal and congenital)
Salmonellosis
Shigellosis
Staphylococcus aureus infection
   Vancomycin-intermediate resistant (VISA)
   Vancomycin-resistant (VRSA)
Streptococcal disease, invasive, group A
Streptococcus pneumoniae
  drug-resistant, invasive disease, all ages
  invasive disease children <5 years
Streptococcal toxic shock syndrome
Syphilis (all forms)
Tetanus
Toxic shock syndrome
Trichinellosis
Tuberculosis
Tularemia
Typhoid fever
Varicella
Yellow fever
West Nile virus disease (all forms)

■Table A2: **Taxonomy of human pathogens, their usual sources, and the main clinical syndromes they cause.**

Pathogens	Usual source	Clinical syndrome
VIRUSES		
DNA VIRUSES		
Herpesviridae		
Alphaherpesvirinae		
Herpes simplex 1	H, Mat	Gingivostomatitis, fever blisters, encephalitis, keratitis, neonatal infection

(continued)

■Table A2:　Taxonomy of human pathogens, their usual sources, and the main clinical syndromes they cause (*continued*)

Pathogens	Usual source	Clinical syndrome
Herpes simplex 2	H, Mat	Genital ulcers, neonatal infection
Varicella zoster virus	H	Chickenpox (varicella), zoster (shingles)
Betaherpesvirinae		
Cytomegalovirus	H, Mat	Infectious mononucleosis, hepatitis, OI – pneumonia, retinitis, enteritis
Human herpes virus 6	H	Fever, roseola, OI – hepatitis, encephalitis
Gammaherpesvirinae		
Epstein–Barr virus	H	Infectious mononucleosis, hepatitis, OI – posttransplant lymphoproliferative disease, Burkitt's lymphoma, other cancers
Human herpes virus 7	H	Fever
Human herpes virus 8	H	Kaposi sarcoma
Adenoviruses		
Multiple serotypes	H	Conjunctivitis, respiratory infection, cystitis, OI
Enteric (40, 41)		Diarrhea
Hepadnaviridae		
Hepatitis B virus	H, Mat	Hepatitis, chronic liver disease, liver cancer
Papovaviridae		
Polyoma viruses	H	OI – progressive multifocal leukoencephalopathy, nephropathy following renal transplant
Papilloma virus	H	Warts – skin, genital, laryngeal, cervical cancer
Parvoviridae		
Parvovirus B 19	H	Erythema infectiosum, aplastic crisis, hydrops fetalis, chronic anemia, OI – hepatitis, encephalitis
Poxviridae		
Chordopoxvirinae		
Orthopoxvirus		
Smallpox virus	H	Smallpox
Vaccinia virus	L	Vaccinia-local, disseminated, encephalitis, myopericarditis
Cowpox virus		
Monkeypox virus	A	Monkeypox
Molluscipox virus		
Molluscum contagiosum	H	Molluscum contagiosum
Parapoxvirus		
Orf virus	A	Orf
Yatapoxvirus		
Tanapoxvirus		

(continued)

(continued)

Pathogens	Usual source	Clinical syndrome
RNA VIRUSES		
Picornaviridae		
Enteroviruses		
Polio viruses	H	Poliomyelitis, encephalitis
Coxsackie, Echovirus	H	Fever, rash, meningitis, encephalitis
Parechovirus	H	Myocarditis, neonatal infection
Hepatovirus		
Human hepatitis A virus	H	Acute hepatitis
Rhinoviruses	H	Upper respiratory tract infection, sinusitis
Caliciviridae		
Noroviruses	H	Diarrhea
Paramyxoviridae		
Measles virus	H	Measles
Mumps virus	H	Mumps
Respiratory syncytial virus	H	Bronchiolitis, pneumonia, URI
Parainfluenza viruses (1,2,3,4)	H	Respiratory tract infection
Human metapneumovirus	H	Respiratory tract infection
Reoviridae		
Rotavirus	H	Diarrhea
Coltivirus		
Colorado tick fever virus	Tick	Colorado tick fever
Coronaviridae	A	Severe acute respiratory syndrome (SARS)
	H	Diarrhea, upper respiratory infection
Astroviridae		
Human astrovirus	H	Diarrhea
Orthomyxoviridae		
Influenza viruses A,B,C	H, A	Influenza
Retroviridae		
Lentivirus		
Human immunodeficiency virus (HIV) 1	H, Mat	HIV infection, AIDS
HIV 2	H, Mat	HIV infection, AIDS
Deltaretrovirus		
Human T-cell lymphotropic virus (HTLV)	H	T-cell leukemia
	H	Tropical spastic paraparesis
Togaviridae		
Rubivirus		
Rubella virus	H, Mat	Rubella, congenital rubella syndrome
Alphaviruses	Mos	Arthropod-borne viruses
Many arthropod-borne viruses		Equine encephalitides

(continued)

■**Table A2:** **Taxonomy of human pathogens, their usual sources, and the main clinical syndromes they cause (*continued*)**

Pathogens	Usual source	Clinical syndrome
Flaviviridae		
Hepacavirus		
Hepatitis C	H	Hepatitis, chronic liver disease
Flavivirus		
Many arthropod-borne viruses	Mos	Yellow fever, dengue, West Nile, Japanese B encephalitis
Arenaviridae		
Lassa fever virus	A	Hemorrhagic fever
Lymphocytic choriomeningitis virus (LCM)	A, Mat	Meningitis, congenital infection
Junin, Machupo, Sabia, Guanarito	A	South American hemorrhagic fevers
Rhabdoviridae		
Lyssaviruses		
Rabies virus virus	A	Rabies – encephalitis
Filoviridae		
Ebola virus	A	Hemorrhagic fever
Marburg virus	A	Hemorrhagic fever
Bunyaviridae		
Bunyavirus		
California, La Crosse encephalitis	Mos	Encephalitis
Many arthropod-borne viruses		
Phlebovirus		
Sandfly fever virus	Fly	Sandfly fever
Rift Valley fever virus	Mos	Rift Valley fever
Hantaviruses		
Hantaan virus	A	Korean hemorrhagic fever
Sin nombre virus	A	Pulmonary syndrome
Nairovirus		
Congo-Crimean hemorrhagic fever virus	Tick	Hemorrhagic fever
Hepatitis D virus	H	Chronic hepatitis associated with HBV

BACTERIA

Obligate intracellular replication, lack cell wall

CHLAMYDIAE

C. trachomatis		
Serovars B, Da, Ia, D-K	H, Mat	Genital tract infection, neonatal conjunctivitis, pneumonia
Serovars A, B, Ba, C	H, Fly	Trachoma
Serovars L1, L2, L3	H	Lymphogranuloma venereum
C. psittaci	A	Pneumonia
C. pneumoniae	H	Pneumonia

(continued)

(continued)

Pathogens	Usual source	Clinical syndrome
RICKETTSIAE		
R. prowazekii	Louse	Epidemic (louse-borne) typhus
R. mooseri (*typhi*)	Flea	Endemic (flea-borne) typhus
R. rickettsii	Tick	Rocky Mountain spotted fever
R. conori	Tick	Mediterranean spotted fever
R. africae	Tick	African tick typhus
Orientia tsutsugamushi	Mite	Scrub typhus
R. akari	Mite	Rickettsial pox
R. sibirica	Tick	Spotted fever
R. australis	Tick	Queensland tick typhus
Coxiella burnetii	A, tick	Q fever (hepatitis, pneumonia)
Ehrlichia	Tick	Ehrlichiosis
Ehrlichia chaffensis		Human monocytic ehrlichiosis
Anaplasma phagocytophilum		Human granulocytic ehrlichiosis
MYCOPLASMAS		
M. pneumoniae	H	Pneumonia, rash, encephalitis
M. hominis	H, Mat	Neonatal pneumonia
M. genitalium	H	Urethritis
Ureaplasma urealyticum	H, Mat	Neonatal pneumonia
SPIROCHETES		
Treponema pallidum subsp. *pallidum*	H	Syphilis
Treponema pallidum subsp. *pertenue*	H	Yaws
Treponema pallidum subsp. *endemicum*	H	Bejel
Treponema carateum	H	Pinta
Leptospira interrogans	A, E	
Multiple serotypes		Leptospirosis
Borrelia		
B. burgdorferi	Tick	Lyme disease
B. recurrentis	Louse	Relapsing fever (louse-borne)
B. duttoni	Tick	Relapsing fever
B. hermsii, *turicatae*, *parkeri*	Tick	Relapsing fever (tick-borne)
Spirillum minus	A	Rat bite fever

Gram-negative bacilli

Enterobacteriaceae – ferment glucose, oxidase-negative, reduce nitrate to nitrite, facultative anaerobes, inhabit the intestine; cause infections arising from the intestine, such as abdominal abscesses, urinary tract infections; nosocomial infections.

(continued)

■Table A2: Taxonomy of human pathogens, their usual sources, and the main clinical syndromes they cause (*continued*)

Pathogens	Usual source	Clinical syndrome
Escherichia coli	A, H, End	Urinary infection, neonatal sepsis, sepsis, NI, specific virulence factors associated with specific forms of enteric infection
Shigella Four species: *S. dysenteriae, flexneri, boydii, sonnei*	H	Diarrhea, dysentery, encephalopathy
Klebsiella pneumoniae and other species	H, End	UTI, pneumonia, NI
Enterobacter	H, End	UTI, NI
Citrobacter	H, End	NI
Serratia	H, End	NI
Proteus	H, End	UTI, NI
Morganella	H, End	UTI, NI
Providencia	H, End	UTI, NI
Hafnia		
Edwardsiella		
Pantoea		
Salmonella		
>2400 serotypes	A	Diarrhea, dysentery, bacteremia
serotype typhi	H	Typhoid fever
Yersinia pestis	A, Flea	Plague
Yersinia enterocolitica	A	Diarrhea, dysentery, pseudoappendicitis

NONFERMENTERS (MANY FAMILIES)

Pathogens	Usual source	Clinical syndrome
Pseudomonas aeruginosa	E	NI, pneumonia especially associated with cystic fibrosis
Burkholderia cepacia	E, H	Pneumonia associated with cystic fibrosis
Burkholderia pseudomallei	E	Melioidosis
Stenotrophomonas maltophilia	E	NI
Acinetobacter species	E	NI
Elizabethkingae meningosepticum	E	Neonatal sepsis, meningitis

SMALL GRAM-NEGATIVE BACILLI (COCCOBACILLI)

Pathogens	Usual source	Clinical syndrome
Bordetella pertussis	H	Pertussis
Brucella (four species)	A	Brucellosis
Capnocytophaga canimorsis	A	Dog-bite wound
Calymmatobacterium granulomatis	H	Granuloma inguinale (Donovanosis)
Campylobacter fetus	A	Sepsis (OI)
Campylobacter jejuni	A	Diarrhea, dysentery
Helicobacter pylori	H	Gastritis
Francisella tularensis	A, arthropods	tularemia

(continued)

(continued)

Pathogens	Usual source	Clinical syndrome
Haemophilus		
Influenzae type b	H	Bacteremia, meningitis, septic arthritis, epiglottitis
Nontypeable	End	Otitis media, sinusitis, pneumonia, conjunctivitis
	H	Brazilian hemorrhagic fever
Haemophilus aphrophilus	End	IE
Haemophilus ducreyi	H	Chancroid
Legionella pneumophila	E	Legionnaires' disease (pneumonia)
Other *Legionella* species	E	"
Actinobacillus actinomycetemcomitans	End	IE
Cardiobacterium hominis	End	IE
Eikenella corrodens	End	Mouth, bite-wound
Kingella kingae	End	Skeletal infections
Streptobacillus moniliformis	A (rat)	Rat bite fever
Bartonellae		
B. bacilliformis	Fly	Oroya fever
B. henselae	A	Cat-scratch disease, bacillary angiomatosis
B. quintana	Louse	Trench fever, bacillary angiomatosis, IE
B. elizabethae	A	IE
NON-ENTEROBACTERIACEAE, FERMENTERS		
Aeromonas hydrophila	E	Water-associated infections
Chromobacterium violaceum	E	Soil-associated infections (OI)
Pasteurella multocida	A	Animal bite-wound infections
Plesiomonas shigelloides		Diarrhea
Vibrios		
V. cholerae	E, H	Cholera
V. parahaemolyticus	E	Diarrhea
V. vulnificus	E	OI – sepsis, oyster-associated

Gram-negative cocci

Pathogens	Usual source	Clinical syndrome
Neisseria		
N. meningitidis	H	Septicemia, meningitis
N. gonorrhoeae	H, Mat	Gonorrhea, neonatal conjunctivitis
Moraxella catarrhalis	End	Otitis media, sinusitis

Gram-positive cocci

CATALASE POSITIVE

Pathogens	Usual source	Clinical syndrome
Staphylococci		
Coagulase-positive; *S. aureus*	H, End	Skin, wound, bacteremia, pneumonia, NI, IE, FB

(continued)

■Table A2:   Taxonomy of human pathogens, their usual sources, and the main clinical syndromes they cause (*continued*)

Pathogens	Usual source	Clinical syndrome
Coagulase-negative; many species	H, End	NI, FB
Including *S. epidermidis*		iv catheters, ventricular shunts
S. haemolyticus		Cystitis
Rothia mucilaginosa		OI – sepsis (neutropenia-associated)
CATALASE NEGATIVE		
Streptococci		
S. pneumoniae	H, End	Otitis media, sinusitis, conjunctivitis, pneumonia, bacteremia, meningitis
S. pyogenes (group A)	H	Tonsillitis, impetigo, wound, puerperal sepsis, toxic-shock like syndrome, acute glomerulonephritis, rheumatic fever
S. agalactiae (group B)	H, Mat	Neonatal sepsis, meningitis, OI – diabetics
S. viridans	End	Dental caries, endocarditis, visceral abscesses, OI – sepsis (neutropenia)
S. bovis (group D)	End	Endocarditis (colonic cancer-associated)
Enterococci		
E. faecalis	End	Endocarditis, NI, FB
E. faecium	"	"
Pediococcus spp.	E	OI – sepsis, NI vancomycin-resistant
Gemella sp.	End	Focal infections, IE
Leukonostoc spp.	E	NI, FB, OI vancomycin-resistant
Gram-positive bacilli, non–spore-forming		
Actinomyces several species (microaerophilic)		
A. israeli	End	Actinomycosis – chronic infection mouth, gut, female genital
A. odontolyticus		
Nocardia		
N. asteroides	E	OI – lung, brain
N. nova		
N. farcinica		
N. otidiscaviarum		
N. brasiliensis	E	Cutaneous infections
N. transvalensis		
Corynebacteria		
C. diphtheriae	H	Diphtheria (throat, larynx, myocarditis, neuropathy)
C. urealyticum	End	Chronic urinary tract infection
C. jeikeium	End	NI, FB

(continued)

(continued)

Pathogens	Usual source	Clinical syndrome
Many others	End	NI, FB
Arcanobacterium haemolyticum	H	Pharyngitis, scarlatiniform rash
Rhodococcus equi	E	OI – pneumonia
Listeria monocytogenes	E, Mat	Bacteremia, meningitis, newborn, elderly, OI
Erysipelothrix rhusiopathiae	A, E	Cellulitis, IE
Gardnerella vaginalis	End	Bacterial vaginosis
Lactobacillus sp.	End	
Rothia denticariosa	End	
Streptomyces somaliensis	E	Mycetoma
Oerskovia spp.	E	IE
Tropheryma whipplei	unknown	Whipple's disease

MYCOBACTERIA

M. tuberculosis	H	Tuberculosis
M. bovis	A	Tuberculosis
M. africanum	H	Tuberculosis
M. leprae	H	Leprosy
M. avium complex	E	Lymphadenitis, OI
M. marinum	E	Water-associated granuloma
M. scrofulaceum	E	Lymphadenitis
Many other species	E	Focal infections, OIs

Gram-positive bacilli, spore-forming, aerobic

BACILLUS

B. anthracis	A, E	Anthrax
B. cereus	E	Acute food poisoning, eye
Several other species		FB, OI

Anaerobic bacteria

GRAM-POSITIVE RODS, SPORE-FORMING (CLOSTRIDIA)

C. tetani	E	Tetanus
C. botulinum	E	Botulism – classic, wound, infant
C. difficile	E, H	Antibiotic-associated colitis (NI)
C. perfringens	E	Food poisoning
	End	Myonecrosis (gas gangrene), hemolysis
Other histotoxic clostridia		Myonecrosis, OI

(continued)

■**Table A2: Taxonomy of human pathogens, their usual sources, and the main clinical syndromes they cause (*continued*)**

Pathogens	Usual source	Clinical syndrome
ANAEROBIC GRAM-POSITIVE RODS, NON-SPOREFORMING		
Bifidobacterium spp.	End	
Eubacterium spp.	End	Dental plaque
Actinomyces spp.	see aerobic Gram-positive rods, above	
ANAEROBIC GRAM-NEGATIVE BACILLI		
Bacteroides	End	Infections arising from mucosae: mouth, gut, female genital tract
Prevotella species	End	As above
Porphyromonas species	End	As above
Fusobacterium species	End	Infections from mucosae, septic thrombophlebitis
ANAEROBIC GRAM-NEGATIVE COCCI		
Veillonella	End	As above
ANAEROBIC GRAM-POSITIVE COCCI		
Peptococcus species	End	As above
Peptostreptococcus species	End	As above
FUNGI		
YEASTS		
Candida species		
C. albicans	End	Mucosal infections – mouth, vagina, NI, FB, fungemia, esophagitis, OI
C. tropicalis	End	
C. pseudotropicalis		
C. parapsilosis		
C. krusei		
C. (Torulopsis) glabrata		
C. lusitaniae		
C. guillermondii		
Cryptococcus neoformans	E	OI – pneumonia, meningitis
Rhodotorula rubra	E	OI
Malassezia furfur	End	Pityriasis versicolor, NI-(catheter-related)
DIMORPHIC FUNGI		
Histoplasma capsulatum	E	Histoplasmosis: pneumonia (bat, bird guano), OI
H. capsulatum var. *duboisi*	E	African histoplasmosis

(continued)

(continued)

Pathogens	Usual source	Clinical syndrome
Coccidioides immitis	E	Coccidioidomycosis: fever, pneumonia, OI
Blastomyces dermatitidis	E	Blastomycosis: pneumonia, skin
Paracoccidioides brasiliensis	E	South American blastomycosis
Other fungi		
Sporothrix schenkii	E	Sporotrichosis (cutaneous, lymphangitis)
Pseudoallescheria boydii	E	OI
Filamentous fungi		
Aspergillus fumigatus, terrae, flavus, niger	E	Aspergillosis – lung, OI, angioinvasive
Zygomycetes		
Mucor	E	Mucormycosis – OI, angioinvasive
Rhizopus	E	Mucormycosis
Absidia	E	Mucormycosis
Cunninghamella	E	Mucormycosis
Penicillium marneffei	E	OI – SE Asia
Dermatophytes		
Trichophyton species	H	Tinea corporis, capitis
Epidermophyton species	H	Tinea corporis, capitis
Microsporum species	H, A	Tinea corporis, capitis

There are many other fungi, living in the environment, and belonging to many families, that can cause infections as a result of injury or immunodeficiency in the host.

PARASITES

Intestinal Protozoa

AMEBAE

Entamoeba histolytica	H	Amebiasis: colitis, liver abscess

FLAGELLATES

Giardia lamblia (intestinalis)	H, A	Diarrhea

SPOROZOA

Cryptosporidium parvum	H, A	Diarrhea
Cyclospora cayetanensis	H	Diarrhea
Isospora belli	H	Diarrhea – OI

(continued)

■Table A2:   Taxonomy of human pathogens, their usual sources, and the main clinical
syndromes they cause (*continued*)

Pathogens	Usual source	Clinical syndrome
MICROSPORIDIA		
Enterocytozoon bieneusi		OI – diarrhea, cholangitis, sinusitis
Encephalitozoon intestinalis		Diarrhea, OI – diarrhea, cholangitis
CILIATES		
Balantidium coli	H, A	Colitis
OTHER		
Blastocystis hominis	H	Diarrhea
Tissue and Blood Protozoa		
AMEBAE		
Naegleria fowleri	E	Meningoencephalitis (fresh water)
Acanthameba	E	Meningoencephalitis, keratitis
Balamuthia mandrillaris	E	Meningoencephalitis
FLAGELLATES		
Leishmania donovani, infantum	Fly	Visceral leishmaniasis
Leishmania mexicana, tropica	Fly	Cutaneous leishmaniasis
Leishmania braziliensis	Fly	Mucocutaneous leishmaniasis
Trypanosomes		
T. cruzi	reduviid bug	S. American trypanosomiasis (Chaga's disease)
T. brucei rhodesiense	Fly	African trypanosomiasis (sleeping sickness)
T. brucei gambiense		African trypanosomiasis
Trichomonas vaginalis	H	Vaginitis
SPOROZOA		
Plasmodium falciparum	Mos	Falciparum malaria (malignant tertian)
Plasmodium vivax	Mos	Vivax malaria (benign tertian)
Plasmodium ovale	Mos	Ovale malaria
Plasmodium malariae	Mos	Quartan malaria
Babesia microti and other species	Tick	Babesiosis
Toxoplasma gondii	A, Mat	Toxoplasmosis: mononucleosis, congenital, OI – encephalitis
MICROSPORIDIA		
Brachiola (Nosema) algerae		Keratoconjunctivitis, skin infection
Nosema ocularum		Keratitis
Vittaforma corneae		Keratitis, disseminated infection

(continued)

(continued)

Pathogens	Usual source	Clinical syndrome
Microsporidium ceylonensis		Keratitis
Microsporidium africanum		Keratitis
Nosema connori		OI – disseminated infection
Encephalitozoon hellem		OI – multiple sites

INTESTINAL WORMS

ROUNDWORMS (NEMATODES)

Enterobius vermicularis (Pinworm)	H	Perianal itching
Ascaris lumbricoides	H-E	Ascariasis, visceral larva migrans, intestinal obstruction
Toxocara canis and cati	A-E	Visceral larva migrans, pneumonitis, ocular granuloma
Baylisascaris procyonis	A-E	Encephalitis
Hookworms		
Necator americanus	H-E	Anemia, hypoalbuminemia
Ancylostoma duodenale	H-E	Anemia, hypoalbuminemia
Strongyloides stercoralis	H-E	Diarrhea, OI – visceral disease
Trichuris trichiura	H-E	Chronic diarrhea, rectal prolapse
Anisakis spp.	A	Gastritis (raw fish)

CESTODES (TAPEWORMS)

Taenia solium	Pig	Tapeworm
Taenia solium larval stage	H	Cysticercosis
Taenia saginata	Beef	Tapeworm
Echinococcus multilocularis	A-E-H	Cysts
Multiceps multiceps	A	Cysts
Echinococcus granulosus	A	Hydatid disease (larval stage)
Diphyllobothrium latum (fish)	Fish	Vitamin B12 deficiency, intestinal obstruction
Spirometra mansonoides	Water, copepod	Eye, visceral disease
Dipylidium caninum		Flea
Hymenolepis nana	H (+/− arthropod)	Anorexia

TREMATODES (FLUKES)

Fasciolopsis buski	Water plants	Intestinal disease
Heterophyes heterophyes	Fish	Intestinal disease
Metagonimus yokagawai	Fish	Intestinal disease

TISSUE AND BLOOD WORMS

TREMATODES (FLUKES)

Paragonimus westermanii	Crustacean	Lung disease
Fasciola hepatica	Sheep-water plants	Liver
Clonorchis sinensis	Fish	Biliary tract
Opisthorcis viverrini	Fish	Biliary tract

(continued)

■Table A2:   Taxonomy of human pathogens, their usual sources, and the main clinical syndromes they cause (*continued*)

Pathogens	Usual source	Clinical syndrome
Schistosomes		
S. mansoni	H-W	Liver fibrosis
S. japonicum	H-W	Liver fibrosis
S. haematobium	H-W	Urinary tract disease
S. mekongi	H-W	Liver fibrosis
NEMATODES		
Wucheraria bancrofti	Mos	Filariasis, elephantiasis
Brugia malayi	Mos	Filariasis
Onchocerca volvulus	Fly	River blindness, subcutaneous nodules
Loa loa	Fly	Subcutaneous nodules, conjunctival disease
Dracunculus medinensis (guinea worm)	W (Copepod)	Skin ulcer, cellulitis
Trichinella spiralis	A	Trichinosis (myositis)
Ancylostoma braziliense and *caninum*	A-E	Cutaneous larva migrans
Gnathostoma spinigerum	Fish	Subcutaneous, visceral swellings
Angiostrongylus cantonensis	Crustacian	Eosinophilic meningitis
Angiostrongylus costaricensis	Slug	Abdominal granulomas

ECTOPARASITES

Mites		
Sarcoptes scabiei	H	Scabies
Eutrombicula alfreddugesi (chigger)	E	Dermatitis
Lice		
Pediculus humanus capitis	H	Head pediculosis
Pediculus humanus corporis	H	Body pediculosis
Phthyrus pubis (crab louse)	H	Pubic pediculosis
Flies		Myiasis
Calliphoridae		
Cuteribridae		
Sarcophagidae		

A = animal, including birds; E = environment; End = endogenous; FB = infections on foreign bodies, such as catheters; H = human; IE = infective endocarditis; L = laboratory; Mat = maternal; Mos = mosquito; NI = nosocomial infection; OI = opportunistic infection; URI = upper respiratory tract infection; UTI = urinary tract infection.

Reading:

Leventhal R, Cheadle RF: Medical Parasitology. A Self-Instructional Text. 5th edition. FA Davis Company, Philadelphia, 2002.

Katz M, Despommier DD, Gwadz RW: Parasitic Diseases. 2nd edition. Springer-Verlag, New York, 1988.

Beck JW, Davies JE: Medical Parasitology. 3rd edition. CV Mosby Company. St Louis, 1981.

Winn W, Jr, Allen S, Janda WM, Koneman EW, Procop GW, Schreckenberger PC, Woods GL: Koneman's Color Atlas and Textbook of Diagnostic Microbiology. 6th edition. Lippincott Williams and Wilkins, Philadelphia, 2006.

Visvesvara GS: In vitro cultivation of microsporidia of clinical importance. Clin Microbiol Rev 2002; 15: 401–413.

List 1: Animate and inanimate sources and infectious agents associated with them.

Abbreviations: CMV = cytomegalovirus; HAV = hepatitis A virus; HBV = hepatitis B virus; HIV = human immunodeficiency virus; HSV = herpes simplex virus; VZV = varicella zoster virus

Human (close (other than sexual) contact, droplet)

Viruses: all herpes viruses, pox viruses, parvovirus, adenovirus, HBV, respiratory viruses, enteroviruses, rhinoviruses, coronaviruses, diarrhea-causing viruses, mumps, measles, papilloma viruses

Chlamydia pneumoniae, Mycoplasma pneumoniae

Streptococcus pyogenes, Streptococcus pneumoniae, Streptococcus agalactiae, Staphylococcus aureus, Neisseria meningitidis, Haemophilus influenzae, Corynebacterium diphtheriae, Arcanobacterium haemolyticum, Mycobacterium tuberculosis, Mycobacterium leprae, Shigellae, *Bordetella pertussis,* Dermatophytes, Lice, *Sarcoptes scabiei*

Human (sexual contact)

HSV, CMV, HIV, HBV, papilloma virus, *Chlamydia trachomatis, Treponema pallidum, Calymmatobacterium granulomatis, Haemophilus ducreyi, Neisseria gonorrhoeae, Trichomonas vaginalis.*

Human (endogenous)

staphylococci, streptococci (especially viridans group), enterococci, *Moraxella catarrhalis, Corynebacterium* spp., *Actinomyces* spp., many Enterobacteriaceae, for example, *E. coli, Haemophilus* spp., many anaerobic bacteria, *Candida* spp.

Ingestion (human feces-contaminated food, water or soil)

HAV, enteroviruses, diarrhea-causing viruses, *Salmonella*, *Shigella*, *Entamoeba histolytica*, *Giardia lamblia*, *Cryptosporidium parvum*, *Taenia solium* (cysticercosis), intestinal flukes, *Ascaris lumbricoides*, hookworms, *Strongyloides stercoralis*, *Enterobius vermicularis*

Ingestion (animal excreta-contaminated food, water, or soil)

Listeria monocytogenes, *Brucella* spp., *E. coli*, *Salmonella*, *Campylobacter*, *Yersinia enterocolitica*, *Mycobacterium bovis* (milk), *Giardia lamblia*, *Cryptosporidium parvum*, *Toxocara*, *Baylisascaris procyonis*, *Echinococcus granulosus*, *Toxoplasma gondii*

Ingestion (uncooked animal tissue)

Bacillus anthracis, *Salmonella* spp., *E. coli*, *Campylobacter*, *Yersinia enterocolitica*, *Toxoplasma gondii*, *Taenia solium* (pig), *Taenia saginata* (beef), *Hymenolepis diminuta* (rat fleas), *Diphyllobothrium latum* (fish), *Trichinella spiralis* (pig, carnivore), *Anisakis* (fish), *Paragonimus* spp., *Gnathostoma spinigerum*.

■**Table A3:   Arthropods as vectors of infectious agents.**

	Viruses	Bacteria	Protozoa	Helminths
Mosquito	Alphaviruses Flaviviruses		Plasmodia	*Wucheraria* *Brugia* *Dirofilaria*
Tick	Colorado tick Congo-Crimean	*Rickettsia* *Coxiella burnetii* *Ehrlichia* *Borrelia duttoni* *Borrelia burgdorferi* *Francisella*	*Babesia*	
Flea		*Yersinia pestis* *Rickettsia typhi*		
Louse		*Borrelia recurrentis* *Rickettsia prowazeki* *Bartonella quintana*		
Fly	Sandfly fever		*Leishmania* *Trypanosoma brucei*	*Onchocerca* *Loa loa*
Triatomid bug			*Trypanosoma cruzi*	
Mite		*Rickettsia akari*		

Animal (contact with animal, animal tissue, animal excreta, bite, scratch)
Ebola virus, Congo-Crimean Hemorrhagic Fever, Rift Valley Fever, Lymphocytic choriomeningitis virus, Lassa fever, Hantaviruses, Rabies virus, *Herpes simiae*, *Chlamydia psittaci*, *Bacillus anthracis*, *Erysipelothrix rhusiopathiae*, *Streptobacillus moniliformis*, *Spirillum minus*, *Pasteurella multocida*, *Yersinia pestis*, *Francisella tularensis*, *Capnocytophaga canimorsus*, *Coxiella burnetii*, *Brucella* spp., *Bartonellae henselae*, *Microsporum canis*

Fresh water (non-enteral exposure)
Leptospira, *Erysipelothrix rhusiopathiae*, *Mycobacterium marinum*, *Legionella* spp., *Naegleria fowleri*, *Acanthamoeba*, *Schistosomes*, *Pseudomonas aeruginosa*, *Aeromonas hydrophila*

Sea water (enteral)
Vibrio cholerae, *Vibrio parahaemoliticus*, *Vibrio vulnificus*

Sea water (non-enteral)
Erysipelothrix rhusiopathiae, *M. marinum*, halophilic vibrios

Inanimate environment (soil, air)
Bacillus cereus, *Rhodococcus equi*, nontuberculous mycobacteria, *Nocardia* spp., Enterobacteriaciae, *Aeromonas hydrophila*, *Chromobacterium violaceum*, *Pseudomonas* spp., *Acinetobacter* spp., *Elizabethkingae meningosepticum*, *Legionella* spp., *Clostridium perfringens*, *Clostridium tetani*, dimorphic fungi, *Cryptococcus neoformans*, *Aspergillus* spp., other filamentous fungi.

Inanimate (human-contaminated)
Enteroviruses, respiratory viruses, *Mycobacterium tuberculosis*, Enterobacteriaceae, hookworms, *Strongyloides*, *Ascaris*

Mother
Rubella, CMV, HSV, HBV, HCV, HIV, VZV, enterovirus, lymphocytic choriomeningitis virus, *Treponema pallidum*, *Chlamydia trachomatis*, *Streptococcus agalactiae*, *Listeria monocytogenes*, Enterobacteriaceae, *Mycobacterium tuberculosis*, *Toxoplasma gondii*, *Plasmodium* spp.

Hospital
VZV, respiratory viruses, enteroviruses, diarrhea-causing viruses, measles, filiviruses, Enterobacteriaceae, *Pseudomonas aeruginosa*, *Stenotrophomonas maltophilia*, *Acinetobacter* spp., *Staphylococcus aureus*, coagulase-negative staphylococci, enterococci, *Clostridium difficile*, *Candida* spp., *Aspergillus* spp.

Blood

HBV, HCV, HIV, CMV, EBV, West Nile virus, *Treponema pallidum*, *Yersinia enterocolitica*, *Listeria monocytogenes*, Trypanosomes, *Plasmodium* spp., *Babesia* spp., *Toxoplasma gondii*, Filaria

Tissue

Prions, CMV, HIV, West Nile virus, rabies virus, contaminating bacteria

General References:

Pickering LK (editor): Red Book: 2003 Report of the Committee on Infectious Diseases. 26th edition. American Academy of Pediatrics, Elk Grove Village, IL.

Pickering LK (editor): Red Book: 2006 Report of the Committee on Infectious Diseases. 27th edition. American Academy of Pediatrics, Elk Grove Village, IL.

Fisher RG, Boyce TE: Moffett's Pediatric Infectious Diseases. A Problem-Oriented Approach. 4th edition. Lippincott, Williams and Wilkins, Philadelphia, 2005.

Long SS, Pickering LK, Prober CG (editors): Principles and Practice of Pediatric Infectious Diseases. 2nd edition. Churchill Livingstone, New York, 2003.

Feigin RD, Cherry JD, Demmler GJ, Kaplan SL: Textbook of Pediatric Infectious Diseases. 5th edition. WB Saunders, Philadelphia, 2004.

Jenson HB, Baltimore RS: Pediatric Infectious Diseases. Principles and Practice. 2nd edition. WB Saunders, Philadelphia, 2002.

Mandell GL, Bennett JE, Dolin R (editors): Principles and Practice of Infectious Diseases. 6th edition. Elsevier Churchill Livingstone, Philadelphia, 2005.

Index